D1031960

WITHDRAWN

TOURO COLLEGE LIBRARY
Midtown

Clinical Pragmatics

Many children and adults experience significant breakdown in the use of language. The resulting pragmatic disorders present a considerable barrier to effective communication. This book is the first critical examination of the current state of our knowledge of pragmatic disorders and provides a comprehensive overview of the main concepts and theories in pragmatics. It examines the full range of pragmatic disorders that occur in children and adults and discusses how they are assessed and treated by clinicians. Louise Cummings attempts to integrate the fields of pragmatics, language pathology and cognitive science by examining the ways in which pragmatics can make a useful contribution to debates about cognitive theories of autism. The reader is encouraged to think in a critical fashion about how clinicians, experimentalists and theorists deal with pragmatic issues.

LOUISE CUMMINGS is Reader in Linguistics in the School of Arts and Humanities at Nottingham Trent University.

Clinical Pragmatics

Louise Cummings

TOURO COLLEGE LIBRARY
Midtown
WITHDRAWN

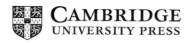
CAMBRIDGE
UNIVERSITY PRESS

MW

CAMBRIDGE UNIVERSITY PRESS
Cambridge, New York, Melbourne, Madrid, Cape Town, Singapore, São Paulo, Delhi

Cambridge University Press
The Edinburgh Building, Cambridge CB2 8RU, UK

Published in the United States of America by Cambridge University Press, New York

www.cambridge.org
Information on this title: www.cambridge.org/9780521888455

© Louise Cummings 2009

This publication is in copyright. Subject to statutory exception
and to the provisions of relevant collective licensing agreements,
no reproduction of any part may take place without
the written permission of Cambridge University Press.

First published 2009

Printed in the United Kingdom at the University Press, Cambridge

A catalogue record for this publication is available from the British Library

Library of Congress Cataloguing in Publication data
Cummings, Louise.
    Clinical pragmatics / Louise Cummings.
        p. ; cm.
    Includes bibliographical references and index.
    ISBN 978-0-521-88845-5 (hardback)   1. Speech disorders.
    2. Speech therapy.   3. Pragmatics.   I. Title.
    [DNLM: 1. Language Disorders.   2. Communication Disorders.
    WL 340.2 C971c 2009]
    RC423.C86 2009
    616.85'5–dc22   2009007868

ISBN 978-0-521-88845-5 hardback

Cambridge University Press has no responsibility for the persistence or
accuracy of URLs for external or third-party internet websites referred to
in this publication, and does not guarantee that any content on such
websites is, or will remain, accurate or appropriate.

6/13/11

In fond memory of my grandparents
Nan & Bob Cummings
Ruby & James Stewart

Contents

Preface

When different disciplines converge on the study of a set of phenomena, one of several things can happen. In one scenario, these disciplines can begin to embrace the concepts, theories and methodologies of those fields of enquiry that are concerned to explain the same phenomena. The result is a genuinely interdisciplinary enquiry which leads to theoretical and other gains that were not realised within any single discipline. In another scenario, the same disciplines can acknowledge shared explanatory interests and can even engage with the concepts and frameworks of neighbouring areas of enquiry. However, to all intents and purposes, there is only the appearance of interdisciplinary enquiry and research proceeds largely along disciplinary lines. In yet another scenario, individual disciplines operate alongside each other with little interest in how other fields of enquiry are attempting to explain essentially the same phenomena. For much of the thirty-year history of clinical pragmatics, the disciplines that have come together to give rise to this field of study (largely pragmatics and language pathology) have displayed the characteristics of the second and third scenarios outlined above. The result has been considerable disarray, with clinical studies undertaken more often than not because they can be done, not because they should be done. No one has gained from this situation, least of all our child and adult clients with pragmatic disorders.

This book addresses what is currently known about a range of pragmatic disorders in children and adults. Pragmatic disorders are now a significant area of clinical language study. Yet, for all their interest to clinical researchers and practitioners, there has been much in the short history of clinical pragmatics that has been problematic. While clinical studies have proceeded apace, they have often done so in a theoretical vacuum. The result has been a large, sprawling body of findings that bear little relation to each other and are not even faithful to the pragmatic concepts that they purport to explain. There have been significant clinical implications of the type of enquiry that has sought to rush ahead with repeated (and often repetitive) studies in the absence of a rationally motivated basis. At best, these studies provide an uncertain foundation upon which to devise reliable pragmatic assessments and plan effective pragmatic interventions. We must acknowledge that one inevitable consequence of this adverse impact on assessment and intervention is that pragmatically disordered clients have for too long not been receiving the type of high-quality clinical services that we have now come to expect for clients with other language disorders (e.g. specific language impairment, aphasia, phonological disorder).

As well as surveying our current state of knowledge of developmental and acquired pragmatic disorders, this book also assumes a deeply critical purpose. Few contributions to clinical pragmatics have even attempted a rational appraisal of the phenomena that investigators have simply assumed to be pragmatic. A research programme that purports to study certain pragmatic notions, but then misrepresents those notions, is neither advancing its own theoretical ends nor revealing anything of significance about the pragmatic competence of a particular clinical population. A similar rational appraisal is necessary of theoretical developments in areas such as developmental psychopathology and cognitive science, areas which should be actively embraced by researchers who are seeking a theoretical explanation of pragmatic disorders. Interdisciplinary exchanges between these disciplines and clinical pragmatics should be facilitated wherever possible, but they must also be handled with great care. For at the same time as they have the potential to throw new light on certain problems, their mismanagement can subvert the very explanatory gains that they were intended to achieve. A further purpose of this book is thus to examine the nature of these interdisciplinary exchanges, many of which have gone unnoticed by clinical pragmatists, and to suggest ways in which these exchanges may contribute to our understanding of pragmatic disorders.

Acknowledgements

I wish to acknowledge with gratitude the assistance of the following people: Judith Heaney for her careful preparation of the bibliography and compilation of the text; Sian Griffiths and other staff at the Boots and Clifton libraries of Nottingham Trent University for their assistance in locating literature; and Helen Barton of Cambridge University Press, for her receptive response to my proposal of this book. The assistance of each of these individuals has been invaluable. Lucy Dipper's detailed comments on an earlier version of the manuscript were particularly constructive. I am very grateful to her for her thorough review of the manuscript on behalf of Cambridge University Press.

Much of the research for this book was undertaken while I was a Visiting Fellow in the Centre for Research in the Arts, Social Sciences and Humanities (CRASSH) at the University of Cambridge. I am grateful to the Director of CRASSH, Mary Jacobus, for her support and encouragement. During my time at Cambridge, Wolfson College provided me with an environment that was particularly conducive to conducting research. I extend my gratitude to its President and Fellows.

Finally, I have been supported in this endeavour by family members and friends who are too numerous to mention individually. I am grateful to them for their kind words of encouragement during my many months of writing.

Chapter 3 originally appeared in Seminars in Speech and Language. Chapter 7 originally appeared in Language and Communication. Both have been extensively reworked for this volume.

1   Clinical pragmatics: theory and practice

1.1   Introduction

The emergence of clinical pragmatics as a field of study in its own right is confirmed by several developments. A number of books, which have either used the title 'clinical pragmatics' or have clinical pragmatics as their central theme, have been published in the last fifteen years.[1] In the same time, academic journals have dedicated special issues to the discussion of clinical pragmatics.[2] Entries on clinical pragmatics are now as likely to appear in encyclopaedias and other reference texts as are entries on phonetics and syntax.[3] Symposia and conferences now routinely dedicate sessions to clinical pragmatics.[4] A greater level of academic interest in clinical pragmatic issues is scarcely imaginable. The question I want to address in this book is whether this interest has advanced our understanding of pragmatic disorders to a significant extent and if the assessment and treatment of these disorders has been facilitated by research in clinical pragmatics. So my task is in part a critical one – a critical evaluation of our current state of knowledge in clinical pragmatics as well as of the application of this knowledge to the assessment and treatment of pragmatic disorders in children and adults. Yet, such a critical evaluation can only reasonably proceed in the context of a wider examination of the clinical studies that have been conducted in the field. One consequence of the intense research activity that has been undertaken in clinical pragmatics is that theorists and clinicians must assimilate the findings of a large and disparate group of studies. Some order must be imposed on these studies if we are to derive new insights from them for our understanding and management of pragmatic disorders. So another part of my task in this book is to reflect on the findings of clinical pragmatic studies that have been undertaken to date. To this end, I conduct a survey of what these studies have revealed about a range of developmental and acquired pragmatic disorders in Chapters 2 and 3.

Before I can embark upon a survey and critical evaluation of clinical pragmatics, it is incumbent on me to address a number of preliminary issues. Since its emergence as a distinct area of enquiry, the field of pragmatics has been bedevilled by discussions about its definition and scope. While these discussions have brought several theoretical issues into sharp focus,[5] they have also had the unintended consequence of creating considerable uncertainty about exactly where the limits of the discipline should lie. In Chapter 7, I argue that this same uncertainty and confusion pervades the related discipline of clinical pragmatics. In the full knowledge that no definition of clinical pragmatics will be wholly adequate on all occasions, I provide a working definition of clinical pragmatics in the next section. This definition will at least have the merits of orientating the reader to the types of issues that are of concern to theorists and practitioners in the field. Pragmatics is still a relatively recent development in both the history of linguistics and the clinical communication sciences. Its 'late' emergence explains certain features of pragmatics itself and of the neighbouring discipline of clinical pragmatics. For example, while developmental stages in the acquisition of phonology and syntax are well documented, we lack comparable milestones in the acquisition of pragmatics. Also, while interventions for phonological disorder in children are theoretically motivated and clinically effective, pragmatic interventions in children consist of a rather ad hoc group of techniques which have no clear theoretical basis and can demonstrate few clinical outcomes. Some sense of the rather limited state of our knowledge in certain areas of clinical pragmatics can be gleaned by examining developments in the past. For this reason, a brief overview of the emergence and development of clinical pragmatics will be presented.

Discussions about the scope of pragmatics notwithstanding, a book of this type is only possible to the extent that we are prepared to accept certain phenomena as pragmatic in nature. Concepts such as speech act and implicature are part of the original Searlean and Gricean reflections that launched pragmatics and, by general consensus, are core pragmatic notions. Topic management, conversational turn-taking and coherence in narrative production are clearly drawing on many of the same competences that are needed to generate and recover implicatures, even though these notions did not receive the direct attention of early theorists such as Austin, Searle and Grice. In short, as the field of pragmatics has developed, an increasing number of linguistic and nonlinguistic behaviours have been described as pragmatic. I will argue in Chapter 7 that this multiplication of pragmatic behaviours has gone too far and that behaviours that are not in any sense pragmatic are now being included in clinical pragmatic studies. In the meantime, however, an account must be given of the nature of different pragmatic concepts, as it is these concepts that are the focus of investigation in the studies reviewed in Chapters 2 and 3. Few theories in pragmatics motivate the studies that have been undertaken of children and adults with pragmatic disorders. This lack of theoretical rationale is in large part responsible for the rather ad hoc nature with which many clinical pragmatic studies have been undertaken. As well as surveying the work that has been undertaken in clinical pragmatics, a further purpose of this book is to highlight those areas in which improvements can be made. One of these areas – the most important one, in my opinion – is that clinical pragmatic investigators need to demonstrate a much stronger sense of theoretical rationale for the particular studies that they undertake. To this end, I will examine significant theoretical approaches within pragmatics in this chapter.

A large range of disciplines converge on the study of disordered pragmatics in children and adults. Speech-language pathologists, educationalists, cognitive and neuroscientists, linguists, psychologists and psychiatrists are just some of the investigators with a professional interest in how the pragmatics of language is disrupted by a brain injury or other problem that has its onset in the developmental period or during adolescence or adulthood. An equally extensive knowledge base is required in order to assimilate the findings of clinical pragmatic studies and to appreciate the implications of these findings for an individual's wider communicative functioning. For example, studies that are investigating the neurocognitive substrates of pragmatic phenomena will only have full significance for a reader who is versed in the neuroanatomical structures that subserve various cognitive and language functions (e.g. the connection between damage to the prefrontal cortex and executive dysfunction). In the same way, the implications of theory of mind deficits in autistic children for communicative functioning in those children will be largely lost on the reader who fails to appreciate that much pragmatic interpretation involves mental state attribution. In short, an extensive knowledge base that includes information about neuroanatomy and neuroimaging techniques, cognition, developmental psychology, language acquisition and processing, and brain injury, amongst many other things, is needed in order to do the work of clinical pragmatics. We will return to the issue of the different disciplines that inform clinical pragmatics in section 1.5 below.

Finally, it is important to be clear from the outset that theorists and clinicians recognise a distinction between primary and secondary pragmatic disorders. In a significant number of children and adults, pragmatic impairments may be related to structural language deficits. For example, the child with specific language impairment or the adult with agrammatic aphasia may be unable to produce indirect requests. However, this inability may not be related to any impairment of pragmatic competence as such – an individual may know that a particular conversational interaction demands the use of an indirect speech act – but may simply reflect the fact that the child or adult lacks the syntactic and semantic structures to formulate indirect requests. In such a case, clinicians and theorists use the term 'secondary' to describe an individual's pragmatic disorder – the disorder is secondary to an impairment of structural language. This type of pragmatic disorder is quite different from the child or adult who doesn't understand that conversational interaction with a teacher or an employer demands the use of polite language forms such as indirect requests.

The child or adult in this case exhibits a primary pragmatic disorder. A final point of note is that the emphasis in clinical studies of pragmatics has been on the deficits or impairments displayed by children or adults. Diagnostic categories such as pragmatic language impairment (formerly semantic-pragmatic disorder) also reflect the preoccupation of clinicians and theorists with the study of deficits and disorders. However, it is worth remarking that even in the most pragmatically impaired clients, some pragmatic skills often remain intact. The preservation of pragmatic skills is frequently overlooked by investigators in their rush to analyse deficits. This book will attempt to redress the balance by giving emphasis whenever possible to aspects of intact pragmatic functioning.

1.2   The scope of clinical pragmatics

In this section, I will endeavour to delineate the types of problems and clients that are studied by workers in clinical pragmatics. Some communication problems have few, if any, adverse implications for language pragmatics. For example, the client who stutters or the adult with a voice disorder will certainly experience problems with communication. However, these problems are not related to any deficit in pragmatic competence. The client with a pragmatic disorder is in a very different situation to the adult with a voice disorder. He or she will be unable to use language to achieve various communicative purposes. These purposes may include relating a story to a friend, ordering a meal in a restaurant, asking for times at a train station or making a promise to be home early. A wide range of cognitive and linguistic skills are needed to perform these seemingly mundane communicative activities. For example, in order to relate a story to a friend, a speaker must be able to secure the attention of a listener, recall the events in the story, link these events in a coherent manner and monitor a listener's state of understanding. These individual skills draw on cognitive processes such as memory and attention, a cognitive capacity to have a theory of other minds and linguistic abilities that are necessary for the construction of grammatical and meaningful utterances. The disruption of one or more of these processes and abilities will lead to communicative failure in that the speaker will not be able to relate, or at least will not relate particularly effectively, a story to a friend. The particular cognitive and linguistic processes that are the cause of this failure are the concern of practitioners and researchers in the field of clinical pragmatics.

Although the child who stutters or the adult with a voice disorder will not struggle with the cognitive and linguistic processes outlined above, there are a substantial number of children and adults for whom these processes are severely disordered. The development of language skills is markedly delayed in the Down's syndrome child with mental retardation. Such a child will lack some of the syntactic and semantic structures that are needed to formulate speech acts. This same child will also exhibit problems with receptive language, so that he or she will be unable to decode the linguistic constructions in which speech acts and other pragmatic phenomena are couched. Similarly, it is now widely acknowledged that autistic children lack the theory of mind skills that are present in normally developing four-year-olds. The ability to attribute beliefs and other mental states to the minds of others is the same cognitive skill that is necessary for pragmatic interpretation – we cannot recover the intended implicature of a speaker's utterance, for example, if we cannot view our interlocutor as someone who entertains certain mental states (viz., communicative intentions). Owing to their underlying cognitive deficit in theory of mind, autistic children can be expected to struggle with language pragmatics. We will see in Chapter 4 that a substantial number of studies are demonstrating the presence of severe and persistent pragmatic deficits in this population of children. The Down's syndrome child and the autistic child both experience developmental pragmatic disorders even though the specific cause of these disorders differs in these cases (language impairment related to mental retardation in the child with Down's syndrome and theory of mind deficits related to cognitive dysfunction in the autistic child). In Chapter 2, we examine the pragmatic deficits that occur in mental retardation and autistic spectrum disorder as well as deficits in two other clinical populations – children with developmental language disorder and emotional and behavioural problems.

Even in the case where pragmatic language skills have developed along normal lines (see section 1.5), an individual may still present with disordered pragmatics. An adult may sustain a right-hemisphere stroke subsequent to which he or she may experience difficulties interpreting non-literal language. The fifteen-year-old boy who is involved in a road traffic accident may have significant cognitive and communication problems related to frontal lobe pathology as part of a traumatic brain injury. The twenty-five-year-old male may present for the first time with pragmatic breakdown during an acute psychotic episode that marks the onset of schizophrenia. In each of these cases, the onset of the brain injury or other event (e.g. cerebrovascular accident) that causes pragmatic disorder takes place during adolescence or adulthood, when the acquisition of most pragmatic skills is likely to be complete. Like developmental pragmatic disorders, acquired pragmatic disorders may be related to linguistic and cognitive problems. For example, the nonfluent aphasic speaker may have such restricted linguistic output that he or she may be unable to implicate anything at all. Also, the verbal output of the fluent aphasic speaker may contain so much jargon that there are few, if any, grammatical and meaningful utterances that a listener can use to recover implicatures. Cognitive deficits in schizophrenic adults are increasingly being linked to the discourse and pragmatic problems of this clinical population. For example, discourse coherence deficits such as non sequiturs, tangential responses and derailment have been significantly correlated with working memory deficits in schizophrenic clients (Melinder and Barch 2003). In Chapter 3, pragmatic deficits in schizophrenia, traumatic brain injury and right-hemisphere damage will be examined at length. We will also discuss two other clinical populations in that chapter – adults with left-hemisphere damage and neurodegenerative disorders, principally Alzheimer's disease.

Thus far, a brief overview has been given of the types of problems and clients that are studied by workers in clinical pragmatics. On the basis of this overview, I want to introduce the following working definition of the field of clinical pragmatics:

Clinical pragmatics is the study of the various ways in which an individual's use of language to achieve communicative purposes can be disrupted. The cerebral injury, pathology or other anomaly that causes this disruption has its onset in the developmental period or during adolescence or adulthood. Developmental and acquired pragmatic disorders have diverse aetiologies and may be the consequence of, related to or perpetuated by a range of cognitive and linguistic factors.

This definition contains a number of features that require some elaboration. First, the notion of a 'communicative purpose' is necessarily open-ended. An individual's purpose in communicating may be to inform a friend of a forthcoming event, to warn residents to leave a burning building or to protest against the actions of a colleague. But, equally, a speaker may choose to communicate in order to maintain or develop a social relationship with an interlocutor, to distract a listener from his or her current preoccupations or to advise a friend that a particular course of action is ill-advised. In short, the purposes for which we communicate are indefinably large and are no more amenable to circumscription than are the grammatical or meaningful sentences in a language. Second, this definition states that communicative purposes are achieved through the 'use of language'. This emphasis on language is intended to counteract a widespread tendency in clinical pragmatic studies to label a whole range of behaviours, including nonlinguistic behaviours, as pragmatic. Certainly, nonlinguistic behaviours such as gesture and eye contact can facilitate a listener's interpretation of a speaker's utterance. The speaker who maintains eye contact with his or her listener, for example, is more likely to be viewed by that listener as a cooperative communicator who will contribute only those utterances that will facilitate an exchange. This assumption of cooperation is the basis of the rational framework by means of which, Grice contends, speakers generate and listeners recover implicatures during conversation with each other. However, a behaviour that contributes to the successful interpretation of a speaker's utterance is not thereby pragmatic in nature (syntactic and cognitive processes also play a significant role in the interpretation of utterances, yet we wouldn't think of labelling these processes 'pragmatic'). The notion of pragmatics that I want to employ in this book is one that is more deeply rooted in language use than many practitioners and researchers in clinical pragmatics have tended to adopt. This point is sufficiently important to warrant further discussion.

Even a brief survey of studies that have been conducted in the area of clinical pragmatics reveals a tendency amongst investigators that is at once puzzling and revealing. This is the tendency to construe pragmatics in such broad terms that it is not clear what this term is intended to exclude. In fact, the term 'pragmatics' has now become coextensive in many (if not most) clinical studies with the notion of communication itself (these studies, and the same pernicious tendency at work in techniques of pragmatic assessment and treatment, are critically evaluated in Chapter 7). I argue in Chapter 7 that this tendency on the part of clinical pragmatic investigators to identify pragmatics with communication has its origin in the Chomskyan distinction between competence and performance, a distinction which served to force pragmatics into the domain of performance. Only knowledge that enabled us to produce grammatical and meaningful sentences warranted, according to Chomsky, the title of 'linguistic competence'. In this book, I want to reverse the tendency set in motion by Chomsky's famous competence/performance distinction by arguing for the integration of pragmatics within our linguistic competence. Specifically, I want to argue that the knowledge that permits communicators to issue threats and warnings, establish the presuppositions of an utterance, produce coherent narratives and recover the implicatures of an utterance is part of our linguistic competence in the same way that the knowledge that enables us to form grammatical, meaningful sentences is part of our linguistic competence. Under this conception, pragmatics is about the knowledge that allows a speaker to employ a linguistic utterance to achieve a certain communicative effect. The fact that other behaviours may attend the employment of this utterance should not detract from the centrality of the linguistic utterance to pragmatics.

This conception of pragmatics has an important precedent in the philosophical views of John Searle. Searle identifies in Chomsky the same conception of the distinction between competence and performance that, I am arguing, is responsible for an unfortunate tendency in clinical pragmatic studies – the tendency to reject any role for pragmatics within a theory of competence by confining pragmatics to an account of language performance. In his essay 'Chomsky's revolution in linguistics', Searle (1974) describes Chomsky's reluctance to countenance a role for a theory of speech acts within his grammar. Chomsky's reluctance, Searle argues, can be explained by several reasons, the first of which he captures as follows:

He (Chomsky) has a mistaken conception of the distinction between performance and competence. He seems to think that a theory of speech acts must be a theory of performance rather than of competence, because he fails to see that competence is ultimately the competence to perform, and that for this reason a study of the linguistic aspects of the ability to perform speech acts is a study of linguistic competence. (1974: 31)

Searle believes that Chomsky's characterisation of a speaker's linguistic competence as 'his ability to produce and understand sentences' is at best misleading, because 'a person's knowledge of the meaning of sentences consists in large part in his knowledge of how to use sentences to make statements, ask questions, give orders, make requests, make promises, warnings, etc., and to understand other people when they use sentences for such purposes' (1974: 28). Any account of our knowledge of how to use sentences for these various purposes, Searle argues, necessarily involves a notion of competence that extends beyond the rather limited conception that Chomsky is prepared to countenance to include a theory of speech acts. By the same token, the reader should be aware that in describing pragmatic language skills and, equally importantly, pragmatic disorders, I am making statements about a speaker's linguistic competence and not merely describing features of language performance. Our knowledge of how to use language to perform a range of speech acts (and do much else besides) is a core component of our linguistic competence that is on a par with our knowledge of how to form grammatical, meaningful sentences. I believe that it is only when we locate pragmatics fully within a speaker's linguistic competence that the various errors that have occurred in the identification of pragmatic phenomena can begin to be corrected. I will return to this issue in Chapter 7.

Third, the above definition deliberately avoids linking developmental and acquired pragmatic disorders to specific chronological periods (i.e. the developmental period, adolescence and adulthood). This linkage has been avoided for an important reason. Pragmatic aspects of language are still being acquired long after syntactic and semantic structures are established in a child's language system. It is now known that pragmatic development can extend well into adolescence (see section 1.5). This creates something of a classification problem for investigators, as it is not always clear in a particular case if a pragmatic disorder is developmental or acquired in nature. For example, a fifteen-year-old who develops a pragmatic disorder following traumatic brain injury is likely to have both developmental and acquired components to his or her disorder. Compared to stages in pragmatic development, chronological periods denoted by terms such as 'adolescence' and 'adulthood' are of secondary importance in determining whether an individual has a developmental or acquired pragmatic disorder. This is why a clear understanding of stages in pragmatic development is important in the study of pragmatic disorder and why the lack of extensive research in this area has adverse implications for clinical pragmatics. Fourth, I have acknowledged through the use of 'other anomaly' in the above definition that not all pragmatic disorders can be linked to the presence of cerebral injuries and pathologies. Indeed, in a disorder such as specific language impairment (SLI) in children, there is a distinct absence of neurological aetiology (in fact, a neurological aetiology must be excluded in order for a diagnosis of SLI to be made). The reader should therefore be aware that while a neurological aetiology is implicated in many of the pragmatic disorders that will be examined in this book, other aetiologies or indeed no clear aetiology at all may underlie these disorders.

Fifth, the above definition emphasises the role of cognitive and linguistic factors in pragmatic disorders. We described earlier how a pragmatic disorder may be secondary to structural language problems. The child with Down's syndrome, for example, who does not have inversion of subject pronouns and auxiliary verbs as part of his or her syntactic repertoire, will not have the syntactic structures required to form indirect requests such as 'Can you open the window?' The same indirect request is likely to be problematic for the agrammatic aphasic adult who has considerably reduced expressive syntax. However, such an adult will be aware of the politeness constraints that operate in conversation and that an indirect request of this type is more appropriate in a formal setting than the direct, but less polite form 'Open the window!' The dependence of pragmatics on other language subsystems is to be expected – after all, we can only produce and comprehend speech acts, generate and recover implicatures and frame coherent narratives if we have access to certain syntactic and semantic structures. The link between pragmatic disorders and cognitive deficits is now well established. An increasing number of pragmatic impairments in both children and adults are being linked to theory of mind deficits. Working memory and executive function deficits have also been found to be associated with pragmatic disorders. The ability to attribute mental states to others, to engage in flexible thinking, to reason deductively and non-deductively and to retrieve information from memory are key cognitive skills that underpin pragmatic interpretation. Given the dependence of pragmatic phenomena on cognition, I will return to the topic of cognition time and again in the chapters of this book. In the meantime, the reader should be aware that in order to understand disordered pragmatics, one must understand how pragmatics is related to other linguistic and cognitive domains.

1.3   The emergence of clinical pragmatics

The impetus for a new discipline of clinical pragmatics shares certain interesting similarities with the origins of pragmatics itself. These origins are standardly taken to reside in the language philosophies of H.P. Grice, J.L. Austin and John Searle.[6] The work of each of these theorists can be seen as a critical reaction to the view of language that was dominant amongst philosophers in the early part of the twentieth century. For his part, Austin challenged the idea that a declarative sentence is always used to describe, either truly or falsely, some state of affairs (what he called the descriptive fallacy). Many declarative sentences, Austin argued, do not describe or report anything. Nor can we sensibly ask if they are true or false. Rather, the act of uttering these sentences constitutes the performance of an action. These so-called performatives include examples like 'I baptise this child Fred Brown' and 'I pronounce you man and wife', in which the mere utterance of these statements constitutes an act of baptism and marriage, respectively. In *How to do things with words*, Austin (1962) states that performative utterances:

A. do not 'describe' or 'report' or constate anything at all, are not 'true or false'; and

B. the uttering of the sentence is, or is a part of, the doing of an action, which again would not *normally* be described as saying something. (1962: 5; italics in original)

The view that language could be used to do things ushered in a new branch of linguistic enquiry. At the centre of this new field of pragmatics was the language user whose linguistic goals in everyday communicative situations were as likely to involve making requests and expressing promises as they were to involve describing events and other states of affairs. Linguistic phenomena that were proving problematic for the logical frameworks employed by semanticists could be more readily explained by this new field of study. In his William James lectures in 1967, Grice proposed a new and revolutionary analysis of sentences such as *Some students pass their exams*. Grice proposed a distinction between what a sentence *says* and what it may be taken to conventionally *implicate*. While a logician and a natural language user may both *say* the same thing, it is a convention of natural language not shared by logic that sentences may also carry implications beyond what they say. In the above sentence, for example, a speaker may be taken to implicate that not all students pass their exams. This is the case even though there is no inconsistency in logic between the sentences *Some students pass their exams* and *All students pass their exams*. As well as conventional implicature, Grice introduced a further category of implicature which has had a profound influence on the development of pragmatic theory. Known as conversational implicature, we will see subsequently that this type of implicature has been one of the most extensively investigated pragmatic phenomena in the clinical literature.

It was not long before practitioners and clinical researchers began to realise that the assessment and treatment of language disorders in children and adults required something of a pragmatic turn. In the same way that theorists such as Austin and Grice had revealed the inadequacy of semantic and logical frameworks in analysing how speakers actually use language, clinicians and researchers set about dismantling some rather unhelpful assumptions about language that had defined for many years how language disorders should be assessed and treated. These assumptions had their origin in a semantic conception of language and meaning. Under this conception, single words and sentences were regarded as the only units of meaning (the notion of discourse was completely overlooked) and meaning was based entirely on language (words and sentences had an invariant meaning that was not influenced by how speakers used these linguistic entities). The effect of these assumptions on clinical practice was that disproportionate emphasis was placed on structural language skills, often at the expense of any consideration of how clients used their language skills in a range of communicative situations. Also, despite the fact that normal language users do not produce utterances in a linguistic vacuum, assessment and treatment of language skills proceeded by and large on the basis of single word and single sentence productions. In attempting to eliminate these assumptions, or at least reduce their significance, clinicians and researchers embraced new methods of pragmatic assessment and treatment, redefined notions of treatment efficacy in pragmatic terms and even devised new nosological categories to reflect the clinical significance of impairments of pragmatic language skills. We discuss some of these developments below.

One of the first clinical areas to reflect this growing interest in pragmatics was the classification of developmental language disorders. Even as the philosophical ideas of Austin and Grice were having an impact on linguistics, clinicians were increasingly being called upon to assess and treat children in whom the principal communicative impairment was not related to any deficit in structural language. The appearance in clinics of children who were not obviously autistic yet who shared some of the bizarre communicative patterns of autistic children led clinicians and researchers to revise classifications of developmental language disorders. To reflect the disproportionately poor use of language by these children, Rapin and Allen (1983) in the US, and later Bishop and Rosenbloom (1987) in the UK, used the term 'semantic-pragmatic disorder'. Although there were differences between these researchers in the application of this term, its emergence in the clinical literature marked the transition of pragmatics from a largely neglected area of clinical enquiry to an aspect of language that was now of diagnostic significance. Today, pragmatics continues to exert its presence in nosological discussions of developmental language disorder. For example, Dorothy Bishop and her colleagues are very actively involved in examining the relationship of pragmatic language impairment – the modern day successor of semantic-pragmatic disorder – to specific language impairment and autism spectrum disorder (see Bishop (2000a) for further discussion). Yet, these discussions would not be possible were it not for the pragmatic insights of early investigators who undertook to think about language and communication disorder in a radically different way.

The new clinical emphasis on pragmatics also came to be reflected in techniques of language assessment, particularly amongst adult clients. The emergence of pragmatics encouraged clinicians to examine how clients used their language skills in communication with others. Such examination required that clinicians assess the impact of a much wider range of factors on a client's language skills than had traditionally been possible. Factors such as context could not be successfully assessed by language batteries such as the Boston Diagnostic Aphasia Examination (Goodglass *et al.* 2001) and the Western Aphasia Battery (Kertesz 2006).[7] Much less were such formal language assessments able to examine the effect of social factors, such as politeness constraints, on clients' linguistic choices or how patterns of language use varied with different conversational partners. Single word and sentence testing formats began to assume less significance in assessment alongside methods that employed the techniques of conversation analysis and discourse analysis. Today, these techniques are included as standard in assessments of the language skills of adults with acquired communication disorders.[8] Although many such assessments are conducted informally according to procedures that are devised by clinicians, there are now a number of published resources that employ the methodology of conversation analysis to assess language impaired adults. One such resource is the Conversation Analysis Profile for People with Aphasia (Whitworth *et al.* 1997). A related profile – the Conversation Analysis Profile for People with Cognitive Impairment (Perkins *et al.* 1997) – is designed for use with clients who have generalised cognitive impairment, such as occurs in dementia or head injury.

The position of pragmatics in clinical practice and research is now secured. Pragmatics is a standard part of the assessment and treatment protocols of developmental and acquired language disorders. Its role in communication impairment continues to be widely investigated by clinical researchers. With a substantial body of work of a pragmatic nature already undertaken in clinical studies, the field of clinical pragmatics needs a thoroughgoing critical assessment of its achievements to date more than it needs findings from further studies. The time is now right to survey the field and consider its substantial successes, but also be cognizant of its failures. The chapters of this book are intended to make a significant contribution towards achieving that end.

1.4   Concepts and theories in pragmatics

One of the most striking features of the development of a distinct discipline of clinical pragmatics has been the proliferation of phenomena that investigators have been prepared to label as pragmatic. From early studies that restricted themselves to an examination of one or two speech acts (Rom and Bliss 1981; Prinz and Ferrier 1983; Abbeduto *et al.* 1988), the field has witnessed an almost exponential growth in so-called pragmatic concepts. Nowadays, clinical pragmatic studies of children and adults are as likely to examine referential communication, the production of narrative discourse, topic management in conversation and the comprehension of sarcasm as they are to examine traditional pragmatic notions such as speech acts. In this section, I present the reader with an overview of the different concepts and topics that feature in clinical pragmatic studies of the type reviewed in Chapters 2 and 3. Owing to constraints of space, this overview will not be exhaustive. However, it will provide the reader with an orientation to the most significant concepts that have featured in clinical pragmatic research in the last thirty years. While there has been a staggering increase in the range of pragmatic concepts investigated in clinical pragmatic studies, the same cannot be said of theories in pragmatics. Nevertheless, a small number of studies have sought to interpret their findings within theoretical frameworks such as relevance theory (Sperber and Wilson 1986, 1995). Also, I argued in section 1.1 that researchers in clinical pragmatics need to develop a much stronger theoretical rationale for the studies they undertake than has been in evidence to date. For both these reasons, I will also introduce the reader in this section to prominent pragmatic theories that have relevance to the work of clinical pragmatics.

1.4.1   Speech acts

The notion of a speech act has its roots in the language philosophies of Austin and Searle (for discussion, see Chapter 1 in Cummings 2005). Austin's and Searle's contribution was to demonstrate that language could be used to do much more than merely report or describe states of affairs. Rather, language could be used to make promises, issue threats and warnings, extend invitations, offer suggestions and do a wide range of other things besides. Some of these actions performed through language can be signalled by the use of performative verbs (e.g. 'I promise to be home early' and 'I bet you £10 that your horse doesn't finish' are a promise and a bet, respectively, and contain the explicit performative verbs 'promise' and 'bet'). However, these same actions are just as likely, and probably more likely, to be performed in ways that don't involve the use of performative verbs (e.g. 'I'll be home early' and '£10 your horse doesn't finish' are equally likely to be understood by listeners in particular contexts as committing their speakers to a promise and a bet, respectively). A speech act that contains a performative verb poses little interpretative challenge to a listener, as the speaker's communicative intention in producing the utterance is explicitly signalled. An altogether more difficult task of interpretation is presented by the utterance that has a declarative form but is serving to warn rather than merely inform a listener (e.g. 'Big Jim is in the park') or by the utterance that has an interrogative form but is serving to make a request rather than ask a question (e.g. 'Can you pay your bill at the desk?'). To determine the communicative intentions behind the utterance of such indirect speech acts, the listener must be able to establish that the utterance's literal meaning is unlikely to represent the speaker's intended meaning within a particular context (a hotel manager, for example, is unlikely to be asking a guest about his or her ability to pay a bill). In a normal scenario, a process of interpretation that starts out from the literal meaning of the utterance combined with salient aspects of context will lead the listener to the speaker's intended meaning.[9]

Of course, in children and adults with pragmatic disorder this normal scenario does not obtain. The child with mental retardation, for example, may lack the linguistic decoding skills that are needed to establish the literal meaning of an utterance. Theory of mind (ToM) deficits may preclude the autistic child or adult from recognising the communicative intention behind a speaker's use of an utterance. The various cognitive and linguistic processes that are involved in pragmatic interpretation are adequately exemplified by the case of speech acts. For this reason, and the fact that it is relatively easy to assess a client's comprehension of speech acts in a clinical setting, speech acts have become one of the most extensively investigated pragmatic phenomena in clinical studies. As well as examining comprehension of speech acts, clinical pragmatic studies have examined the production of a range of speech acts by children and adults. In order to use speech acts effectively, a speaker must make judgements about the formality of context (an indirect request may be more appropriate than a direct request), an addressee's mental states (a speaker who utters 'Big Jim is in the park' to someone who doesn't know Jim has hardly produced a felicitous warning) and one's own ability to execute the action contained in the speech act (a promise to help someone move house when the speaker knows he will be out of the country on holiday falls short of being a felicitous promise). These judgements, which are effortless for the pragmatically intact speaker, can be problematic for speakers with pragmatic disorder (one can imagine how an autistic child with ToM deficits will be unable to frame a speech act with his addressee's state of knowledge in mind). A skilled clinician can usually successfully elicit a range of speech acts from clients in the setting of a clinic. For example, a clinician can prompt a child to request his or her favourite toy by placing it out of reach. The ability to produce speech acts is an important aspect of pragmatic competence that has been extensively examined in clinical studies.

1.4.2   Implicatures

The notion of implicature has also been dominant in clinical pragmatic studies. Grice's treatment of implicature is discussed at length in Chapter 1 in

Cummings (2005). Grice was interested in examining the set of rational expectations that speakers and listeners operate with in conversation with each other, expectations that allow A in the following exchange to conclude that B does not want to accept his invitation to dinner:

A: Do you want to come round to my place tonight for dinner?
B: John's mother is visiting this evening.

Grice's theory of conversational implicature seeks an explanation of this exchange and of the central role of cooperation within it. Grice couches his definition of the cooperative principle in a speaker-directed imperative:

Make your conversational contribution such as is required, at the stage at which it occurs, by the accepted purpose or direction of the talk exchange in which you are engaged. (1975: 45)

In itself, the cooperative principle doesn't state exactly what is 'required' of a conversational contribution. Specificity is conferred on this principle through a series of four maxims: the maxim of quality (do not say that which you believe to be false or that for which you lack adequate evidence); the maxim of quantity (make your contribution as informative as is required, but do not contribute more information than is required); the maxim of relation (make you contribution relevant to the exchange); and the maxim of manner (be brief and orderly; avoid ambiguity and obscurity of expression). The cooperative principle and maxims can be used to account for the above exchange between A and B as follows. As a response to A's question, B's utterance is superficially irrelevant. The superficial irrelevance of B's response is noted by A, who assumes that B is attempting, at a minimum, to be cooperative within the exchange. On the basis of this assumption of cooperation A goes on to infer that B is attempting to communicate a declination of A's invitation.

The implicature generated by B's response in the above exchange is described by Grice as a particularised conversational implicature. It is so-called because it depends on a particular context (John is B's husband; John's mother is B's mother-in-law; B's mother-in-law lives in a different city from B and visits infrequently; B likes her mother-in-law and feels a sense of obligation to be present when she visits, etc.). However, in a different context – imagine A knows that B dislikes her mother-in-law – a very different implicature may be generated by B's response. In that case, B may be taken to implicate that she will be happy to accept A's invitation to dinner, possibly as a means of avoiding having to spend time with her mother-in-law. Particularised conversational implicatures are the type of implicature that is most often investigated in clinical pragmatic studies. However, Grice proposed another main category of implicature called generalised conversational implicature, one type of which – scalar implicature – has also been examined by clinical investigators. A scalar implicature is demonstrated by the example below, in which the sentence in A may be taken to implicate B:

A: There will be eight of us on the committee.
B: There won't be more than eight of us on the committee.

Scalar implicatures are so-called because linguistic features are arranged along a scale according to their information content. The affirmation of one feature on the scale (in the example above, number eight) implicates that all the informatively stronger features on the scale (e.g. nine, ten, eleven, etc.) do not hold (Segerdahl 1996: 102).

1.4.3   Presuppositions

Levinson (1983) states that 'the technical sense of presupposition is restricted to certain pragmatic inferences or assumptions that seem at least to be built into linguistic expressions' (168). Some of these 'linguistic expressions' are factive verbs (e.g. 'She *regretted* divorcing her husband' presupposes that she divorced her husband), cleft constructions (e.g. '*It was* Henry who let John's tyres down' presupposes that someone let John's tyres down), definite descriptions (e.g. 'The car knocked over *the girl in the red dress*' presupposes that there exists a girl in a red dress) and change-of-state verbs (e.g. 'Have you stopped fox hunting?' presupposes that the addressee did at one time hunt foxes). Although each of these presuppositions appears to be 'built into' a particular linguistic expression, we can readily envisage contexts in which they can be cancelled. For example, there is no logical inconsistency in a speaker saying 'Sue regretted divorcing her husband until she woke up and realised that she hadn't actually divorced him at all'. It is this reliance on context that makes presupposition such a central pragmatic notion. Notwithstanding its significance to pragmatics, presupposition has received little direct examination by clinical investigators.[10] Possible reasons for this neglect include misunderstanding amongst clinical researchers about the exact status of presupposition (especially its relationship to notions such as entailment) and methodological concerns about how this notion can be best assessed. Problems with the use of presuppositions are often only revealed through extended analyses of conversational exchanges and other types of discourse. Yet conversation and discourse analyses are not always the method of choice for investigators who have one eye on time and another eye on scientific desiderata such as the standardisation of techniques and the replication of findings.

Although presuppositions have seldom been the focus of clinical studies, a presuppositional ability is necessary to other pragmatic phenomena that have been examined by investigators. During discourse production a speaker must make a number of judgements about the information that should be explicitly conveyed to a listener (new information) and the information that the listener already knows (given or old information) and that it would be inefficient for the speaker to directly convey. These judgements made, presupposition becomes the speaker's principal mechanism for dealing with given information.[11] Lexical choices and even the structure of utterances reflect the information that a speaker is presupposing in his or her production of an utterance. The use of the definite article 'the' as opposed to the indefinite article 'a' in the utterance 'The party will start at 8pm sharp' reflects a belief on the part of the speaker that the listener knows the specific referent of the noun accompanying the definite article. The cleft construction 'It was Sarah who drowned in the lake' presupposes the speaker's belief that the listener knows someone drowned in the lake – this information is given – while at the same time conferring prominence on the individual, Sarah, who suffered this particular fate by placing her name before the tragic event in question (compare this cleft construction to the utterance 'The person who drowned in the lake was Sarah' which conveys the same information but places 'Sarah' in a much less prominent position in the utterance). Normal speakers can readily manipulate presuppositions and given and new information and perform the lexical and syntactic processes that reflect these different types of information. The question of whether these same presuppositional and linguistic processes are problematic for children and adults with pragmatic disorder is still open and cannot de definitively addressed on the basis of research that has been conducted to date.[12]

1.4.4   Deixis

Deixis is a significant concept in the field of pragmatics. In earlier work, I stated that deictic terms 'describe entities within the wider social, linguistic or spatiotemporal context of an utterance' (Cummings 2005: 22). Although extensive discussion of these terms was undertaken in that work, some of them can be demonstrated in the present context by means of the following examples. Consider the utterance 'I've lived here for ten years, but will move out tomorrow'. To establish the referents of the personal pronoun 'I', the adverb 'here' and the calendrical term 'tomorrow' in this utterance, a listener must know certain things. He or she must know who the speaker of this utterance is, where the speaker is located at the point of utterance and the day on which this utterance is produced. A named individual, who is the speaker of the utterance, is the referent of the pronoun 'I'. A specific address is likely to be the intended referent of 'here' (an aspect of linguistic context, namely the verb 'move out', supports this particular referent over a referent such as 'Hull' or 'England'). If the utterance is spoken on 20 July 2007, 'tomorrow' will refer to 21 July 2007. The words 'I', 'here' and 'tomorrow' are examples of person, spatial and temporal deixis, respectively. Other forms of deixis in language include socially deictic expressions. The tu/vous pronoun distinction in French encodes certain social attributes of the listener, namely familiarity to the speaker and social distance from the speaker, respectively. Discourse deictic terms refer to a part of wider discourse, where discourse may be understood as either a written or oral text. Discourse deixis, which includes expressions such as 'the last chapter' and 'the next section', may be used by writers to orientate readers to particular points in a larger piece of writing (e.g. 'In the next section I develop this point in detail').

Notwithstanding its centrality to pragmatics, deixis has been almost entirely neglected by workers in clinical pragmatics. This is particularly surprising given reports of pronoun problems in a clinical population with significant pragmatic disorder, namely, children with autism. Jordan (1989) examined the use and understanding of the personal pronouns 'you' and 'me' in eleven autistic children. There were no significant differences between these children and normally developing children and mentally handicapped children matched by receptive vocabulary age on the comprehension of these pronouns. However, only two autistic children displayed the same pattern of responses using these pronouns as all but four of the twenty-two control children in the study. Autistic children used incorrect case pronouns or proper names for self or other reference. Interestingly, they displayed almost no pronoun reversal.[13] Jordan interprets these findings 'in the light of significant difficulties in the acquisition of person deixis in autistic children' (1989: 169). In one of the few other clinical studies to investigate deixis, Varley (1993) examined the use of deictic forms in the conversational speech of fluent and nonfluent aphasic subjects and subjects with right-hemisphere damage. Significantly more deictic expressions were used by subjects with fluent aphasia than by other clinical groups and by a group of non-brain-damaged control subjects. Subjects with nonfluent aphasia used significantly fewer deictic forms than these other groups. Deictic use did not correlate significantly with performance on lexical tests. Nor was there an inverse relationship between deictic use and number of clause elements at the level of the group. Clearly, further clinical studies of deixis must be undertaken before any conclusions can be drawn about the role of this concept in pragmatic disorder.

1.4.5   Context

The notion of context is so central to pragmatics that most definitions of the field make explicit reference to it (see Chapter 7). By its very nature, context is a broad concept that involves physical, linguistic, epistemic and social elements. For example, in the exchange between A and B in section 1.4.2, repeated below, physical context includes features such as the day and time of speaking, other people present, the physical setting in which the exchange is conducted (office, restaurant, etc.):

A: Do you want to come round to my place tonight for dinner?
B: John's mother is visiting this evening.

An aspect of physical context, namely time, is explicitly signalled by both A and B in their use of the indexical expressions 'tonight' and 'this evening', respectively. The immediate linguistic context that A uses to recover the implicature of B's response is the question posed by A himself. However, earlier parts of the conversation between A and B may also contribute linguistic context that may be relevant to the implicature that A derives from B's response. For example, B may have communicated at the start of the conversation that her mother-in-law is in declining health and will soon be unable to undertake journeys. With this piece of linguistic context in mind, A may even more strongly conclude that B is implicating that she cannot come for dinner as it is important that she meet her mother-in-law. The epistemic context describes the shared background knowledge and beliefs between speaker and listener in an exchange (the term 'doxastic' may be used when beliefs are at issue). For example, A and B clearly share all sorts of knowledge about who John is, what dinner is, where A lives, and what part of the day is being referred to by the word 'evening'. At least equally important to the success of the above exchange is the knowledge and beliefs that A and B have about each other's mental states. In this way, A could not have derived an implicature from B's utterance if he did not know that B knows that one can only commit oneself to come for dinner if there are no other competing engagements. By the same token, B could not have implicated her declination of A's dinner invitation if she did not know that A knows that family commitments often take precedence over other engagements. Finally, it is a feature of social context, specifically some degree of social distance between A and B, that leads B to decline A's dinner invitation indirectly rather than by means of the more direct, but less polite response of simply 'No!'

Clinical studies have employed diverse methodologies to examine the processing of context by children and adults with pragmatic disorders. In general, context tends to be construed within these studies in terms of a single sentence or a short passage (i.e. linguistic aspects of context are examined to the exclusion of other aspects of context). Subjects must be able to draw upon this sentence or passage in order to achieve the disambiguation of a word or sentence or the correct pronunciation of a homograph. This procedure was recently employed in a study by Norbury (2005) of lexical ambiguity resolution in nine- to seventeen-year-olds with language impairment, autistic spectrum disorder (ASD) plus language impairment and ASD with verbal abilities in the normal range. Norbury investigated the ability of these children to process context in order to determine the correct meanings of ambiguous words in two conditions. These conditions examined contextual facilitation and suppression. Accuracy and response times to picture judgements were recorded in each condition. As an example of the stimuli used in the context facilitation condition, children were required to make picture judgements following a neutral sentence (sentence (1) below) and following a biased sentence context (sentence (2) below):

Sentence (1): He *ran* from the bank – picture *money*
Sentence (2): He *stole* from the bank – picture *money*

Although all groups of children responded quickly and more accurately to words that followed a biased context, children with language impairment, and ASD plus language impairment, did not use context as efficiently as their peers without language impairment. Moreover, subjects with language impairment, either in isolation or with ASD, produced errors in the suppression condition that reflected poor contextual processing. Similar techniques have been used to investigate deficits in context processing in subjects with schizophrenia (Bazin *et al.* 2000; Sitnikova *et al.* 2002).

A substantial number of investigations have addressed epistemic aspects of context such as listener knowledge. Speakers are constantly required to make judgements about their listeners' state of knowledge. We cannot give a motorist directions to a particular location, explain how a game is played to a child or tell a story to a friend if we are not able to establish the motorist's, child's and friend's current state of knowledge. An assessment of listener knowledge is conducted effortlessly by most speakers in everyday situations. We can readily assume, for example, that a motorist will understand what it means to turn left at a roundabout even if he doesn't know the exact route to his desired location. Normal speakers also have little difficulty in tailoring their directions, explanations and stories in a way that takes account of their listeners' knowledge. For example, a pedestrian knows that it is not necessary to describe to a motorist what it means to turn left at a roundabout, even if he needs to be told how to get onto the motorway. The same linguistic and cognitive skills that permit normal speakers to give informative directions to a motorist are often lacking in children and adults with pragmatic disorder. Investigators use a range of techniques to assess these skills in pragmatically impaired subjects. For example, Brenneise-Sarshad *et al.* (1991) assessed the effect of two listener conditions – a knowledgeable listener condition and a naïve listener condition – on the content of narrative discourse in aphasic subjects. In both conditions, aphasic subjects told stories based on black-and-white line drawings to a listener. Only in the knowledgeable condition did the listener view the drawings along with the aphasic subject. Referential communication tasks also require a speaker to tailor information according to a listener's state of knowledge.[14] These tasks have been used in clinical studies of a range of clients including those with dementia related to Alzheimer's disease (Carlomagno *et al.* 2005; Feyereisen *et al.* 2007).

1.4.6   Non-literal language

Irony, metaphor, idiom and proverb are frequently topics of investigation in clinical pragmatic studies. An expression's ironic, metaphorical, idiomatic and proverbial meaning is not the result of a compositional analysis of the literal meanings of the component parts of the expression. The speaker who utters 'What glorious weather we're having!' in the middle of a snow storm is clearly doing so with considerable ironic intent. By the same token, the grandmother who says 'The children were angels during their stay' does not intend to communicate that the children *were* angels, merely that they exhibited certain attributes of angels – their behaviour was blameless, they were kind, etc. Also, the speaker who utters 'Sally always spills the beans' and 'As usual, Fred was last to hit the sack' is communicating something about Sally's lack of discretion and Fred's bedtime routine, respectively. Similarly, expressions such as 'A stitch in time saves nine' and 'John is caught between a rock and a hard place' are not communicating anything about sewing and rocks, but rather that dealing with things at the time prevents them escalating into bigger problems and that John is confronting two equally undesirable options. Perhaps unsurprisingly, these different types of non-literal language have been shown to be problematic for children and adults with pragmatic disorder. Impaired proverb interpretation is a hallmark of schizophrenia (Kiang *et al.* 2007). Metaphor comprehension has been found to be impaired in patients with right-hemisphere damage (Rinaldi *et al.* 2004). Individuals with Asperger's syndrome – a high functioning variant of autism – have been observed to have difficulty interpreting irony (Martin and McDonald 2004). Idiom comprehension has been found to be impaired in subjects with right brain damage and in subjects with left brain damage (Papagno *et al.* 2006).

1.4.7   Conversation

More often than not, conversation is the context in which pragmatic language skills are manifested. The dyadic nature of conversation is integral to most pragmatic phenomena. A speaker cannot successfully implicate anything unless there is a listener who is able to recover the speaker's intended implicature. In response to the question 'Do you want to go out tonight?' a speaker may respond 'I'm feeling really tired'. However, this response can only be taken to implicate that the speaker does not want to go out if a listener is present to recover this particular implicature. The exchange of a range of speech acts requires the presence of a speaker and a listener. For example, the utterances 'I bet you £10 he will pass the test', 'Do you have the time?' and 'The river has burst its banks' can only function as a bet, an indirect request for the time and a warning to residents to leave their homes if the presence of a speaker and a listener can be assumed. Deictic expressions such as 'you' and 'I' (personal deixis), 'today' and 'next week' (temporal deixis) and 'here' and 'there' (spatial deixis) presuppose the existence of a speaker and a listener in relation to which events, objects and people are organised spatially and temporally. A speaker can only successfully presuppose certain information in an utterance when he knows that information is shared with a listener. For example, it makes little sense for a speaker to utter 'It was the teenager who smashed the window' if he is aware that his listener doesn't know that the window is broken. Clearly, implicatures, speech acts, deictic expressions, presuppositions and a range of other pragmatic phenomena are only able to function to the extent that the dyadic structure that is typical of conversation can be presumed to hold.

With so many pragmatic concepts dependent on the dyadic structure of conversation, it is unsurprising that conversational phenomena should feature extensively in clinical pragmatic studies. The speaker who lacks awareness of the turn-taking rules of conversation may fail to respond to an indirect request to be given the time, for example. A similar failure to acknowledge the exchange structure of conversation may lead to conversational domination by a speaker. Even when a speaker is aware of the need to contribute turns in conversation and to yield his turn to other speakers, the turns that he contributes may be irrelevant to or otherwise fail to develop the topic under discussion.[15] Conversational irrelevance is a feature of many pragmatic disorders in children and adults, including adults with schizophrenia, individuals with an autistic spectrum disorder and children with pragmatic language impairment.[16] As well as failing to develop a topic in conversation, speakers with pragmatic disorder may select topics for discussion that are of little interest to other conversational participants. The autistic child may discuss one of his restricted interests (e.g. trains) during conversation for a length of time and to a level of detail that is not appropriate. Cognitive, behavioural and psychiatric problems (e.g. depression[17]) that attend brain injury and disease can reduce a client's conversational initiative and cause him or her to assume a passive role in conversation. These problems may manifest themselves during conversation in a failure to select topics for discussion, the assumption of the role of responder in conversation and the relinquishment of responsibility to others for opening and closing conversations. The onset of dementia related to Alzheimer's disease, for example, is frequently noted to reduce an individual's initiative to engage in conversation.[18] Similarly, adults with traumatic brain injury may display reduced conversational initiative and increased passivity during conversation.[19] These conversational problems, and others like them, are increasingly the focus of investigation in clinical pragmatic studies.

1.4.8   Discourse

Discourse production and comprehension draw upon many of the pragmatic language skills that we have examined thus far. To see this, consider the case of a speaker who is relating a story to a friend. As described in section 1.4.4, this speaker must be able to assess his or her listener's state of knowledge. This assessment will determine the type of information that can either remain implicit in the speaker's narrative (on the assumption that a listener can supply it) or that can be presupposed by that narrative. For example, on being told a story about a friend's birthday party, a listener can reasonably be expected to infer certain things (that guests were present, gifts were exchanged, refreshments were available, etc.) even though none of these details are explicitly presented by the speaker. Similarly, if a speaker knows that his or her listener witnessed an armed burglary at the local shop a week earlier, the utterance 'It was the city side gang who raided the shop' can mark this prior listener knowledge as a presupposition (the presupposition that someone raided the shop). A narrative that fails to take account of listener knowledge by leaving certain information implicit and by presupposing other information will be inefficient for the speaker (who will have to state every detail explicitly) and unrevealing for the listener (who will be told many things he or she already knows). As well as considering listener knowledge, a speaker who is relating a story to a friend must attend to the coherence and cohesion of his or her narrative. Coherence is a function of many interrelated factors, including the relevance of utterances to the topic under discussion and the logical representation of events (e.g. relating events in temporal sequence, displaying clear cause–consequence relations). A coherent discourse may still not display cohesion, if there are few of the linguistic devices that allow a speaker to link utterances together (e.g. the use of pronouns such as 'he' and 'him' to make reference to an earlier named individual).

With notions such as relevance, presupposition and listener knowledge so integral to discourse, it is clear that there is much in discourse that is of significance to workers in clinical pragmatics. This fact has not been lost on clinical practitioners and researchers who are increasingly including discourse analytic techniques in the assessment of clients and examining different aspects of discourse performance in research studies. Narrative is by far the most extensively investigated form of discourse in clinical studies. McInnes *et al.* (2004) state that 'narratives are functionally important in children's everyday communication, for example, in describing the day's events or in telling stories, and are a clinically useful indicator of their pragmatic competence' (306).

Narrative discourse is most often elicited in a clinical context in one of two ways. A speaker may be asked to retell a story that he or she has just been told. Alternatively, a speaker is encouraged to generate a story using a wordless picture book or a comic strip. Procedural discourse can be elicited by asking subjects to say in four or five steps how they would go about doing a particular task (e.g. buying groceries). Narrative and procedural discourse tasks have been used in studies of adults with temporal lobe epilepsy (Bell *et al.* 2003), aphasic subjects (Williams *et al.* 1994; Li *et al.* 1995; Weinrich *et al.* 2002), subjects with closed head injury (Hartley and Jensen 1991), adults with right-hemisphere damage (Tompkins *et al.* 2000) and psychotic patients (Ribeiro and Pinto 2009). As well as revealing discourse deficits – Hartley and Jensen (1991) found, for example, that closed head injured subjects use fewer cohesive ties per utterance than normal subjects – studies have also found preservation of pragmatic skills in subjects. Using an analysis of personal narratives, Ulatowska and Olness (2007) demonstrated that aphasic adults are able to achieve discourse coherence.

1.4.9   Relevance theory

Relevance theory (Sperber and Wilson 1986, 1995) is undoubtedly one of the most prominent theories in pragmatics. Within a relevance-theoretic approach to communication the entire framework of Gricean maxims is superseded by a principle of relevance. This principle, Sperber and Wilson contend, achieves a necessary simplification of Grice's framework, while at the same time losing none of the explanatory power of that framework: 'All of Grice's maxims can be replaced by a single principle of relevance – that the speaker tries to be as relevant as possible in the circumstances – which, when suitably elaborated, can handle the full range of data that Grice's maxims were designed to explain' (Wilson and Sperber 1991: 381). Relevance is a guiding principle of communication. In this way, speakers and listeners bring to each conversational interaction the 'standing assumption' that each party has tried to make their contributions as relevant as possible and is interpreting the contributions of others with relevance in mind:

We also assume that a speaker who thinks it worth speaking at all will try to make his utterance as relevant as possible. A hearer should therefore bring to the processing of every utterance the standing assumption that the speaker has tried to be as relevant as possible in the circumstances. It is this assumption that we call the principle of relevance. (1991: 382)

However, the principle of relevance is also intended to apply to the domain of cognition in general. The processing that is warranted by this principle proceeds in a cost–benefit fashion. What this amounts to is that when the cost that is required to process a proposition for its contextual effects exceeds the benefit that is obtained from these effects, further relevance processing of that proposition ceases. This process can be demonstrated by the following example:

A: Will you join me for lunch?
B: We'll be at the bank for some time.

For Sperber and Wilson, B's response is a logical form (a semantic representation) which must be referentially completed, disambiguated and enriched in order to obtain the propositional form that is expressed by the utterance. Contrary to minimalist accounts of the semantic content of the utterance (Borg 2004), Sperber and Wilson argue that relevance plays a role in establishing the referent of the pronoun 'we', disambiguating the noun 'bank' and enriching the phrase 'some time'. So in relevance theory, the fully developed logical form of an utterance, known as the explicature, is already the product of pragmatic factors. It is quite clear, however, that in producing the utterance in the above exchange, B is not intending to communicate only that he or she will be spending some minutes (or hours) at the side of a river (or at the local bank or at the blood bank, depending on disambiguation). Rather, B is intending to communicate a declination of A's lunch offer. In relevance-theoretic terms, B implicates this declination by guaranteeing A that his or her utterance is optimally relevant when its explicature is processed in a context that is part of A's stored knowledge. Here, again, the principle of relevance guides A to process the explicature of B's utterance in the least effortful processing context within which an implicature can be obtained. That context is one in which a single proposition is accessed within A's stored knowledge (if one is to spend a considerable period of time at the local bank, then one will not be able to join someone elsewhere for lunch). More costly contexts in which the explicature of B's utterance can be processed, involving several propositions in A's stored knowledge, are effectively excluded by the principle of relevance. For a more detailed discussion of relevance theory, the reader is referred to Chapters 1 and 4 in Cummings (2005).

A small, but growing, number of studies are beginning to apply Sperber and Wilson's relevance-theoretic framework to the study of children and adults with language impairment and pragmatic disorder.[20] Schelletter and Leinonen (2003) used the assumption of optimal relevance in relevance theory to explain specification of referents by children with specific language impairment. Loukusa et al. (2007a) used relevance theory in an investigation of the ability of children with Asperger's syndrome and high-functioning autism to use context to answer questions and give explanations of those answers. Dipper et al. (1997) looked to relevance theory to explain bridging inference problems in subjects with right-hemisphere damage. Happé (1993) based predictions about the processing of figurative language (simile, metaphor and irony) in autism on relevance theory. Leinonen and Kerbel (1999) used relevance theory to explain data obtained from three children with reported pragmatic difficulties. Episodes of communicative 'oddness' were assessed by both authors and were accounted for in terms of breakdown of key relevance-theoretic notions such as explicature. These investigations exemplify an important, mutually beneficial interaction between pragmatic theory and clinical studies. Pragmatic theory can help us move beyond merely describing pragmatic impairments in children and adults – the overriding tendency in clinical studies to date – to providing a coherent explanation of those impairments. As well as serving to explain the performance of pragmatically impaired children and adults, pragmatic theories such as relevance theory can receive much needed validation from the study of subjects with pragmatic disorders. The study of these subjects provides theories in pragmatics with 'a natural empirical test bed' (Bara and Tirassa 2000: 10), which may lead theorists to revise or even reject certain theoretical proposals. These same interactions between pragmatic theory and clinical studies are amply demonstrated in Bruno Bara's cognitive pragmatics theory, to which we now turn.

1.4.10   Cognition and pragmatics

It will not have escaped the reader that cognitive approaches to pragmatics and specific clinical disorders feature extensively in this book. Relevance theory, which we have just examined, is essentially conceived from within the framework of cognitive psychology.[21] In Chapters 2 and 3, developmental and acquired pragmatic disorders are related to a range of cognitive skills and deficits in children and adults. In Chapter 4, I discuss the pragmatic adequacy of three cognitive theories of autism – theory of mind (ToM), executive function theory and weak central coherence theory. The cognitive substrates of acquired pragmatic disorders will be examined in Chapter 5. Given this extensive coverage of cognitive issues, the reader could be forgiven for thinking that I have a specific cognitive theory of pragmatics that I wish to expound in this book. The fact is I have no such theory. Nor do I believe a satisfactory cognitive theory of pragmatics or of clinical disorders such as autism exists. However, I do consider that the relationship between pragmatics and cognition is of such fundamental significance to an investigation of pragmatic disorder that no pragmatic study, theoretical or clinical, can reasonably neglect the very real connections that exist between pragmatic phenomena and cognition. For this reason, I will discuss a number of cognitive approaches to pragmatics in this book. One of these approaches – cognitive pragmatics theory – uses the findings of neuropsychological research into subjects with cognitive impairments (e.g. adults with closed head injury) to constrain a competence theory of human intentional communication that has been developed on independent grounds. Another approach to be examined in Chapter 5 – Asa Kasher's modular pragmatics – uses a prominent perspective in cognitive science to address the question of the relationship of pragmatics to cognition. I will examine cognitive pragmatics theory in the present context.

Cognitive pragmatics theory (Airenti *et al.* 1993a, 1993b) seeks to explain the cognitive processes that underlie intentional verbal and nonverbal communication. On the assumption that the same competence is involved in our use of linguistic and extralinguistic communication acts, the proponents of this framework sought to replace the traditional roles of 'speaker' and 'hearer' with 'actor' and 'partner', respectively. Central to this theory is the idea that a partner in communication establishes an actor's communicative intention by identifying the particular behaviour game that an actor wishes him to play. A behaviour game is a social structure that is mutually shared by communicative participants. The operation of such games can be demonstrated as follows:

Suppose a colleague of yours says:
    I'd appreciate a coffee.
while you are working together in her office. Her utterance may be interpreted as a request of a pause, with reference to a sort of [WORK-TOGETHER] behavior game. The same statement, uttered in your house after dinner, might be recognized as a typical move of a [DINNER-TOGETHER] behavior game: a guest announces a desire that the host is bound to accomplish. Finally, the same utterance would be puzzling, if someone you've never seen before suddenly pops in your office to produce it: either you are able to find a behavior game related to it (i.e., to understand what the actor wants you to think or do), or it will remain unexplained. (Bara *et al.* 1997: 5–6)

The complexity of the inferential steps (the 'inferential load') that are needed to refer an utterance to the particular behaviour game that is bid by the actor can explain difficulties in speech act comprehension. In this way, direct and conventional indirect speech acts (so-called 'simple speech acts') make immediate reference to an intended behaviour game and are easier for young children to acquire than nonconventional indirect speech acts ('complex speech acts'). Bucciarelli *et al.* (2003) reported that children from the age of 2:6 years find direct and conventional indirect speech acts easier to understand than nonconventional indirect speech acts (for example, the use of the question 'Do you like subzero temperatures?' to get someone to switch on the heating).

A further cognitive factor that accounts for the difference in difficulty of comprehending pragmatic phenomena is the complexity of the underlying mental representations. According to cognitive pragmatics theory, in standard communication default rules of inference are used to comprehend a person's mental states. These rules are involved in our comprehension of direct, conventional indirect and nonconventional indirect speech acts, where what an actor says conforms to his or her private beliefs. The simple mental representations of these so-called standard communicative acts contrast with the more complex mental representations that are involved in the comprehension of nonstandard communication such as deceit and irony. In order to comprehend the ironic intent of an actor who utters 'What a delightful child!' in the presence of a disruptive three-year-old, the partner must not only block the action of default rules, but he or she must be aware that the actor is entertaining a private belief that is diametrically opposed to the belief that is reflected by the utterance. Cognitive pragmatics theory thus predicts that the more complex mental representations involved in deceit and irony will be reflected in greater levels of difficulty in children in acquiring these communicative acts than in acquiring standard communicative acts. The theory also predicts that the comprehension of irony will be more difficult than the comprehension of deceit, because the partner who comprehends an ironic utterance must additionally represent that the actor shares the partner's awareness of a discrepancy between private belief on the one hand and the belief expressed on the other hand. Once again, these predictions were borne out by the results of Bucciarelli *et al.*'s (2003) study in children. These investigators found an increase in difficulty in the comprehension of simple standard communicative acts, simple deceits and simple ironies in their study of children between 2:6 and 7 years of age.

As well as receiving support from investigations of developmental pragmatics, the central tenets of cognitive pragmatics theory are consistent with the findings of studies of neuropsychological subjects. These studies have revealed that the breakdown of pragmatic competence in these subjects follows the developmental pattern observed in normally developing children, i.e. those pragmatic skills that are late acquired are the first skills to decay in these subjects. In a study of thirteen subjects who had sustained a closed head injury, Bara *et al.* (1997) reported a clear order of difficulty in the comprehension of certain pragmatic phenomena. Difficulty increased from direct/indirect speech acts to irony, from irony to deceits and from deceits to failure recovery. The recovery of failure in each of these pragmatic categories was judged to be the most difficult because 'to repair a failure requires that the actor recognize it, identify its causes and plan a suitable alternative strategy' (1997: 26). Similar results were obtained in a later study by Bara *et al.* (2001) of thirty subjects with closed head injury. In this study, sixteen videotaped scenes were used to investigate the comprehension of communicative actions that were realised through extralinguistic means such as pointing or clapping. The performance of these subjects decreased from simple standard acts to complex standard acts, deceits and ironies. As before, subjects' performance was worse on failed than successful communicative actions (see Angeleri *et al.* (2008) for the same order of difficulty in the comprehension *and* production of pragmatic phenomena in twenty-one subjects who sustained a traumatic brain injury). A similar pattern of decay in extralinguistic pragmatic competence was observed by Bara *et al.*

(2000) in a study of fourteen subjects with Alzheimer's disease. These subjects understood nonstandard extralinguistic tasks less well than standard communicative tasks. These studies confirm a central claim of cognitive pragmatics theory, that a unified pragmatic competence mediates both linguistic and extralinguistic communicative acts.

1.5   The multidisciplinary nature of clinical pragmatics

In Cummings (2005), I argued that pragmatics lies at the intersection of a number of disciplines and is, for this reason, a multidisciplinary area of enquiry. In the same way, I now want to claim that a range of different disciplines converge on the study of pragmatic disorder in children and adults. Some of these disciplines are more central to clinical pragmatics than other disciplines. For example, speech-language pathology is the field that is most directly concerned with the assessment and treatment of clients with pragmatic disorder. Meanwhile, psychiatry has a more circumscribed interest in pragmatic disorders with investigators largely concerned to examine the manifestations of these disorders in clients with conditions such as autistic spectrum disorder and schizophrenia. As well as various disciplines converging on the study of pragmatic disorders, workers in clinical pragmatics must have an extensive knowledge of a range of different subject areas in order to understand how the pragmatics of language can be disrupted. Here, again, some disciplines (e.g. linguistics and first language acquisition) have a more central role in this knowledge than other disciplines. What this necessary multidisciplinary knowledge base of workers in clinical pragmatics demonstrates is that investigators must be able to do more than merely identify a speech act or recognise an implicature in order to study pragmatic language disorders. Space limitations preclude an exhaustive review of each of the disciplines that converge on clinical pragmatics. However, in the rest of this section, I discuss some of the problems that can arise when investigators who lack a multidisciplinary knowledge base attempt to characterise pragmatic disorders. I also describe one discipline, or rather subdiscipline, which is integral to the study of pragmatic disorders and about which remarkably little is still known.

As well as contributing to our understanding of pragmatic disorders, the convergence of many disciplines on the study of pragmatic impairment has had an unfortunate consequence. This consequence can be characterised as the tendency to incorrectly represent pragmatic concepts and the processes involved in pragmatic interpretation. In Chapter 7, I relate this tendency to a wider failure amongst theorists to delineate the field of pragmatics. However, there is a very real sense in which these mistaken characterisations stem from a misunderstanding of the nature of certain pragmatic concepts. Many of the studies identified in Chapter 7 as committing errors in the identification of pragmatic phenomena have been undertaken by psychologists whose choice of experimental tasks reveals a misunderstanding of the pragmatic concepts they are claiming to investigate. In this way, a subject who recognises the violation of a Gricean conversational maxim does not thereby recover the implicature of a speaker's utterance (see discussion of Surian *et al.* (1996) in Chapter 7). By the same token, the individual who is able to identify that a speaker entertains a false belief in a test of faux pas recognition performs first-order belief attribution, whereas the recognition of communicative intentions that is integral to pragmatic interpretation demands second-order belief attribution (see discussion of Baron-Cohen *et al.* (1999) in Chapter 7). These mistaken characterisations of pragmatic phenomena reflect, I contend, the disciplinary backgrounds of the investigators who have pursued these studies (psychologists are ideally placed to conduct experimental studies but are perhaps less well informed of the nature of pragmatic concepts such as implicature). Different disciplinary backgrounds have also been credited with influencing the diagnoses of children with pragmatic language impairment.[22] Clearly, diverse disciplines can only meaningfully contribute to the study of pragmatic disorder to the extent that workers in these disciplines have a knowledge base that extends beyond their own area of enquiry.

The multidisciplinary knowledge base that is integral to the study of pragmatic disorder must include, at a minimum, a sound understanding of the developmental stages that children go through on their way to acquiring full pragmatic competence. As the dearth of developmental studies of pragmatics demonstrates, we are still some way off attaining a comprehensive knowledge of the stages in pragmatic development. A significant factor in the lack of developmental research that has been undertaken in pragmatics is an inability on the part of investigators to agree on the particular knowledge and skills that are integral to the development of pragmatics.[23] Ninio and Snow (1996) identify three areas which represent 'the major achievements of language learners within the domain of pragmatics' (13). These areas are: (1) the development of rules that govern the communicative uses of speech, (2) the development of skills required for conversation and (3) the development of skills that are needed to produce extended discourse and genre-specific forms. However, these developmental achievements notably exclude other areas, such as the acquisition of rules of politeness and deictic forms, which most investigators would wish to include within the domain of pragmatics. Clearly, this is not the context in which to attempt an extensive review of our knowledge of pragmatic development. However, two issues that are relevant to discussion in subsequent chapters will be considered in this section. The first is the question of which behaviours amongst an infant's early communicative repertoire are to count as pragmatic. The second issue relates to the observation that many pragmatic language skills are still being acquired well into adolescence and after the point at which syntactic and semantic aspects have become well established within a child's language system.

In Chapter 7, I describe a tendency among investigators in clinical pragmatics to identify nonverbal behaviours such as gesture as pragmatic in nature. In that chapter, I attribute this tendency to the erroneous identification of pragmatics with communication, nonverbal communication specifically included. This identification, I want to argue, appears plausible given the view of some investigators that 'children's early language is continuous with their preverbal communicative system' (Ninio and Snow 1996: 49). Labelled the continuity hypothesis, 'this view implies that the communicative intents expressed by the first words are identical to those expressed with gestures or vocalizations by preverbal children' (Ninio and Snow 1996: 49). As the discussion in section 1.2 was intended to demonstrate, the notion of pragmatics that this view entails – that nonlinguistic behaviours may be labelled 'pragmatic' – is not one that I wish to endorse in this book. My own view of pragmatics is much closer to that espoused by Ninio and Snow (1996) in their comprehensive study of pragmatic development in children. These investigators argue that regardless of the difficulty of applying this criterion in practice, a linguistic code must be present if an utterance is to count as 'an instance of meaningful language use':

> The expression used (or at least the phonetic target) is verbal and not merely vocal: It consists of conventional or semiconventional forms accepted in the speaker's speech community. This criterion distinguishes between language and nonlinguistic vocal productions. Words and sentences – that is, forms that are conventionally and arbitrarily restricted in phonetics – are included, as are semiconventional exclamations, onomatopoeia, nicknames, and so forth. In other words, meaningful speech involves the use of a conventional and arbitrary vocal *code*. Of course, we recognize the difficulty of applying this criterion in practice, given the gradual transition between preverbal babbling and early conventional words on all phonetic and phonological analyses; nonetheless, the criterion of a linguistic code is one we maintain in principle. (1996: 17)

The requirement that a linguistic code be present means that a number of behaviours that might otherwise be informative (e.g. facial expressions and gestures convey all sorts of information about a speaker's emotional state and thoughts) still do not qualify as pragmatic in nature. In developmental terms, early speech too falls short of achieving anything pragmatic: 'beginning speakers are mostly using speech simply to ensure the basic interpersonal achievement of intersubjectivity. Speech is not used at this initial stage for anything truly pragmatic, such as making requests more intelligible, bringing inner states or emotions to the knowledge of the interlocutor, or telling a story about a personal experience' (Ninio and Snow 1996: 70). We described in section 1.2 how Searle's philosophical reflections serve to locate pragmatics squarely within a speaker's linguistic competence. Ninio and Snow's developmental study of pragmatics, it can now be seen, emphasises the centrality of a linguistic code to pragmatics.

These important features of pragmatics, which have been swept aside in the relatively short history of the discipline, should now be actively embraced by workers in clinical pragmatics.

Studies of language development have tended to focus almost exclusively on preschool and young school-age children. This poses a problem for the study of pragmatic development, as many of the skills that we identify as being pragmatic in nature are still being acquired during adolescence and beyond. Levorato and Cacciari (2002) examined the development of figurative language across four age groups: children aged 9;6 and 11;3 months, adolescents aged 18;5 months and adults. These investigators found that the ability to use figurative language required 'a long developmental time span'. Although the ability to produce certain conventional figurative expressions is achieved by fifteen years of age (according to Levorato and Cacciari's (1995) Global Elaboration Model), the metalinguistic ability that is needed to make innovative figurative expressions communicatively appropriate and conceptually sensible continues to evolve up to adulthood. Complex speech acts are still undergoing development during adolescence and adulthood. Nippold *et al.* (2005) examined persuasive writing[24] in children, adolescents and adults whose mean ages were eleven, seventeen and twenty-four years, respectively. Older subjects advanced more reasons in support of their position (an average of 12.72 reasons at age twenty-four compared to 6.80 reasons at age eleven) and also approached controversies in a more flexible manner. Nippold *et al.* describe, for example, how an eighteen-year-old boy was able to express both sides of an issue, while a twenty-five-year-old woman evidenced this same flexible attitude and also offered solutions to the problems raised by the issue. It is interesting that some 35 per cent of adults only offered a one-sided opinion on the controversy and did not acknowledge other perspectives in their writing. Notwithstanding the importance of adolescence to the development of pragmatic language skills, it remains the case that little is known about the maturation that occurs in these skills during this time.[25]

1.6   Primary and secondary pragmatic disorders

In section 1.1, I characterised the distinction between primary and secondary pragmatic disorders as follows. Some pragmatic disorders are related to deficits in structural language. For example, the speaker with aphasia or the child with specific language impairment may be fully aware that a particular communicative context demands the use of an indirect speech act. Yet, such a speaker may be unable to produce the syntactic structures that are the conventional means of performing indirect speech acts. In English, it is conventional for language users to utter 'Can you tell me the time?' or 'Do you know the time?' when they want a listener to give them the time. However, the syntactic inversion of subject pronoun and auxiliary verb in both these utterances may not be within the expressive syntactic repertoire of the aphasic adult or the SLI child. It seems clear in cases of this type that while the child and adult speaker present with a pragmatic disorder – neither is able to use a conventional means of producing certain indirect speech acts (e.g. requests) – the disorder is related more to a deficit in expressive syntax than to any failure of pragmatic competence. Clinicians use the term 'secondary' to describe this type of pragmatic disorder and to distinguish it from a primary pragmatic disorder.[26] The speaker with a primary pragmatic disorder may fail to understand the significance of context features for his choice of linguistic utterance. For example, such a speaker may fail to use an indirect request in a situation that demands it because he is largely unaware of politeness considerations and social constraints that operate in conversation. Expressive language skills, particularly in the areas of syntax and semantics, may be intact or at least not impaired to an extent that the speaker is unable to formulate certain speech acts. Although both speakers may present with the same pragmatic deficit – a failure to use indirect requests – it is only in the speaker with relatively intact structural language skills that the disorder can be characterised as primary.

This characterisation of primary and secondary pragmatic disorders is problematic in a couple of respects. First, it tends to suggest that pragmatic disorder can be classified relatively easily as either primary or secondary in nature. In reality, this is a determination that clinicians and researchers have struggled to make in several clinical populations. Consider the case of specific language impairment in children. These children exhibit significant morphosyntactic and lexical semantic deficits (see section 2.2 in Chapter 2). Given the extent of these children's structural language problems, it is unsurprising that investigators should have sought to relate pragmatic impairments in this population to these problems. However, some researchers have begun to question the validity of this particular assumption.[27] In Chapter 2, we examine the findings of studies that have found evidence of pragmatic impairments in SLI children that cannot be accounted for by any deficits in structural language in these children. Second, the above characterisation of the distinction between primary and secondary pragmatic disorders may lead the reader to think that only one of these types of disorders can occur in a single individual. Once again, however, an examination of subjects with pragmatic disorders suggests that this is not the case. The child with autism, for example, may have limited expressive and receptive language skills and be unable to produce and comprehend certain speech acts as a result (a secondary pragmatic disorder). However, other pragmatic impairments in the same autistic child are less clearly related to deficits of structural language and are primary in nature. For example, the failure to attribute communicative intentions to a speaker, to select topics during conversation that are of interest to a listener and to monitor a listener's understanding of a conversational exchange are all pragmatic deficits that are much more likely to have their origins in mind-reading and imaginative deficits than in any language impairment as such.

1.7   Pragmatic deficits and pragmatic preservation

Traditionally, the emphasis in clinical studies of language has been on characterising specific deficits and impairments in language impaired children and adults.[28] Clinical studies of pragmatics are no exception in this regard with investigators describing deficits in a large range of pragmatic skills. This rather blinkered perspective in clinical pragmatic studies has resulted in the almost total neglect of areas in which subjects still retain intact pragmatic functioning and of the ways in which pragmatic skills may be used to compensate deficits in other aspects of language. For example, it is frequently observed that subjects with deficits in receptive syntax are able to use wider aspects of context such as world knowledge to facilitate the processing of syntactically complex structures. In a language assessment task, an aphasic subject may struggle to select a picture that corresponds to the sentence 'The car is followed by the lorry', but may point to the correct picture in response to the sentence 'The mouse is chased by the cat'. Although both sentences are passive voice constructions, world knowledge can only facilitate comprehension of the second sentence – as language users, we have no expectations about whether cars follow lorries, or vice versa, but it is part of our background knowledge that cats typically chase mice. Such is the power of this deficit-only perspective that it has also led investigators to attribute pragmatic deficits to subjects where none exist. In section 7.3 of Chapter 7, for example, we describe an exchange between a woman with TBI called Pat and her therapist. The analysts of this exchange, Body *et al.* (1999), are so preoccupied with characterising Pat's communicative performance in terms of pragmatic deficits that they completely overlook the pragmatic ingenuity that she displays during her conversational interactions with others.

A few investigators have sought to place significance on preserved areas of pragmatic functioning. Prutting and Kirchner (1987) emphasise preserved pragmatic abilities in their pragmatic protocol.[29] Ulatowska and Olness (2007) examined the preservation of pragmatic abilities in subjects with aphasia. These investigators used the notion of discourse coherence as a framework for understanding pragmatic preservation in the personal narratives of these subjects. Chapman and Ulatowska (1989) examined the ability of aphasic subjects to identify antecedents for ambiguous pronouns in brief narratives. When the referents of these pronouns were not readily identifiable from world knowledge, the aphasic subject had significant difficulty using textual cues to resolve the referents. When referents were recoverable from world knowledge or were explicitly stated, aphasic subjects had little difficulty establishing the referents of pronouns. More recently, Perovic (2006) found that young adults with Down's syndrome had difficulty comprehending reflexives, but not pronouns. While the interpretation of reflexives proceeded on the basis of a syntactic relation between the reflexive and its antecedent, the interpretation of pronouns required an extra-syntactic or pragmatic mechanism. Clearly, the extralinguistic knowledge of these Down's syndrome subjects confers an advantage on their interpretation of pronouns that is not present in their comprehension of reflexives. World knowledge in the form of scripts has also been found to facilitate the training of semantic constructions in subjects with mental retardation. Kim and Lombardino (1991) investigated the effects of script-based and nonscript-based treatment on the training of two semantic constructions in four preschool children with mental retardation. The script-based treatment involved the routines of popcorn-making, pudding-making and milkshake-making and was found to be more effective than the nonscript treatment in facilitating comprehension of the targeted semantic constructions in three of the four subjects.

NOTES

1 Several examples are listed in chronological order: *Clinical pragmatics: unravelling the complexities of communicative failure* (Smith and Leinonen 1992); *Pragmatics in neurogenic communication disorders* (Paradis 1998a) – this book is a special issue of volume 11 of the *Journal of Neurolinguistics*; *Pragmatics in speech and language pathology* (Müller 2000) – this book is volume 7 in the series *Studies in Speech Pathology and Clinical Linguistics*; *Children's pragmatic communication difficulties* (Leinonen *et al.* 2000); *Pragmatic impairment* (Perkins 2008).
2 Three such journals are *Brain and Language*, *Clinical Linguistics & Phonetics* and *Seminars in Speech and Language*. In 1999, *Brain and Language* brought together eleven articles on the theme of Pragmatics: Theoretical and Clinical Issues (Stemmer 1999). In 2005, *Clinical Linguistics & Phonetics* published seven articles on the theme of Clinical Pragmatics: An Emergentist Perspective (Perkins 2005). In 2007, *Seminars in Speech and Language* brought together five papers on the theme of Pragmatics and Adult Language Disorders (Cummings 2007a).
3 Clinical pragmatics appears as an entry in the *Handbook of pragmatics* (Verschueren and Östman 2006) and in *The pragmatics encyclopedia* (Cummings 2009).
4 It is perhaps a sign of the growing significance of clinical pragmatics that some of these symposia and conferences address audiences in fields other than speech and language pathology and communication disorders. For example, clinical pragmatics was the theme of a symposium entitled 'Being Pragmatic' which was organised by the Department of Psychology at the University of Waterloo in June 1999. This symposium was held as part of an annual meeting of academics in the fields of theoretical and experimental neuropsychology. Other professional and academic bodies that have recently dedicated special sessions to discussion of topics in clinical pragmatics include the American Speech-Language-Hearing Association (ASHA). In the 2003 ASHA convention, a short course was conducted on pragmatic disorders (Pragmatic Communication Disorders: Biology to Bedside to Billing).

5 The excellent theoretical discussions that have taken place on the interface between semantics and pragmatics are a case in point. For an account of those discussions, the reader is referred to Jaszczolt (2008).

6 Grice's theory of conversational implicature was first presented in a series of William James lectures at Harvard University in 1967. This theory was published in 1975 as the essay 'Logic and conversation'. The Oxford philosopher J.L. Austin developed speech act theory in the 1930s. This theory was expounded in twelve William James lectures at Harvard University in 1955 and was published in 1962 in the book *How to do things with words* (edited by J.O. Urmson). Searle, a student of Austin's, develops Austin's theory in his 1969 book *Speech acts: an essay in the philosophy of language*.

7 The Boston Diagnostic Aphasia Examination and Western Aphasia Battery were first published in 1972 and 1982, respectively.

8 The *Clinical guidelines* of the Royal College of Speech and Language Therapists (2005) stipulate not only that assessments of aphasia should include 'functional and pragmatic aspects of communication', but that an assessment of the conversation/ interaction patterns of the person with aphasia and their conversation partner 'may include conversation analysis (CA)' (2005: 99, 109).

9 This characterisation of the process by means of which a speaker's communicative intention in producing an utterance is established makes all sorts of theoretical assumptions, none of which I want to defend in the present context. For example, theorists such as François Recanati who adhere to a position called contextualism argue that pragmatic factors intrude into the truth-conditional content of an utterance. So pragmatic interpretation does not 'start out from' the literal meaning of an utterance; rather, the literal meaning already contains input from pragmatics.

10 A search of Medline conducted on 24 July 2007 revealed only five papers that include presupposition in their abstracts. In two of these papers – Rees and Shulman (1978) and Roth and Spekman (1984) – presupposition is discussed within reviews of assessment procedures. In a third paper, Wetzel and Molfese (1992) recorded event-related potentials during the processing of sentences that contained either factive or nonfactive verbs in ten healthy adult subjects. So, in effect, only two studies conducted original investigations of presuppositions in clinical subjects. Rowan *et al.* (1983) examined the presuppositional abilities of language-disordered children. Eisele *et al.* (1998) tested twenty-four children with unilateral left- or right-hemisphere damage on their ability to presuppose the truth of factive sentences.

11 Bock (1977) states that 'the decision to treat something as given information constitutes a pragmatic presupposition on the part of the speaker' (723).

12 This research consists of a small number of studies including investigations of given-new information in aphasic subjects (Cannito *et al.* 1986), language disordered children (Skarakis and Greenfield 1982) and autistic children (McCaleb and Prizant 1985; Dennis *et al.* 2001).

13 Although pronoun reversal has been standardly included in accounts of the linguistic and communicative features of autism (Bartak *et al.* 1975), studies have often failed to find evidence of increased pronoun reversal by autistic children. In a study of the use and comprehension of the personal pronouns 'I', 'you' and 'me', Lee *et al.* (1994) found few instances of pronoun reversal among autistic subjects. Autistic and nonautistic mentally retarded children and young adults matched for chronological age and verbal mental age were able to comprehend these pronouns in test

situations. In a visual perspective-taking task, autistic subjects were significantly less likely to use the pronoun 'me'. In certain photograph-naming tasks, lower ability subjects were more likely to use their own proper names than personal pronouns. Autistic subjects were also less likely in some circumstances to use the pronoun 'you' to refer to the experimenter than controls.

14 In a typical referential communication task, two participants are given the same set of pictures in two different random orders A and B. The participant who received the set in the B order must attempt to replicate the A order based on a series of descriptions given by the other participant. According to one model (the collaborative model) of how this task is achieved, 'when speakers try to identify a referent, they begin with a provisional clause and propose what they believe to be an adequate expression enabling the addressee to recognize it. They take into account the knowledge they assume to be shared with their partner – the common ground – in order to choose the most appropriate formulation of the message' (Feyereisen *et al.* 2007: 4).

15 This is evident in the following conversational exchange taken from Crystal and Varley (1998: 161). In this exchange, a therapist (T) and an autistic child (P) are playing with toy cars. Although the autistic child is contributing turns to the conversation, none of these turns are engaging in any meaningful way with the prior turns of the therapist. To all intents and purposes, the autistic child is keeping up a monologue which just happens to be broken up by the therapist's turns (stress and pitch markings have been removed from this exchange and some other minor modifications have been made):

T: What are you going to do with that car now?
P: I like my car (pushing it on the floor).
T: Look. I've got one like that.
P: In here it goes (pushing car into garage).
T: Don't forget to shut the doors.
P: Find the man now (looking about).

16 Conversational irrelevance in schizophrenia is amply demonstrated by the following extract taken from Thomas (1997: 41): 'Then I left San Francisco and moved to … where did you get that tie? It looks like it's left over from the 1950s. I like the warm weather in San Diego. Is that a conch shell on your desk? Have you ever gone scuba diving?' This violation of the maxim of relevance occurs within what Thomas calls distractible speech in which 'the subject suddenly stops talking in mid-sentence and changes the subject in response to a nearby stimulus' (1997: 41). In the following conversational exchange between a therapist (T) and a child (P) with pragmatic disorder, the child's response is completely irrelevant to the therapist's question: (T) Where do you go to school? (P) Tommy goes to my school because I see him in the hall everyday but we have different teachers and he has a new bicycle (Crystal and Varley 1998: 179).

17 High rates of depressive symptoms are reported in subjects with traumatic brain injury. Bay *et al.* (2007) found significant levels of depressive symptoms in nearly 40 per cent of an outpatient sample of seventy-five persons with mild-to-moderate TBI. Thompson *et al.* (2007) report that depression in Alzheimer's disease is common (15 to 63 per cent) and is associated with significant morbidity and increased mortality.

18 A lack of initiative is commonly reported in individuals with Alzheimer's disease and other forms of dementia. Robert *et al.* (2006) obtained a lack of initiative and interest pathological score for nineteen out of thirty-one patients (61 per cent) with Alzheimer's disease. In a study of 235 community-dwelling persons with Alzheimer's disease, Tractenberg *et al.* (2002) found that loss of initiative was one of several behavioural symptoms that emerged in the greatest proportion of patients between baseline measures and measures taken at twelve-month visits. Bózzola *et al.* (1992) found diminished initiative/growing apathy in 61.3 per cent of eighty patients with Alzheimer's disease who were examined at a dementia clinic. Blair *et al.* (2007) state that reduced conversational initiation is seen in the behavioural variant of frontotemporal dementia.

19 Decreased initiative is a significant problem in many patients following traumatic brain injury (TBI). Zebenholzer and Oder (1998) examined thirty-three patients four and eight years after severe head injury. These investigators found that 67 per cent and 70 per cent of subjects respectively displayed poor initiative at the first and second examination. Lippert-Grüner *et al.* (2006) found that decreased initiative was one of several neurobehavioural deficits in forty-one patients with severe TBI in which there was further deterioration in the post-traumatic follow-up.

20 Many more studies have applied relevance theory to the study of pragmatic phenomena during language comprehension and reasoning tasks in pragmatically intact subjects. Relevance theory has been used to examine scalar implicature (Noveck and Posada 2003; de Neys and Schaeken 2007), the use of context in question answering (Ryder and Leinonen 2003), the binding of pronouns (Foster-Cohen 1994) and the distinction between what is said and what is implicated (Nicolle and Clark 1999) in subjects with no pragmatic disorder. Also, relevance theory has been extensively discussed in relation to the Wason selection task, with investigators both claiming and denying a role for this theory in an explanation of the performance of normal subjects on this task (Sperber *et al.* 1995; Fiddick *et al.* 2000). Van der Henst (1999) used relevance theory to explain the effect of premise order on spatial reasoning in subjects.

21 Such is the cognitive psychological nature of relevance theory that Kempson has described Sperber and Wilson's theory as 'unrepentant cognitive psychology' (1988: 16).

22 Bishop (2000b) remarks that 'when relatively high-functioning children present with subtle deficits affecting a range of different behaviors, one has the impression that the particular diagnosis, and consequently the type of intervention received, may be more a function of the discipline of the specialist who is the point of first referral than of the particular symptom profile. The same child might receive a diagnosis of PDD-NOS [pervasive developmental disorder–not otherwise specified] or atypical autism from a psychiatrist, of developmental language disorder (semantic-pragmatic type) from a speech-language therapist, or right-hemisphere learning disability from a neuropsychologist' (2000b: 274–5).

23 Ninio and Snow (1996) remark that 'what distinguishes pragmatics [from grammar and the lexicon] is the considerable disagreement about exactly what knowledge and skills constitute the domain of pragmatic development' (4).

24 Persuasion is a perlocution in Austin's (1962) characterisation of the acts that are performed through speaking. Following pragma-dialectics (Cummings 2009), I am presenting persuasion (or, rather, persuasive argumentation) as a complex speech

act. Another type of argumentation that has been examined in adolescents is negotiation (Selman *et al.* 1986).

25 Adams (2001) states that 'relatively little is known about normal language development in the older child, especially in the semantic and pragmatic domains' (294). Nippold (1998) remarks that 'little is known about the development of humor in adolescents, and it is unclear to what extent performance in this area improves beyond age 15' (148). In fact, as is the case with many pragmatic language skills, much more is known about the use and appreciation of humour in adolescent and adult subjects with clinical disorders than in normal subjects of similar age. In this way, humour has been investigated in adolescent subjects with high-functioning autism and Asperger's syndrome (Emerich *et al.* 2003) and Williams syndrome (Sullivan *et al.* 2003) and in adult subjects with agenesis of the corpus callosum (Brown *et al.* 2005) and right-hemisphere damage (Winner *et al.* 1998), amongst a range of other disorders.

26 Adams (2001) describes the case of a child aged 7;03 years who had secondary pragmatic deficits which diminished as his language skills improved. This child responded to therapy that was based on phonological principles. More recently, Adams (2005) has challenged the distinction between primary and secondary pragmatic disorders: 'it may be timely to move away from considerations of pragmatic impairments as being primary or secondary to more complex interdependent models' (186).

27 Leonard (1998) argues that 'given the criteria for SLI, it would be natural to assume that any pragmatic difficulties observed in these children were secondary to problems of linguistic form or content ... Indeed, some of the evidence of pragmatic difficulties in children with SLI is of this type. In other instances, however, the basis of the problem is not so clear' (78).

28 This traditional emphasis on deficits and impairments is very clearly exemplified by the following remarks of Damico (1985): 'While description of communicative strengths is important, the primary function of the speech-language pathologist is to discover difficulties that interfere with communication. The question always asked in diagnosis is, "What language errors mark this individual as disordered?"' (169).

29 'The identification of intact abilities is also important from a clinical standpoint. These aspects can provide important information that can be used in designing treatment strategies that build on existing abilities' (Prutting and Kirchner 1987: 113).

2   A survey of developmental pragmatic disorders

2.1   Introduction

In Chapter 1, the extended course that normally developing children pass through on their way to acquiring pragmatic competence was examined. Our knowledge of normal pragmatic development derives from experimental studies that have examined a range of pragmatic phenomena in language-intact children. Amongst other pragmatic skills, these studies have assessed normally developing children's appreciation of scalar implicatures (Noveck 2001; Feeney *et al*. 2004) and their use of speech acts such as apologies and promises (Astington 1988; Ely and Gleason 2006). It was noted in the first chapter that the literature on developmental pragmatics is considerably less extensive than the literature on other aspects of language development. One need only compare the relatively underdeveloped state of our knowledge of the acquisition of speech acts or implicatures to our much greater understanding of the order in which young children acquire grammatical morphemes and speech sounds to see that this is the case. The less advanced state of our knowledge of developmental pragmatics compared to other aspects of language development has had serious consequences for the study of disordered pragmatics. Clearly defined accounts of the acquisition of syntax and phonology in normally developing children have provided investigators with a framework within which to interpret findings of syntactic and phonological impairment in language-disordered children. In pragmatics, no such framework exists. This is as true today as it was nearly thirty years ago when the first clinical studies of pragmatics began to emerge. The result has been a proliferation of clinical pragmatic studies, the findings of which are poorly understood both on their own terms and in relation to normal pragmatic development. In the absence of a theory of developmental pragmatics, or even a clear account of the chronological acquisition of key pragmatic skills, what we are left with is a burgeoning group of studies which is powerless to explain findings of pragmatic disorder and which is cut off from almost everything else in language study.[1]

Notwithstanding the problem of studying developmental pragmatic disorders in the absence of a theory of normal pragmatic development, such a study will be undertaken in the current chapter. In order to conduct the more critical enquiries of later chapters, the reader must have a sense of what clinicians and researchers are treating as a pragmatic disorder (even if, as it has been argued in Cummings (2007b), characterisations of pragmatic disorder are somewhat problematic). We will see shortly that the domain of developmental pragmatic disorders, at least as that domain is represented by clinical studies, is truly immense. In an attempt to impose some order on this sprawling, empirical field, pragmatic disorders will be examined in relation to four clinical populations: (1) developmental language disorders, (2) autistic spectrum disorders, (3) mental retardation and (4) emotional and behavioural problems. In each of these populations, pragmatic competence fails to develop along normal lines. In most cases, this failure of pragmatic development occurs alongside problems in other domains of functioning, so that pragmatic disorder may not be the only or even the most significant deficit in an individual (e.g. children and adults with autistic spectrum disorders have impairments of socialisation and imagination in addition to communication impairments). The presence of these other impairments can mask pragmatic disorders and, in some cases, obscure them altogether (e.g. the child with a severe developmental language disorder may have pragmatic impairments that are obscured by his or her poor structural language skills). Any survey of pragmatic disorders in each of these clinical populations must accordingly be conducted from within a perspective that addresses deficits in a range of other areas in addition to pragmatics. For this reason, we will address the broad phenotype of the children and adults that constitute these clinical populations before proceeding to examine specific aspects of pragmatics in each population.

As well as influencing how a pragmatic disorder is manifested in a particular individual, the additional impairments of language, cognition and intelligence that are present in these clinical populations present a valuable opportunity for the study of a number of key interactions involving pragmatics. One such interaction exists between pragmatics and impairments of structural language of the type seen in developmental language disorder. The child who cannot produce certain syntactic forms, for example, inversion of the subject and auxiliary verb of a sentence (e.g. 'Are you leaving now?'), is not only unable to employ syntactic means to form questions (a significant group of speech acts) but is also unable to use a conventional means of making indirect requests (e.g. 'Can you wash teddy?'). In such a case, there are clear grounds for saying that a child's pragmatic disorder (his failure to use certain speech acts) is a direct consequence of his syntactic impairment, that is, his structural language impairment is a *primary* disorder and his pragmatic impairment is a *secondary* disorder. However, it is clear that not all pragmatic impairments in developmental language disorder are of this type – we will see below, for example, that there is evidence that some children with specific language impairment have pragmatic difficulties that are not related to their difficulties with language form. Another important interaction presented by the study of these clinical populations is that between pragmatics and cognition. Studies are increasingly finding evidence of cognitive deficits, particularly in areas such as speed of information processing and verbal (phonological) working memory, in children with specific language impairment. A cognitive deficit is believed to be responsible for the impairments of socialisation, communication and imagination that characterise the autistic spectrum disorders (different theories of this deficit will be examined in Chapter 4). Global cognitive delay is responsible for the wide-ranging impairments across verbal and nonverbal domains that are experienced by children and adults with mental retardation. Cognitive problems such as sustained attention and impulse control deficits are typical of individuals with attention deficit hyperactivity disorder. The relationship between these cognitive disorders and impairments of pragmatics has been all but neglected. Such studies as have been conducted will be reviewed in the sections below.

2.2   Developmental language disorder

When clinical pragmatic studies began to emerge thirty years ago, children with language disorder were one of the first clinical groups to be investigated. These initial studies were quite limited in scope. Investigations of individual speech acts (usually requests) or groups of speech acts tended to dominate these early studies (Rom and Bliss 1981; Prinz 1982; Prinz and Ferrier 1983). A smaller number of studies examined features other than speech acts, for example, revision behaviours and nonverbal pragmatic behaviours in language-impaired children (Gallagher and Darnton 1978; Rom and Bliss 1983). These studies were problematic in several respects. Definitions of pragmatics were inaccurate in many cases – a study by Hubbell (1977) bizarrely characterises pragmatics as 'the effects of communication on behavior'. With behaviours as diverse as smiling and playing (Rom and Bliss 1983), parental expansions of a child's telegraphic utterances (Schodorf and Edwards 1983) and verbal requests for answers and actions (Rom and Bliss 1981) all being treated as 'pragmatic', it is not clear what these early investigators intended the term 'pragmatics' to exclude. Also, the children who participated in these early studies satisfied different diagnostic criteria for developmental language disorder.[2] It is thus likely that the participants in these studies formed a rather heterogeneous group in which language disorders may have been attributable to aetiologies not permitted within a diagnosis of developmental language disorder. Notwithstanding these various problems, early studies of pragmatic disorder in language-impaired children did produce some significant gains. These studies prepared the way for a major revision in the classification of developmental language disorder. A subgroup of language-impaired children who exhibited significant deficits in the area of pragmatics was labelled as having semantic-pragmatic syndrome by Rapin and Allen (1983) in the US and semantic-pragmatic disorder by Bishop and Rosenbloom (1987) in the UK. Although there were differences in the application of these terms, their emergence in the clinical literature marked the transition of pragmatics from a largely neglected area of clinical enquiry to an aspect of language that was now of diagnostic significance. This diagnostic debate continues today and will be addressed again, as we proceed to survey the pragmatic impairments of this clinical population.

Our starting point in this survey of pragmatic impairments must be a clear description of the clinical population that we have been describing as developmental language disorder. This is no simple task, as is indicated by the large number of terms that have been used in relation to this clinical population over the years. Although the label 'specific language impairment (SLI)' currently has widespread acceptance, it is predated by terms such as speech/language delay, speech/language disorder, speech/language impairment, childhood aphasia, developmental dysphasia, developmental language disorder and language learning disability (Schuele and Hadley 1999). The term 'specific language impairment' reflects the fact that while language development fails to proceed along normal lines in these children, other domains of functioning are within normal limits (i.e. the developmental disorder is *specific* to language). Typically, these children exhibit poor language performance alongside normal nonverbal intelligence. Motor and sensory skills (specifically hearing) are unimpaired and children do not present with the severe socialisation impairments that are evident in autistic spectrum disorders. Language impairment is not secondary to craniofacial anomalies (e.g. cleft lip and palate) and is not the result of a genetic or chromosomal syndrome (e.g. Down's syndrome). In other words, each of the conditions that may put a child at risk of developing a language disorder (hearing loss, mental retardation, etc.) are lacking in the case of the SLI child. The requirement that each of these conditions be excluded as a possible cause of the child's language disorder is why specific language impairment is described as a diagnosis by exclusion.[3]

Epidemiological features of SLI are also integral to a wider description of this clinical population. Tomblin *et al.* (1997) obtained an estimated overall prevalence rate of SLI in monolingual English-speaking kindergarten children of 7.4 per cent. On the basis of this prevalence rate, and using information from the 1990 US Census, Tomblin *et al.* estimate that 273,025 of the 3,689,533 five-year-old children in the United States present with SLI. This disorder, these investigators conclude, is a 'common condition among kindergarten-age children when compared with the prevalence of many developmental disorders' (1997: 1258). Although figures vary from study to study, the prevalence of SLI in males is consistently reported to be greater than that in females. Tomblin *et al.* (1997) obtained prevalence estimates for boys and girls of 8% and 6%, respectively. Cheuk *et al.* (2005) found that males accounted for 75.2% of SLI cases below five years of age referred over a four-year period to the Duchess of Kent Children's Hospital in Hong Kong. Cheuk *et al.*'s figure produces a male:female sex ratio of approximately 3:1. A growing number of studies is revealing an increased prevalence of language and communication impairments in the biological relatives of SLI children (Rice *et al.* 1998a; Tallal *et al.* 2001; Conti-Ramsden *et al.* 2006; Ruser *et al.* 2007). The aggregation of language impairments in the families of SLI children points strongly to the existence of a genetic aetiology of SLI. Further support for a genetic aetiology is provided by findings of higher concordance rates of SLI in monozygotic (identical) than in dizygotic (non-identical) twins (Bishop *et al.* 1995). For further discussion of these findings and of the genetic basis of SLI, the reader is referred to Cummings (2008).

Morphosyntactic deficits are among the most frequently observed linguistic impairments in SLI. Problems with tense-marking morphemes (e.g. past tense –ed) have been extensively reported by investigators. SLI children are late in acquiring these morphemes and use them in fewer obligatory contexts than children with normally developing language (Rice and Wexler 1996; Bedore and Leonard 1998; Rice *et al.* 1998b; Rice *et al.* 2000; Eadie *et al.* 2002; Leonard *et al.* 2003).[4] As well as morphosyntactic deficits, SLI children have also been shown to produce and accept past tense overregularisations (e.g. he falled) and infinitive forms in finite positions (e.g. he fall off). They accept finite form errors in verb phrase complement positions (e.g. he made him fell), use nonfinite forms of lexical verbs and omit auxiliary verbs such as 'be' more often than children with typically developing language (Rice *et al.* 1995; Grela and Leonard 2000; Redmond and Rice 2001).[5] Lexical semantics is another significant area of linguistic impairment in SLI children. During picture and object naming, SLI children produce more errors than children with no language impairment. Moreover, their errors often consist of responses that are semantically or phonologically related to the target word or that are indeterminate (e.g. 'don't know') (Lahey and Edwards 1999; McGregor *et al.* 2002). As well as displaying expressive problems in lexical semantics, SLI children have also been found to perform more poorly than subjects with normally developing language on tasks requiring the recognition of lexical labels and the semantic features of objects and actions (Alt *et al.* 2004). Additional impairments in SLI children include a reduced ability to learn words (Oetting *et al.* 1995), phonological deficits (Aguilar-Mediavilla *et al.* 2002), speech delay (Shriberg *et al.* 1999), stutter-like dysfluencies (Boscolo *et al.* 2002) and problems with reading and writing (Boudreau and Hedberg 1999; Flax *et al.* 2003; Mackie and Dockrell 2004; Catts *et al.* 2005).

Traditionally, it has been assumed that pragmatic language skills are an area of strength in SLI children. Alternatively, investigators have argued that if pragmatic language deficits do exist in SLI children, these deficits are merely secondary to the structural language problems of these children.[6] However, it is becoming increasingly clear that both these positions are mistaken. Pragmatic deficits are present in SLI children. Crespo-Eguilaz and Narbona (2006) examined eighty-six SLI children aged four to nine years. They found that 21 per cent of this sample had problems in the pragmatic use of language. Conversational responses in SLI children have been shown in several studies to be inadequate. Rocha and Befi-Lopes (2006) found that SLI children aged three to six years had a significantly higher average of inadequate answers during interaction with an adult than children aged three to five years with normal language development. Also, while there was a decrease in the use of inadequate answers with increasing age in the children with normal language, SLI children continued to use inadequate answers with increasing age. Similar results were reported for younger SLI children by Befi-Lopes et al. (2004). Bishop et al. (2000) examined SLI children's responses to adult conversational solicitations. They found that SLI children rated as having pragmatic difficulties on a teacher checklist were more likely than controls matched on age and nonverbal ability (CA controls) and language level (LA controls) to give no response and to make very little use of nonverbal responses (e.g. nodding). Children who failed to use nonverbal responses also produced a relatively high level of pragmatically inappropriate responses that could not be explained by limitations of grammar or vocabulary. Bishop et al. conclude that 'this study lends support to the notion that there is a subset of the language-impaired population who have broader communicative impairments, extending beyond basic difficulties in mastering language form, reflecting difficulty in responding to and expressing communicative intents' (2000: 177).

Rinaldi (2000) studied comprehension of two types of ambiguity in sixty-four students with specific developmental language disorder who were aged eleven-plus to fourteen-plus years. The two forms of ambiguity – inconsistent messages of emotion and multiple meanings in context – are evident in a range of communicative intent (e.g. sarcasm, idiomatic expression, deceit and humour). Students with language disorder were less able to use context to understand implied meanings than either of two comparison groups (non-impaired students who were matched for chronological age and language age). When non-impaired children did not know a non-literal meaning, they were more able than language-disordered children to rule out literal interpretations. These findings were statistically significant. This study, Rinaldi argues, also challenges the view that semantic and pragmatic disorders necessarily co-occur (just such a view is the basis of the diagnostic category of semantic-pragmatic disorder; see below for further discussion). Ten of the sixty-four students with specific developmental language disorder attained age-appropriate or near age-appropriate scores on an assessment of word comprehension (the language measure used, which is in effect a test of semantic comprehension). Notwithstanding intact semantic comprehension in these students, they still had difficulty on one or both pragmatic comprehension procedures. This particular finding, along with the findings of the Bishop *et al.* (2000) study reported above, lend support to the view that pragmatic difficulties in SLI are not merely a consequence of structural language problems.

Laws and Bishop (2004) examined pragmatic aspects of language in four groups of subjects: children and adults with Williams syndrome, children and adults with Down's syndrome, children with specific language impairment and typically developing children. Pragmatic language skills were assessed in these groups by means of the Children's Communication Checklist (CCC) (Bishop 1998), which was completed by teachers and speech and language therapists in the case of SLI children. All three clinical groups scored significantly less than controls on the pragmatic composite (PC) of the CCC. However, there were no statistical differences in PC scores among the three clinical groups. Although the mean PC score of the SLI group (133.4) was slightly above the cut-off point of 132 for pragmatic impairment, seven children with SLI (41 per cent of the SLI group) scored 132 or less on the pragmatic composite and thus had pragmatic difficulties. SLI children showed significantly more evidence of stereotyped conversation than controls. It is clear from the results of this study that SLI children have impaired pragmatic language skills compared to subjects with normal language and that pragmatic language impairments are at least as severe in SLI children as those found in other clinical populations. Botting (2004) found that eleven-year-old children with SLI were less impaired on the pragmatic scale of the CCC than same-aged children with a definite diagnosis of autistic spectrum disorder (ASD), children with a clinical history of primary pragmatic language impairment (PLI) and children who had low performance IQ and language impairment (LilowIQ). Only 15% of SLI children scored on or below the 132 cut-off point for pragmatic language impairment, compared to 22% LilowIQ children, 37% PLI children and 60% ASD children. When a higher threshold of 140 was adopted, 29% of SLI children had pragmatic language impairment. It is possible that the superior pragmatic skills of the SLI children in Botting's study compared to those of the SLI children studied by Laws and Bishop may indicate some improvement of pragmatic skills with increasing age (the SLI children studied by Laws and Bishop were aged 4;05–7;02 years, with a mean age of 6;00 years; the mean age of the SLI children studied by Botting was 10;11 years).

All pragmatic interpretation involves the use of inferencing. Botting and Adams (2005) examined this key skill in twenty-five children with SLI and twenty-two children with primary pragmatic difficulties (PD), all of whom were aged eleven years at the time of study. Subjects participated in an inferential comprehension task, during which they were asked a series of literal and inferential questions. Inferential questions required subjects to compute logical (text connecting) inferences, bridging (gap filling) inferences and elaborative inferences. Children in both clinical groups scored more poorly than age-matched peers on this task, but showed no significant differences from younger children aged seven and nine years. Perhaps of most significance is the finding that SLI children performed similarly to the children with primary pragmatic difficulties on this inferential comprehension task – the mean scores of the SLI and PD children were almost identical (15.2 and 15.1, respectively). This similarity in performance of these two groups extends more widely than this study. Botting and Adams remark that 'other studies examining inferential ability have also struggled to measure any difference between those known to have pragmatic language difficulties and those with more typical SLI' (2005: 60).[7] This raises the possibility that in relation to this key skill for pragmatic functioning, SLI children may share certain primary pragmatic deficits with PD children.

Clearly, pragmatic deficits are present in SLI children or at least in a subgroup of SLI children. The existence of this subgroup has been the focus of debate since the term 'semantic-pragmatic syndrome' was first used by Rapin and Allen in 1983 to characterise a group of children that had until then evaded clinical description. These children spoke aloud to no one in particular, displayed inadequate conversational skills, exhibited poor maintenance of topic and verbosity and answered besides the point of a question in the presence of unimpaired phonology and syntax. They also displayed comprehension deficits for connected speech, made atypical word choices and had word-finding deficits (Rapin 1996). Rapin and Allen (1983) applied the term 'semantic-pragmatic syndrome' to children with known organic aetiologies (primarily hydrocephalus[8]), to children with no brain damage and to children with and without mental retardation. When Bishop and Rosenbloom introduced their term 'semantic-pragmatic disorder' four years later in 1987, it was used to describe a subtype of specific language impairment.[9] Today, Bishop takes the view that semantic-pragmatic disorder does not form a distinct syndrome. Rather, pragmatic difficulties that were previously identified with semantic-pragmatic disorder are more accurately a 'variable correlate' of SLI. In this way, it is possible to find pragmatic difficulties in children with structural language problems (the type of child that Rapin (1996) describes as having a phonologic-syntactic deficit disorder) and in fluent children who have good structural language skills (the type of child identified as having semantic-pragmatic disorder). Also, pragmatic difficulties do not co-occur with semantic problems, as the term 'semantic-pragmatic disorder' suggests, but can also be found in children who have no word-finding or vocabulary problems. To capture this pattern of pragmatic deficits across a range of other language impairments and competences, a pattern that cuts across earlier classificatory labels, Bishop proposes to institute the label 'pragmatic language impairment' as a more satisfactory successor to 'semantic-pragmatic disorder'.

Studies have confirmed the clinical validity of pragmatic language impairment (PLI).[10] There is clear evidence that PLI does indeed operate as a 'variable correlate' of SLI. As the studies above demonstrate, pragmatic impairments that cannot be accounted for by deficits in structural language have been found in SLI children. Rinaldi's (2000) observation that ten of her subjects with specific developmental language disorder had difficulty with the pragmatic comprehension procedures in her study, despite attaining age-appropriate or near age-appropriate performance on the British Picture Vocabulary Scale (Dunn *et al.* 1982), is a clear indication that at least some pragmatic impairments in SLI children are not merely the consequence of deficits in structural language (i.e. these impairments are primary in nature). Further support for the primary nature of some pragmatic deficits in SLI is provided by Bishop *et al.*'s (2000) finding that the SLI children in their study had problems with conversational responsiveness that could not be readily explained in terms of limited grammar or vocabulary. At the same time, SLI children with deviant structural language have also been found to have pragmatic impairments. The children with typical SLI in Norbury and Bishop's (2002) study of inferential processing had language scores at least one standard deviation below the normative mean on two or more standardised language assessments. In addition to these structural language problems, these children exhibited the same inferential processing deficits as two groups of pragmatically impaired children (both of these groups scored 118 on the pragmatic composite of the Children's Communication Checklist, a score which is considerably below the 132 threshold for pragmatic language impairment). Clearly, inferential processing deficits of the type found in children with pragmatic impairment are also found in children with structural language problems. As we learn more about the types of pragmatic deficits that occur in SLI children, it may emerge that a descriptive category of pragmatic language impairment is poorly suited to capture these particular deficits. But to the extent that pragmatic deficits can be present in a range of SLI children, and in developmental disorders other than SLI (children in one of Norbury and Bishop's two pragmatically impaired groups had autism), it is clear that the term pragmatic language impairment has some initial clinical validity.

Studies that are attempting to delineate further the category of children with pragmatic language impairment are now addressing the relationship of PLI and SLI to autism. Although SLI and autism have traditionally been viewed as distinct developmental disorders (indeed, diagnostic criteria for SLI have standardly been taken to exclude the presence of autism), our increasing knowledge of the phenotypes of both populations is beginning to reveal a more complex picture than was previously assumed to be the case. In this way, Conti-Ramsden *et al.* (2006) report a prevalence rate of autism spectrum disorders in a sample of seventy-six children (aged fourteen years) with a confirmed history of SLI of 3.9 per cent. This prevalence figure, Conti-Ramsden *et al.* remark, is about ten times higher than the rate of ASD in the general population. Recently, Bishop (2003a) has examined the significance of three factors which indicate a much greater convergence between SLI and autism than traditional accounts of these disorders have suggested: (1) structural language impairments in autism are similar to those found in SLI,[11] (2) the presence of symptoms in some children that are intermediate between SLI and autism, and (3) the presence of a high rate of language impairments in the relatives of people with autism (see section 2.3). On the basis of these factors, Bishop considers if autism is a type of SLI plus – the presence of additional impairments in autism is, according to this view, the only factor differentiating these disorders. However, she concludes that a more plausible explanation of these facts is to treat structural and pragmatic language impairments as 'correlated but separable consequences of common underlying risk factors' (2003a: 213). Bishop and Norbury (2002) investigated the presence of autistic disorder in PLI children. Although many of the PLI children displayed some autistic features, only five out of thirty-one PLI children (16 per cent) met criteria for autistic disorder on all three assessments used in the study. These investigators caution against taking the presence of pragmatic difficulties in children to indicate the presence of autism or PDD,NOS (pervasive developmental disorder, not otherwise specified). Botting and Conti-Ramsden (1999) studied ten children with PLI. Four of these PLI children, these investigators believed, might be better characterised as having autism or Asperger's disorder. Clearly, much work remains to be done on the exact nature of the relationship of SLI and PLI to disorders on the autistic spectrum.

In recent years, researchers have begun to investigate the cognitive basis of SLI. A key motivation for some of these studies has been the desire to obtain a better understanding of the genetics of SLI – in the absence of clearly defined phenotypes of developmental language disorder, a 'cognitive measure of phenotype'[12] may prove to be a more productive starting point in an investigation of the genetics of SLI than the various clinical criteria that have guided identifications of the disorder to date. Another important reason for conducting studies of the cognitive basis of SLI is that these studies can lead to the modification or refinement of the clinical criteria that we use to diagnose SLI. For example, the criterion that nonverbal intelligence should be normal in SLI children begins to appear problematic if a range of cognitive deficits can be shown to exist in these children (in this case, SLI isn't completely 'language specific' after all).[13] A further impetus for these cognitive studies can be captured thus: if the linguistic impairments of SLI are the result of cognitive deficits, might our intervention efforts not be more beneficially directed at improving these deficits than in treating the language impairments that are caused by them? Regardless of the rationale for these investigations, there is now an extensive set of studies which claims to find evidence of particular cognitive deficits in SLI. In the rest of this section, the findings of many of these studies are reviewed. The implications of these findings for our understanding of the cognitive basis of pragmatic impairment in developmental language disorder will also be considered.

One of the most commonly reported cognitive deficits in SLI children is reduced speed of processing. Fazio (1998) found poorer recognition of serial patterns in SLI children than age-matched peers under short presentation conditions. However, under long presentation conditions the performance of SLI children was similar to that of age-matched peers. The serial memory deficits of these SLI children were not specific to phonological processing – recognition of common objects, which could be easily recoded into a phonological form, was not impaired relative to visual tasks that were less likely to be recoded. Fazio concludes that serial memory in these SLI children was affected by the duration of presentation and that '[t]he findings from this study are further support for general speed of processing problems in children with SLI' (1998: 1380). Weismer and Hesketh (1996) investigated the effect of rate of linguistic input on performance in a novel word-learning task in sixteen children with SLI and sixteen normal language controls matched on mental age. Rate effects were most evident on production of novel words – SLI children produced significantly fewer words that had been produced at fast rate during training than normal language children. Weismer and Hesketh conclude that 'findings from the present study are consistent with the claim that processing capacity limitations, especially temporal processing constraints, appear to be at least one component of the difficulty that these children are experiencing' (1996: 188). Miller et al. (2001) examined the mean response times of SLI children and children with normal language on tasks involving linguistic and nonlinguistic activities. They found that SLI children responded more slowly across all task conditions and also when linguistic and nonlinguistic tasks were analysed separately. Miller et al. state that 'the results of the group analyses support the hypothesis that speed of processing in children with SLI is generally slower than that of children with normal language' (2001: 416). Other studies that report speed of processing problems in SLI children include Lahey and Edwards (1996), Edwards and Lahey (1996), Schul et al. (2004) and Miller et al. (2006).[14] Studies have also found evidence of deficits in rapid auditory processing in infants at risk of SLI (Benasich and Tallal 2002; Choudhury et al. 2007).[15]

Amongst the cognitive deficits investigated by SLI researchers are impairments of verbal (phonological) short-term and working memory. In a study of twenty SLI children aged seven to eleven years, Archibald and Gathercole (2006a) found that the majority had dual deficits in verbal short-term and working memory. Montgomery (2000) examined the effect of a verbal working memory task on sentence comprehension in SLI children.[16] In this task, children tried to recall words under three processing load conditions – a no-load condition, a single-load condition (words were recalled according to the physical size of word referents) and a dual-load condition (words were recalled by the semantic category and physical size of word referents). Redundant (longer) and nonredundant (shorter) sentences were used in the comprehension task. Montgomery found that SLI children recalled fewer words than normally developing, age-matched controls in the dual-load condition and comprehended fewer redundant and nonredundant sentences than these controls. These results were taken to indicate that SLI children have less functional verbal working memory capacity (i.e. ability to coordinate storage and processing functions) than age-matched peers. Briscoe et al. (2001) found that the mean scores of SLI children on tests of phonological short-term memory were significantly poorer than those of age-matched controls. Weismer et al. (1999) used the Competing Language Processing Task, developed by Gaulin and Campbell (1994), to examine verbal working memory capacity in SLI children. These children performed similarly to normal language controls on true/false comprehension items, but displayed significantly poorer word recall than these controls. These researchers conclude that 'findings from this investigation indicate that children with SLI evidence greater deficits in verbal working memory capacity than normal language peers' (1999: 1258). Other studies that have found similar memory deficits in SLI children include Marton and Schwartz (2003), Gillam et al. (1998), Hoffman and Gillam (2004) and Hick et al. (2005). Short-term and working memory abilities in the visuospatial domain have been found to be at age-appropriate levels in SLI children (Archibald and Gathercole 2006b).[17]

Although reduced processing speed and problems with verbal short-term memory have been extensively studied in SLI, they are not the only cognitive deficits to be examined. Other deficits, including problems in shifting attention between stimuli (Niemi et al. 2003; Lum et al. 2007), have also been reported in SLI. While these cognitive deficits have been shown to be related to the structural language impairments of SLI children,[18] their relevance to the pragmatic impairments of these children is altogether more difficult to assess. We have no idea, for example, how findings of reduced processing speed in SLI are supposed to relate to the inferential processes that are integral to pragmatic interpretation. If these processes are not part of a specific language module, such as grammar, but rather are a feature of cognition in general – as they are held to be in relevance theory (Sperber and Wilson 1986, 1995)[19] – then they may exhibit the same slowed processing that occurs in SLI.[20] In the absence of experimental studies which demonstrate that pragmatic inferential processes in SLI children do indeed proceed more slowly than these same processes in normal language children, we can only speculate about the likely cognitive substrates of pragmatic impairments in developmental language disorder.

A large part of the difficulty we confront when we come to consider the cognitive basis of pragmatic impairments in developmental language disorder is this: researchers in pragmatics are as unsure today as they were when Grice first proposed the concept of implicature of exactly what type of inferential mechanism is believed to operate when we recover the implicature of an utterance or establish the referent of a deictic expression. Of course, we can say that this mechanism must be capable of integrating information from a range of sources (e.g. memory, visual perception and linguistic decoding all play a role in establishing the referent of *she* in the utterance 'She is outstanding'). This inferential mechanism must also be responsive to the emergence of new information within the wider context of utterance, a feature that is necessary given what we know about the cancellability of implicatures.[21] But apart from tentative suggestions in this direction, nobody is beginning to understand what such an inferential process might look like.[22] In the absence of a clear idea of the type of inferential mechanism that is at work in utterance interpretation, it is difficult to see how we can proceed to establish the cognitive substrates of pragmatics in language intact subjects, let alone language disordered subjects (we are, in effect, attempting to find the cognitive substrates of a 'we know not what'). While this is clearly an unsatisfactory situation, it is not one that is going to be resolved any time soon.

A group of cognitive deficits that is likely to hold special significance for the study of pragmatic impairments in developmental language disorder are those characterised by researchers as 'theory of mind'. In brief, theory of mind (ToM) describes the ability to attribute mental states such as beliefs both to one's own mind and to the minds of others. Belief attribution is a key cognitive skill in all forms of pragmatic interpretation – consider, for example, how difficult it would be to derive the implicature of a speaker's utterance if we could not attribute beliefs to this speaker about what he or she may be intending to implicate. ToM is known to be compromised in children and adults with autistic spectrum disorder (we will examine ToM deficits in autistic spectrum disorder in detail in section 2.3 of this chapter and in Chapter 4). However, ToM abilities are usually described as being intact in SLI. To the extent that SLI children perform poorly on the false belief tests that are used to assess theory of mind, their poor performance is usually accounted for by deficits in structural language. In this way, Miller (2004) found that the performance of SLI children in their study on tests of false belief was similar to that of age-matched controls when the linguistic complexity of false belief tests was low. These same children performed more poorly than age-matched controls on a test of sentence complement comprehension (a child must be capable of producing and understanding sentence complement structures of the form shown in square brackets if he is to perform a false belief task: Patty thinks [the cookies are in the cupboard]). Moreover, sentence complement performance was found to correlate with false belief for all children. Similar results were obtained by Miller (2001).

Miller takes these findings as providing support for a view proposed by Jill de Villiers and colleagues (de Villiers and de Villiers 2000; de Villiers and Pyers 2002). According to these researchers, the mastery of sentence complement structures is the key developmental event in the language domain which makes it possible for a child to develop false belief: 'We wish to argue that the child needs the full syntax of mental verbs plus sentential complements in order to *represent* in his own mind the belief states of other people, not simply to *encode* them for reporting about them in speech' (de Villiers and Pyers 2002: 1056; italics in original). There is now growing empirical support for the idea that language may be integral to the development of a naïve psychology of other minds in SLI children. Johnston *et al.* (2001) collected longitudinal language samples from twenty-six SLI children aged 4;4 years. These investigators examined the use of cognitive state predicates such as *know*, *pretend* and *think* by these children. Each of these predicates 'refer directly or by implication to the knowledge state of the speaker, listener or a third party' (2001: 355). Johnston *et al.* found that SLI children used cognitive state predicates less frequently than mental age peers and with no greater frequency or variety than younger, language peers aged 2;11 years. Moreover, it was language level on a test of grammatical knowledge that best predicted the use of cognitive state predicates by the SLI children. The exact nature of the relationship between language and ToM development in normal and SLI children requires further investigation. Whatever is shown ultimately to be the nature of the relationship between these two key areas of development, the central role of ToM skills such as belief attribution in utterance interpretation means that this is an investigation that workers in pragmatics can ill afford to neglect.

2.3   Autistic spectrum disorder

For a significant number of children and adults, impairments of communication occur alongside deficits in socialisation and imagination. To describe impaired functioning across these three domains, Wing and Gould in 1979 coined the expression 'triad of impairments'. Today, this expression captures the main behavioural features of a group of disorders, which clinicians have variously labelled as autistic spectrum disorders (ASDs) or pervasive developmental disorders (PDDs). While ASD and PDD are both in current use in the clinical literature, in this section we will follow the dominant tendency in

British literature and use the term 'autistic spectrum disorder'. In the absence of biological markers for the autistic spectrum disorders, clinicians have developed detailed behavioural criteria for the diagnosis of ASDs. These criteria are included in the *Diagnostic and statistical manual of mental disorders* (American Psychiatric Association) and the *International classification of diseases* (World Health Organisation). They are continually revised as more becomes known about the phenotype of autism and other ASDs.[23] The most recent edition of the *Diagnostic and statistical manual* – DSM-IV-TR (American Psychiatric Association 2000) – recognises five pervasive developmental disorders: autistic disorder, Rett's disorder, childhood disintegrative disorder, Asperger's disorder and pervasive developmental disorder, not otherwise specified (PDD, NOS). The International Classification of Diseases includes eight categories of pervasive developmental disorder.[24] Although these disorders have much in common – most notably, some combination of deficits in socialisation, communication and imagination – they also differ in relation to factors such as age of onset, developmental history and prognosis. For discussion of these factors in relation to each ASD, the reader is referred to Cummings (2008).

Epidemiological investigations of ASDs have resulted in varying estimates of the prevalence and incidence of these disorders. In its review of autism research, the Medical Research Council found that the average prevalence from all studies published by the year 2000 is 10 per 10,000 for autistic disorder and 2.5 per 10,000 for Asperger syndrome (Medical Research Council 2001). Considerably lower prevalence rates are reported for other PDDs.[25] Using data recorded in the UK General Practice Research Database, Kaye *et al.* (2001) reported an incidence rate for autism of 2.1 cases per 10,000 person years among children aged twelve and under who were newly diagnosed in 1999. Studies have reported an increase in the incidence of ASDs in recent years. Powell *et al.* (2000) found that incidence rates for classical childhood autism increased by 18 per cent per year between 1991 and 1996. A much larger increase (55 per cent per year) was seen for other ASDs. While the exact cause of this increase in ASD cases remains unknown, factors which may contribute to it include changing diagnostic thresholds and better case ascertainment. Boys with the autism phenotype typically outnumber girls by at least four to one (Skuse 2000). Males constitute an even greater proportion of Asperger's syndrome cases. Gillberg (1989) reports a male to female sex ratio for Asperger's syndrome of between nine and ten to one.

Genetic, neurobiological and psychological factors have been advanced as causal explanations of autism. Psychological theories of autism will be examined in Chapter 4. Here, we discuss possible genetic and neurobiological aetiologies of autism. That genetic factors play a key role in the aetiology of autism is suggested by several lines of evidence. First, twin studies have revealed a high concordance rate for autism in monozygotic (identical) twins (Bailey *et al.* 1995). Also, the rate of autism in the siblings of autistic singletons is considerably higher than the prevalence of the disorder in the general population (Szatmari *et al.* 1998). Second, there is evidence that relatives of autistic individuals may display some of the features of the behavioural phenotype of autism, such as social and language impairments. Ruser *et al.* (2007) found that 15 per cent of the parents of children with autism in their study had severe communication deficits. Landa *et al.* (1992) found that autism parents in their study exhibited atypical pragmatic behaviours more often than controls. Bailey *et al.* (1995) report concordance rates for a broader phenotype of social and/or language abnormalities of 92% and 10% in monozygotic and dizygotic twins, respectively. Third, autism is often associated with medical conditions,[26] many of which involve single gene disorders or chromosomal abnormalities. These conditions include untreated phenylketonuria, tuberous sclerosis, fragile X syndrome, Turner's syndrome, duplication and inverted duplication of chromosome 15q11q15 and FRAXE. Advances in neuroimaging and neuropathology have transformed our understanding of the brain mechanisms in autism. In its review of autism research, the Medical Research Council (2001) describes three areas that postmortem and structural MRI studies have shown consistently to be abnormal in autism: (1) brain weight is increased, (2) decreased Purkinje cell number and (3) developmental abnormalities of the inferior olive. However, the functional significance of each of these findings is still not entirely clear at the present time. For further discussion of genetic and neurobiological aetiologies of autism, the reader is referred to Cummings (2008).

From the earliest vocalisations, the development of communication is markedly deviant in autism. In a study of early vocal behaviours in young children with autism, Sheinkopf *et al.* (2000) found that autistic children did not have difficulty with the expression of well-formed syllables (i.e. canonical babbling). These children did exhibit, however, significant impairments in vocal quality (i.e. atypical phonation). In specific terms, they produced a greater proportion of syllables with atypical phonation. Atypical early vocalisations foreshadow later problems in speech and language development in autistic children.[27] Speech and language are late to emerge. In a study by Bartak *et al.* (1975), 58 per cent of autistic children had no single words by twenty-four months and no phrase speech by thirty months (it is worth noting that 42 per cent of cases had a diminished or abnormal babble). If speech and language do develop, problems in both domains are normally evident. In a study of thirty children with high-functioning autism (HFA), Gibbon *et al.* (2004) found normal articulation in twenty-four subjects and articulation disorders in six subjects.[28] Among these six subjects, disorders ranged from mild to severe. 'Atypical' substitutions accounted for 53 per cent of the errors in this group and these subjects rarely produced errors in the 'almost mature' category. The HFA subjects with normal articulation produced a majority of errors (49 per cent) that were 'almost mature'. None of these children

produced more than one 'atypical' substitution. Articulation errors in the autistic population have also been found to extend into adolescence and beyond
(Shriberg *et al.* 2001).

Prosody plays an important role in several communicative functions, one
of which is the expression of emotions or the speaker's affective state. The
presence of impaired social and emotional functioning in autism has led investigators to enquire if prosodic disturbances might not also feature amongst
the communication deficits in this disorder. Paul *et al.* (2005) examined the
production and perception of three prosodic elements (stress, intonation and
phrasing) in a group of ASD subjects. Each of these elements was examined in
two prosodic functions: a grammatical and a pragmatic/affective function. The
performance of twenty-seven ASD subjects with diagnoses of HFA, Asperger's
syndrome and PDD,NOS on a series of prosodic tasks was compared with that
of thirteen typically developing subjects. Paul *et al.* found significant differences between the ASD and typically developing groups in the grammatical
production of stress, as well as in the pragmatic/affective perception and production of stress. The difference between the two groups on the grammatical
perception of stress also showed a trend towards significance. The standard
view of language impairment in autism is that although pragmatic deficits are
common and constitute a significant barrier to effective communication, structural language is relatively intact.[29] Recent studies, however, are beginning
to challenge this standard view. Kjelgaard and Tager-Flusberg (2001) found
significant impairments of vocabulary, syntax and semantics in a subgroup of
autistic children whose language was defined as borderline or impaired. The
pattern of these impairments combined with other features of the performance
of these children (viz. good articulation skills and a difficulty with nonsense
word repetition) led Kjelgaard and Tager-Flusberg to conclude that there is a
distinct subgroup of autistic children with specific language impairment (SLI):
'Although, by definition, SLI may not be diagnosed in children who meet criteria for autism, in fact, our data suggest that some children with autism may
have a parallel or overlapping SLI disorder, as indicated by their pattern of
impaired performance on diagnostic language measures' (2001: 304).[30]

While structural language impairments have tended to be overlooked in
autistic spectrum disorder, an area that has attracted considerable clinical and
research interest is pragmatics. It is frequently commented that autistic individuals fail to use language in either an appropriate or effective way in a range
of communicative situations. Pragmatic aspects of language that are disordered
in ASD include the comprehension and production of speech acts, the use and
understanding of non-literal language and a range of conversational skills (e.g.
turn-taking). Speech acts have received relatively little attention in research
into pragmatic deficits in autism. Among the studies that have been conducted,
some have construed 'speech acts' so widely that it is not clear what the term

is intended to exclude.[31] One study has attempted to relate the speech acts used by autistic individuals to the mental states of these speakers. Ziatas *et al.* (2003) examined assertive speech acts in autistic children and children with Asperger's syndrome. SLI children and normally developing children acted as comparison groups. It was found that autistic children used significantly lower proportions of assertions involving explanations and descriptions than the SLI or normally developing children. Autistic children also used significantly lower proportions of assertions involving internal states and explanations than the children with Asperger's syndrome. When mental assertions were analysed further, it was found that children with autism and Asperger's syndrome referred predominantly to desire and made few references to thought and belief. SLI and normally developing children, however, used a higher proportion of references to thought and belief. Ziatas *et al.* relate these findings to ToM impairments in the autistic children (theory of mind and other cognitive deficits in autism will be examined further in Chapter 4).

Non-literal language presents autistic individuals with a particular problem of interpretation. To see why this is the case, one need only consider how normal speakers and listeners interpret non-literal language. To understand when an utterance is being used to implicate something beyond that which is stated, a listener must be able to establish the speaker's communicative intention in producing the utterance. In order to arrive at this intention, a listener must be able to make certain inferences about the belief and other mental states of the speaker. The ability to make inferences about the mental states of others – to have a 'theory' of other 'minds' – is known to be lacking or at least impaired in individuals with autism. One consequence of this impairment in autism is difficulty in the use and understanding of irony and humour in language. Martin and McDonald (2004) found that individuals with Asperger's syndrome (AS) performed significantly more poorly than controls on tasks requiring the interpretation of ironic jokes. AS subjects were more likely to conclude that the protagonist in stories was lying than telling an ironic joke. A further aim of this study was to test which, if either, of two theories could best explain the pragmatic performance of AS subjects. The two theories in question were weak central coherence (WCC) and theory of mind (ToM). WCC did not appear to be related to pragmatic interpretation. By contrast, second order ToM reasoning – where the subject is required to indicate what the protagonist believes about the listener's knowledge – was significantly associated with the ability to interpret non-literal utterances. Martin and McDonald conclude that 'the ability to infer the mental states of others plays a significant role in the interpretation of non-literal language, such as irony, in individuals with AS' (2004: 326).

Surian (1996) examined the detection of utterances that violate Grice's maxims by children with autism. The detection of these violations is the first step in the recovery of the implicature of an utterance and autistic children with ToM deficits may reasonably be expected to experience difficulty with this particular task. Surian found that most of the autistic children in the study performed at chance on this detection task, while SLI and normal children all performed above chance. Moreover, the performance of autistic children on the detection task was related to their ability to attribute false beliefs. This study provides further support for the role of ToM deficits in the pragmatic difficulties of autistic children. Other studies have found evidence of a role for deficits in executive function (e.g. cognitive flexibility) in the pragmatic impairments of autism. Emerich *et al.* (2003) investigated the ability of adolescents with high-functioning autism or Asperger's syndrome to comprehend humorous material. Typical subjects and subjects with HFA or AS were required to choose funny endings for cartoons and jokes. Results confirmed the presence of a breakdown in the comprehension of humorous material in autistic subjects. For cartoon and joke tasks combined, adolescents with autism performed significantly more poorly than typical adolescents. Only on the joke task was there a significant difference between autistic adolescents and typical adolescents. On the cartoon task, autistic subjects chose significantly more straightforward endings than other endings. There was no significant difference in the endings chosen on the joke task, but the humorous non sequitur ending was selected most often by autistic adolescents. Both these endings, Emerich *et al.* remark, are consistent with impairment in cognitive flexibility. It was concluded that the autistic subjects in this study had difficulty with surprise and coherence aspects of humour.

It is widely recognised that autistic children struggle to comprehend the teasing behaviour of other children and cannot use teasing effectively in social interaction. An examination of the skills that are involved in teasing makes it clear why this is the case. The comprehension of teasing requires an ability to understand intention, non-literal communication, pretence and social context (Heerey *et al.* 2005). During teasing, the teaser must convey and the recipient decipher conflicting intentions – the teaser's intention to be critical of the recipient and the intention to convey this criticism in a playful and affectionate manner. In order to establish these intentions, the recipient must be able to attribute belief and other mental states to the teaser. We described above how autistic subjects had particular difficulty with this theory of mind skill. Equally, teasing requires mastery of non-literal communication: 'Much of the playful content of a tease is nonliteral, seen in similes, prosodic variations … and grammatical devices … that indirectly render the provocation less hostile' (Heerey *et al.* 2005: 56). However, we have just seen how the use and understanding of non-literal language is compromised in autism. Aspects of social context, such as the social relationship between speaker and hearer, can affect how a particular utterance is interpreted (e.g. as teasing or as hostile behaviour). Teasing is an appropriate verbal behaviour within certain social relationships (e.g. between same-age children) but is largely inappropriate in relationships that involve greater social distance between the speaker and hearer. Studies have shown that autistic subjects are unable to use features of context within the interpretation of utterances (Loukusa *et al.* 2007a). In short, teasing and other aspects of social communication depend on a range of cognitive and pragmatic language skills. To the extent that these skills are impaired in autism, autistic children and adults can be expected to experience significant problems with teasing and social communication in general.

Discourse skills have been extensively studied in autism. Some of these studies have attempted to relate aspects of discourse performance to theory of mind skills in autistic subjects. Colle *et al.* (2008) examined the use of referential expressions (temporal expressions and anaphoric pronouns) by twelve adults with HFA or Asperger's syndrome during a story-retelling task. These investigators predicted that there would be no significant differences in the general narrative abilities of the HFA and AS subjects, but that AS subjects would use fewer personal pronouns, temporal expressions and referential expressions which require ToM abilities. Both of these predictions were confirmed. Hale and Tager-Flusberg (2005) examined discourse skills – specifically, the use of topic-related contingent utterances – and theory of mind in fifty-seven autistic children. Over one year, autistic children made significant gains in the ability to maintain a topic of discourse. Theory of mind contributed unique variance in the contingent discourse skills of these children beyond the significant contribution made by language skills. Capps *et al.* (2000) found that the narrative abilities of thirteen children with autism were linked to performance on measures of theory of mind and to an index of conversational competence.[32] Diehl *et al.* (2006) analysed the narratives of seventeen children with high-functioning ASDs. The narratives of these children were similar to those of typically developing children in terms of story length and syntactic complexity. ASD children were also able to use the gist of a story to aid its recall. However, these children produced narratives that were significantly less coherent than the narratives of the typically developing children.

Specific conversational skills have also been studied in autism. Volden (2004) examined the repair abilities of nine high-functioning ASD children when confronted with communication breakdown indicated by a stacked series of requests for clarification (RQCLs). The repair abilities of the ASD children were similar to those of language age-matched control children in a number of respects. ASD children were able to respond to RQCLs and employed a variety of repair strategies. Like control children, ASD children varied their repair strategy as a breakdown persisted by adding more information. However, ASD children were also significantly more likely than controls to use an inappropriate response when faced with an RQCL. Capps *et al.* (1998) compared the behaviour during semi-structured conversation of fifteen children with autism to fifteen children with developmental delays matched for language ability. Autistic children less often offered new, relevant contributions than developmentally delayed controls. They also produced fewer narratives of personal experience and more often failed to respond to questions and comments than controls. Some studies have produced unexpected conversational findings. Verbosity is included routinely in accounts of communication deficits in Asperger's syndrome. Klin and Volkmar (1995) state that some authors view verbosity as one of the most prominent differential features of the disorder. However, Adams *et al.* (2002) found that children with Asperger's syndrome were no more verbose during conversations that differed in emotional content than a control group of children with severe conduct disorder. Verbosity, Adams *et al.* remark, was 'not a reliable character-istic of the group as a whole' (2002: 679).

Most studies have characterised pragmatics as an area of dysfunction in aut-ism. In a few studies, however, unacknowledged areas of pragmatic compe-tence in autism have been addressed. Echolalia has typically been described as a meaningless behaviour that is performed in the absence of comprehension.[33] Barry Prizant and colleagues were the first researchers to demonstrate that this characterisation of echolalia is somewhat simplistic and that echolalic utter-ances can actually serve a range of communicative functions for autistic chil-dren. Prizant and Duchan (1981) classified the immediate echolalic behaviours of autistic children according to several functional categories. In some of these categories – for example, turn-taking – echolalia has an interactive function (in the case of turn-taking, echolalic utterances function as turn fillers in an alternating verbal exchange). In other categories, the function of echolalia is noninteractive – in rehearsal, for example, the autistic child repeats the previ-ous utterance as a means to aiding its processing (of course, other instances of immediate echolalia serve no identifiable purpose and are categorised as 'non-focused'). Delayed echolalic utterances can function interactively by providing information and requesting objects. For example, the autistic child may utter 'Do you want juice?' as a means of saying he's thirsty and would like a drink. Delayed echolalic utterances can also function noninteractively by regulating the child's own actions (in this case, echolalic utterances are produced at the same time as a particular motor activity). To the extent that these functional categories of immediate and delayed echolalia can be shown to be valid,[34] it is clear that the echolalic utterances of autistic children are performing a number of important pragmatic functions. Dobbinson *et al.* (2003) have extended the study of the interactional significance of echolalia to the use of formulaic utter-ances by autistic subjects.

2.4   Emotional and behavioural disorders

In this section, we examine the pragmatic problems that occur in children with emotional and behavioural problems. The category of emotional and behavioural problems contains several different disorders, each of which has its own diagnostic criteria in DSM-IV-TR. Gimpel and Holland (2003) describe five categories of emotional and behavioural problems: (1) externalising problems, which involve acting-out, defiant and noncompliant behaviours; (2) internalising problems, which involve withdrawal, depression and anxiety; (3) disorders linked to abuse and neglect (e.g. post-traumatic stress disorder); (4) pervasive developmental disorders (e.g. Rett's disorder); and (5) other problems (e.g. sleep problems, feeding disorder). We discussed pervasive developmental disorders in the previous section and will not return to them in the present section. Rather, we examine the three emotional and behavioural disorders (EBD) that have received most attention in the clinical linguistic literature (even this has been rather limited in extent). These disorders are attention deficit hyperactivity disorder (ADHD), conduct disorder (CD) and selective mutism (SM). ADHD and CD are both externalising problems that frequently co-occur in affected individuals (see Lalonde *et al.* (1998) below); selective mutism falls within Gimpel and Holland's category of other disorders. We describe each of these disorders in brief before proceeding to consider the language and pragmatic characteristics of children with these emotional and behavioural disorders. We will also discuss the findings of the small, but growing, body of literature on cognitive deficits in EBD children.

Attention deficit hyperactivity disorder is diagnosed in DSM-IV-TR when an individual shows six or more symptoms of inattention that have persisted for at least six months to a degree that is maladaptive and inconsistent with developmental level. In addition to these inattention symptoms, individuals must also show six or more symptoms of hyperactivity-impulsivity. Some hyperactive-impulsive or inattentive symptoms must be present before seven years of age and impairment from these symptoms must be evident in two or more settings (e.g. at school and at home). Clinically significant impairment in social, academic or occupational functioning must be clearly demonstrated and the symptoms must not occur during pervasive developmental disorder, schizophrenia or other psychotic disorder. Nor should they be better accounted for by another mental disorder (e.g. mood disorder). There are three main subtypes of ADHD – a combined type, a predominantly inattentive type and a predominantly hyperactive-impulsive type. In a study of 100 youths diagnosed with ADHD, Lalonde *et al.* (1998) found that the combined, inattentive and hyperactive-impulsive subtypes of ADHD accounted for 78%, 15% and 7% of these subjects, respectively. These investigators also found that subjects with the inattentive subtype of ADHD showed lower rates of comorbid oppositional defiant disorder[35] than those ADHD subjects with the combined subtype (33% and 85%) and hyperactive-impulsive subtype (33% and 100%). ADHD subjects with the hyperactive-impulsive subtype displayed a higher prevalence of conduct disorder than those with the inattentive subtype

(57% and 0%) and combined subtype (57% and 8%). ADHD is estimated to affect between 3% and 7% of school-age children and occurs more frequently in males than females – male-to-female sex ratios can range from 2:1 to 9:1 (American Psychiatric Association 2000). Biederman *et al.* (2007) state that approximately 50% to 75% of ADHD children satisfy criteria for the disorder as adolescents and adults.

For a diagnosis of conduct disorder to be made in accordance with DSM-IV-TR criteria, an individual must exhibit 'a repetitive and persistent pattern of behaviour in which the basic rights of others or major age-appropriate societal norms or rules are violated' (Biederman *et al.* 2007: 98). Such an individual must exhibit three or more of the following criteria in the past twelve months, with at least one criterion present in the last six months: aggression to people and animals; destruction of property; deceitfulness or theft; serious violations of rules. The behaviour disturbance in conduct disorder must cause clinically significant impairment in social, academic or occupational functioning. Criteria for antisocial personality disorder must not be met if the individual is eighteen years or older. There are three subtypes of conduct disorder – a childhood-onset type (onset of at least one criterion prior to ten years of age), adolescent-onset type (absence of criteria prior to ten years) and unspecified onset (age at onset unknown). In general population studies, the prevalence of conduct disorder varies from less than 1% to more than 10% (American Psychiatric Association 2000). Prevalence rates are higher in males than in females. DSM-IV-TR criteria require the individual with selective mutism (formerly elective mutism) to display a consistent failure to speak in certain social situations (e.g. at school) even though speaking occurs in other situations. The disturbance should last at least one month (not the first month of school) and should interfere with educational or occupational achievement or with social communication. The failure to speak must not be the result of a lack of knowledge of or comfort with the language required in a social situation. The disorder should not be better explained by a communication disorder (e.g. stuttering) and must not occur during a pervasive developmental disorder, schizophrenia or other psychotic disorder. Selective mutism is the least common of the disorders we will examine with less than 1 per cent of individuals in mental health settings displaying the disorder (American Psychiatric Association 2000).

The aetiology of ADHD, conduct disorder and selective mutism is still uncertain. Investigators have identified factors that place children at risk of developing ADHD. In individuals with ADHD there may be a history of multiple foster placements, child abuse or neglect, infections (e.g. encephalitis), neurotoxin exposure (e.g. lead poisoning), mental retardation and drug exposure in utero (American Psychiatric Association 2000). Low birth weight has also been found to be a risk factor for ADHD (Hultman *et al.* 2007). A genetic aetiology is suggested by the finding that the biological parents of ADHD children experience elevated rates of ADHD. Sprich *et al.* (2000) found ADHD in 18 per cent of biological parents of ADHD probands in their study. Only 6 per cent of adoptive parents of ADHD probands were diagnosed with ADHD. Genetic and environmental factors have been found to increase the risk of children and adolescents developing conduct disorder. Children who have a biological or adoptive parent with antisocial personality disorder or a sibling with conduct disorder are at an increased risk of the disorder. Also, conduct disorder appears to be more common in children whose biological parents have mood disorders, alcohol dependence, schizophrenia or a history of ADHD or CD (American Psychiatric Association 2000). Parental psychopathology, parenting strategies (viz., non-physical punishment), childhood maltreatment, poor mother–child communication and prenatal exposure to smoking have been found to be associated with conduct disorder (Drabick *et al.* 2006; Monuteaux *et al.* 2006; Vostanis *et al.* 2006; Young *et al.* 2006). Risk factors for conduct disorder in girls include the timing of menarche, physical abuse at home and a broken primary family (Burt *et al.* 2006; Ilomaki *et al.* 2006). While risk factors for conduct disorder have been extensively investigated, much less is known about the factors that predispose a child to selective mutism. Elizur and Perednik (2003) found that within their sample of nine immigrant and ten native children with selective mutism, the disorder appeared to be associated with social anxiety/phobia disposition, neurodevelopmental delay/disorder and family immigration. Marital discord was a general risk factor for selective mutism. Black and Uhde (1995) report a first-degree family history of social phobia and selective mutism in 70% and 37%, respectively, of families of children with selective mutism. Such a finding suggests a role for genetic factors in the aetiology of selective mutism.

Few studies have undertaken an examination of language and communication skills in children with emotional and behavioural disorders.[36] This is despite the fact that those studies which have been undertaken indicate quite clearly that many of these children experience significant language and communication impairments. In a review of studies of language skills in EBD children, Benner *et al.* (2002) found that 71 per cent of children formally identified with EBD experienced clinically significant language deficits.[37] Cohen *et al.* (1998) report that 40 per cent of 380 children aged seven to fourteen years who had been referred to child psychiatric services had a language impairment that had never been suspected. Tirosh and Cohen (1998) found that 5.2 per cent of a cohort of 3,208 children aged between six and eleven years had attention deficit hyperactivity disorder. Amongst these ADHD children, a language impairment rate of 45 per cent was reported. Steinhausen and Juzi (1996) found speech and language disorders in 38 per cent of a sample of children with elective mutism.[38] These disorders included articulation disorders, expressive and receptive language disorders, stuttering and cluttering. Studies are also revealing that language skills are related to academic performance in EBD children. Nelson *et al.* (2006) found that language skills exerted a significant proximal effect and distal effect on academic skills in students with emotional disturbance. Children with previously identified and unsuspected language impairments in Cohen *et al.*'s (1998) study had significantly poorer academic achievement than normal language children (reading disability was present in 54% and 17% of these children, respectively). Given the high prevalence of language deficits in EBD children and the potential for these deficits to adversely affect academic performance, it is clear that greater investigation of language and communication in EBD children is warranted. In the paragraphs below, we consider what is known about the language impairments of EBD children.

Perhaps unsurprisingly, expressive language and speech disorders have been commonly reported in children with selective mutism. Steinhausen and Juzi (1996) reported expressive language disorders in 28% of their sample of children with elective mutism. Articulation disorders were present in 20% of this sample. Only 2% of these children experienced receptive language disorders. In a study of thirty-seven children with elective mutism, Andersson and Thomsen (1998) reported that almost 50% had speech difficulties. The children with selective mutism studied by McInnes *et al.* (2004) had normal receptive language skills, but produced shorter, linguistically simpler narratives than children with social phobia (SP). Specifically, SM children produced fewer words and communication units than SP children. They also used fewer subordinate clauses and produced proportionately fewer left-branching clauses, even in a home setting, than children with social phobia. Manassis *et al.* (2003) found that SM children scored significantly lower than SP children on a test of speech sound discrimination. There was also a trend towards lower scores in the SM children on a test of receptive vocabulary. Gray *et al.* (2002) examined two sets of twins with selective mutism. Twins A1 and A2 displayed notable articulation difficulties and deficits in oromotor coordination. Their low average to below average expressive language skills were significantly poorer than their average to above average receptive language skills. The receptive and expressive language performance of twins B1 and B2 was in the impaired to borderline range and was much more uniformly depressed than in twins A1 and A2. All twins displayed a general tendency to respond in one-word sentences or short utterances. Two- to three-word responses were occasionally offered by twin B2. Poor grammar and sentence construction characterised her occasional sentence length responses (e.g. 'bicycle is you ride in it').[39]

Studies are increasingly describing language impairments in ADHD and conduct disordered children. Al-Haidar (2003) found coexistent expressive language disorder in 28.3 per cent of ADHD patients under nineteen years of age who attended a child psychiatric clinic. Redmond (2004) reported that conversation-based measures of utterance formulation differentiated ADHD children from SLI and typically developing children. Specifically, ADHD children used significantly more mazes and longer mazes than SLI and typically developing children (mazes included false starts, fillers, revisions and repetitions). Using a systemic functional linguistic perspective, Mathers (2005) conducted an analysis of grammatical intricacy of storytelling, recount and procedural discourse in ADHD children across both spoken and written modes.[40] Non-ADHD controls attained higher grammatical intricacy scores than ADHD children on spoken texts and significantly higher scores on written texts. ADHD children also failed to show the differences in grammatical intricacy across spoken and written versions of the same text that were evident in the texts produced by non-ADHD control subjects. Mathers states that 'one explanation … might be that ADHD children failed to adjust their choice of linguistic resources to suit the change in modality, or in sociolinguistic terms, they showed no adaptation to contextual change' (2005: 223). Such a finding is also suggestive of the presence of pragmatic impairment in ADHD (see below). Davis et al. (1991) found that adolescent male institutionalised delinquents performed worse than nondelinquent peers on both informal and standardised language measures. Differences between delinquent and nondelinquent subjects were significant on the percentage of utterances with error from the Clinical Discourse Analysis (Damico 1985) and the Adolescent Language Quotient, a global language quotient from the Test of Adolescent Language-2 (Hammill et al. 1987). The relationship between adolescent delinquency symptoms and language impairment has been investigated by Brownlie et al. (2004). These investigators found that boys diagnosed with language impairment at five years scored higher than controls at nineteen years of age on parent-rated delinquent behaviour.

Pragmatic language skills in children with emotional and behavioural disorders have received relatively little attention in the clinical literature. This is despite the fact that conversational behaviours are included among the diagnostic features of at least one of these disorders in DSM-IV-TR. Inattention, hyperactivity and impulsivity in ADHD are associated with several conversational problems. According to DSM-IV-TR, the individual with inattention displays frequent shifts in conversation, does not listen to others and does not keep his or her mind on conversations (86). Hyperactivity may be expressed by excessive talking (86). The impulsive individual may blurt out answers before questions have been completed, may 'make comments out of turn, fail to listen to directions, initiate conversations at inappropriate times [and] interrupt others excessively' (86).[41] Humphries et al. (1994) compared teacher evaluations of the language functioning of ninety-five boys aged 6.5 to 13.8 years. Thirty of these boys had attention problems, thirty-three were learning disabled and thirty-two displayed average achievement. Significantly more boys with attention problems were rated as having pragmatic difficulties than either learning disabled boys or boys of average achievement. Compared with other groups, boys with attention problems had greater difficulty maintaining a conversation than in initiating a conversation. This pragmatic difficulty was positively associated with teacher ratings of impulsivity in boys with attention problems.

Bishop and Baird (2001) found that the overall pragmatic composite on the Children's Communication Checklist (CCC) for children with ADHD was as low as for children with Asperger's syndrome or PDD,NOS. When parent and professional ratings were combined, 73% of ADHD children scored below the 132 cut-off point indicative of impairment (this compares with 77% of children with Asperger's syndrome and 61% of PDD,NOS children). ADHD children obtained particularly poor scores on the scale measuring inappropriate initiation. Geurts et al. (2004) also used the CCC to examine pragmatic language skills in ADHD children. These investigators found that ADHD children demonstrated pragmatic deficits compared to normal controls. McInnes et al. (2003) examined a community sample of ADHD boys aged nine to twelve years. Despite having normal language skills for their age, these boys displayed comprehension deficits when listening to spoken expository passages. Specifically, these boys were able comprehend factual details in expository and narrative passages as well as normal children, but had significantly more difficulty than normal children in making inferences from expository information. Explanations of the poorer inferential comprehension of these ADHD subjects aside,[42] it is clear that a deficit in the inferential processing of language is likely to have an adverse impact on the pragmatic language skills of these subjects. Bignell and Cain (2007) examined pragmatic language skills in a nondiagnosed population of seven- to eleven-year-old children with problems of inattention and hyperactivity. These investigators found that groups of children with poor attention and poor attention/high hyperactivity were impaired in their comprehension of figurative language and in pragmatic aspects of communication, as measured on the CCC. Children in a high hyperactivity group did not display communication impairments, but were impaired in their comprehension of figurative language.

Little is known about the pragmatic language skills of children with conduct disorder or selective mutism. Gilmour et al. (2004) used the Children's Communication Checklist to investigate pragmatic abilities in 142 children who were referred for clinical investigation. Of these children, fifty-five had a predominant diagnosis of conduct disorder, eighty-seven had an autistic spectrum condition and sixty displayed typical development. Males predominated in the conduct disorder group in a ratio of 9:1. Pragmatic language impairments and other behavioural features similar to those found in autism were observed in two-thirds of the conduct disordered children. Fifty-four children, who had been excluded from elementary schools, were surveyed in a further study. Over two-thirds of these children were found to have comparable deficits. Gilmour et al. conclude that 'severe deficits in pragmatic abilities and autistic-like behaviours can coexist with psychiatric conditions other than autism, especially in boys' (2004: 967). McInnes *et al.* (2004) examined narrative skills in seven children with selective mutism. Although no significant differences were found in the use of story elements by these children and children with social phobia, large effect sizes suggested that in a larger sample, performance differences in the following areas would be demonstrable statistically: inclusion of internal responses and initiating events in home-elicited samples of narrative, and inclusion of settings and internal responses in clinic-elicited samples of narrative.[43,]

Cognitive deficits have been reported in children with emotional and behavioural disorders, although the role of these deficits in the language and pragmatic impairments of EBD children is still unclear. McInnes *et al.* (2003) found that ADHD children exhibited significantly poorer verbal working memory, spatial span and spatial working memory than normal children. These investigators remark that these findings add 'to the growing evidence that working memory deficits are a consistent cognitive correlate of ADHD' (2003: 437). Geurts *et al.* (2004) examined five major domains of executive functioning in ADHD children: inhibition, visual working memory, planning, cognitive flexibility and verbal fluency. ADHD children displayed executive function deficits in inhibiting a prepotent response and verbal fluency. In a study of ninety-nine children aged six to twelve years, Oosterlaan *et al.* (2005) found that ADHD was associated with deficits in working memory and planning. No executive function deficits were associated with oppositional defiant disorder/conduct disorder (ODD/CD) in these children. In children with comorbid ADHD and ODD/CD, the presence of ADHD was responsible for executive function deficits. Oosterlaan *et al.* conclude that 'these results suggest that EF deficits are unique to ADHD' (2005: 69). For further discussion of executive functioning in ADHD and ODD/CD, the reader is referred to Sergeant *et al.* (2002). Fewer studies have examined ToM deficits in ADHD and ODD/CD children. Buitelaar *et al.* (1999) found that ADHD children performed significantly worse than normal children and similarly to autistic and PDD,NOS children on second-order ToM tasks. Subjects with conduct disorder in this study performed as well as normal subjects on these tasks. Charman *et al.* (2001) found no difference between boys with ADHD and typically developing boys on an advanced ToM measure. Clearly, further research is needed to establish the presence and extent of any ToM deficit in children with ADHD or conduct disorder.

2.5   Mental retardation

A substantial number of children and adults fail to develop normal communication skills because of significant retardation of cognitive, mental or intellectual development. Several terms have been used to describe this group of individuals, some of which are no longer considered to be acceptable.[44] The term 'mental retardation' lacks the ambiguity of other terms[45] and will accordingly be employed in the present context. Traditionally, intelligence quotients (IQs) have been used to indicate the severity of 'impaired intelligence' in mental retardation.[46] Today, definitions of mental retardation are as likely to be based on functional descriptors and on the level of support that is required by affected individuals as they are on measures of intelligence. In this way, the Department of Health in the UK uses functional descriptors in its definition of learning disability. One such descriptor (impaired social functioning) states that the learning disabled individual must exhibit a reduced ability to cope independently.[47] Also, the American Association on Mental Retardation (2002) states that 'mental retardation is a disability characterized by significant limitations both in intellectual functioning and in adaptive behavior as expressed in conceptual, social, and practical adaptive skills. This disability originates before age 18' (Luckasson *et al.* 2002: 8).[48] One of five 'assumptions' that are judged to be essential to the application of this definition is stated as follows: an important purpose of describing limitations is to develop a profile of needed supports. This broadening of the definition of mental retardation has occurred alongside a more proactive approach to medical and therapeutic interventions for individuals with mental retardation.

In this section, we give a brief overview of the population of children and adults who have mental retardation. We begin by examining epidemiological features of this population both in the UK and the US. A vast range of medical aetiologies can result in mental retardation, including genetic and chromosomal syndromes, head injuries and infections. We describe the diverse aetiologies that make the population of individuals with mental retardation so heterogeneous. The heterogeneity of this population also makes any general characterisation of its language impairments all but impossible. Accordingly, we review the findings of several studies that have examined aspects of receptive and expressive language in subjects with mental retardation. Researchers have also attempted to characterise the pragmatic skills and deficits of mentally retarded children and adults. We consider below what studies have revealed about pragmatic functioning in mental retardation. Finally, we examine what is known about the relationship between specific cognitive deficits and language impairments in mentally retarded subjects.

In the UK, the Department of Health estimates that around twenty-five people per 1,000 population have mild/moderate learning disabilities – that is, some 1.2 million people in England alone. The Department estimates that a further 210,000 people have severe/profound learning disabilities. Within this figure, there are 65,000 children and young people, 120,000 adults of working age and 25,000 older people. As part of the Metropolitan Atlanta Developmental Disabilities Surveillance Program, the Center for Disease Control (CDC) in the

US tracked the number of children with mental retardation in a five-county area in metropolitan Atlanta. This study revealed that between 1991 and 1994, on average about 1 per cent of children between the ages of three and ten years had mental retardation. The CDC also found that mental retardation was more common in older children (six to ten years) than in younger children (three to five years), in boys than in girls and in black children than in white children. In 1993, the CDC used data from the Department of Education and the Social Security Administration to determine prevalence rates for mental retardation in children and adults in the United States. This study showed that an estimated 1.5 million persons aged between six and sixty-four years in the US had mental retardation and that the overall rate of mental retardation was 7.6 cases per 1,000 population. The mental retardation rate was higher for children (11.4 cases per 1,000) than for adults (6.6 cases per 1,000). Shea (2006) estimates that there are currently approximately six million American children and 560,000 Canadian children under the age of fourteen years with mental retardation.

Despite improvements in genetic screening and other diagnostic techniques, it remains the case that no cause can be found for mental retardation in approximately 30% of severe cases and in 50% of mild cases (Sebastian 2002). Known aetiologies include genetic and chromosomal disorders, infections, trauma, metabolic disorders and toxic agents. Mental retardation can be part of a syndrome which is caused by an abnormal number of chromosomes (e.g. in Down's syndrome), deletions of parts of chromosomes (e.g. the short arm of chromosome 5 in cri du chat syndrome) or submicroscopic deletions (microdeletions) of DNA (e.g. Prader-Willi syndrome and Angelman syndrome). Some forms of mental retardation are inherited. Inheritance can occur through the X chromosome, as in fragile X syndrome. Other disorders involve autosomal-dominant inheritance (e.g. tuberous sclerosis). Most of the metabolic disorders that cause mental retardation have an autosomal-recessive pattern of inheritance. The best known and most common of these disorders is phenylketonuria. Maternal infections can put an unborn baby at risk of mental retardation. Prior to the rubella vaccine being licensed for use in the US in 1969, congenital rubella was a significant cause of mental retardation.[49] Other maternal infections that can cause mental retardation through their adverse effect on prenatal neurodevelopment are cytomegalovirus, toxoplasmosis, listeriosis, herpes simplex virus type 2 and human immunodeficiency virus (HIV). A number of substances can have teratogenic effects on the developing foetus. Chief amongst these toxic agents is ethanol (alcohol), which can cause foetal alcohol syndrome when consumed by women during pregnancy. Foetal lead exposure has also been found to have an adverse effect on neurodevelopment (Hu et al. 2006).

Each of the aetiologies described above occurs in the prenatal period. However, events in the perinatal and postnatal period can also put the neonate at risk of brain damage and mental retardation. Complicated deliveries (e.g. breech delivery) present a greater risk of perinatal asphyxia. Although birth asphyxia can cause neonatal brain injury, it is a less common cause of mental retardation than was previously thought to be the case (Paneth and Stark 1983; Gonzalez de Dios and Moya 1996). Mental retardation is one of the sequelae of bacterial meningitis. In a study of outcomes of bacterial meningitis in 1,602 children, Baraff *et al.* (1993) found that 4.2 per cent had mental retardation. Accidental and non-accidental brain injury in the postnatal period can also result in mental retardation. Koskiniemi *et al.* (1995) examined the long-term outcome of severe brain injury sustained in thirty-nine children of preschool age. Seven children (18 per cent) attended a school for the mentally retarded. The central nervous system in children can also be damaged by tumours that originate within it (e.g. posterior fossa tumours) or that infiltrate it, usually during the advanced stage of acute lymphocytic leukaemia. Significant improvements in survival rates in these neoplastic conditions are largely attributable to the use of radiotherapy and chemotherapy. However, as more children survive these conditions, it is becoming increasingly clear that radiotherapy and chemotherapy can induce structural and functional changes in the central nervous system that can lead to long-term negative sequelae. Intellectual impairment has been observed to occur in children who have undergone cranial irradiation, with reported incidences ranging from 25 to 60 per cent (Murdoch *et al.* 1999). For further discussion of each of these aetiologies of mental retardation, the reader is referred to Cummings (2008).

Structural language deficits are commonly reported in children and adults with mental retardation. Roberts *et al.* (2007a) compared expressive syntax and vocabulary skills in thirty-five boys with fragile X syndrome (FXS) and twenty-seven younger typically developing boys matched for nonverbal mental levels. The FXS boys used shorter, less complex utterances and produced fewer different words than typically developing boys during conversational speech. Noun phrases, verb phrases and sentence structure were less complex in the FXS boys in the study. However, FXS boys did not use fewer questions and negations than typically developing boys. Persson *et al.* (2006) examined the language skills of nineteen children with 22q11 deletion syndrome who were aged five to eight years. Only one of these children had an average sentence length within normal limits. Five children produced subordinate clauses within normal limits. Grammatical errors were present in a median of 4 per cent of utterances. The receptive vocabulary score for the group was moderately low. A complete consonant inventory was present in about 50 per cent of the children. A phonological process analysis indicated that phonological development was delayed rather than deviant. Language skills have been extensively investigated in Down's syndrome (DS). Chapman (2006) states that people with Down's syndrome exhibit 'expressive language deficits relative to comprehension that are most severe for syntax, and, in adolescence, strengths in comprehension vocabulary, improvements in expressive syntax, but losses in comprehension of syntax' (61). Thordardottir *et al.* (2002) found that developments in syntax can continue into late adolescence in Down's syndrome. The DS adolescents in their study did not differ from MLU-matched typically developing children in their use of conjoined and subordinate sentence forms. The structural language impairments and skills of children and adults with mental retardation are examined further in Cummings (2008).

Pragmatic language skills have been extensively investigated in the population of children and adults with mental retardation. Below, we examine the findings of studies that have examined particular aspects of pragmatics in this population. First, we describe how Abbeduto and Hesketh (1997) characterise the pragmatic development of individuals with mental retardation. Conversational turn-taking, these investigators argue, is an area of relative strength. However, it has yet to be established if mentally retarded individuals can deal with contextual variations in the rules that govern turn-taking. Mentally retarded individuals have particular difficulty formulating their utterances in such a way as to make clear their intended referents.[50] The expression and understanding of speech acts such as questions and requests are also delayed. When expressing speech acts, individuals with mental retardation have difficulty with linguistic politeness. They are also delayed in learning how to signal when an utterance has not been understood and in learning how to respond to these signals in others. Although the quality of their contributions to a topic is not clear, individuals with mental retardation are able to produce utterances that are on topic. Several of these pragmatic language skills will be examined again subsequently.

Given the heterogeneity of the population of mentally retarded individuals, investigators have been inclined to examine the pragmatic language skills of these individuals on a syndrome-by-syndrome basis. In a recent study of pragmatic skills and social relationships in Williams syndrome (WS), Laws and Bishop (2004) observed significant levels of pragmatic language impairment in seventeen of nineteen WS subjects examined. Parents of WS individuals were asked to complete the Children's Communication Checklist (Bishop 1998), or an adult form of the checklist where the WS subject was over eighteen years of age. The same checklists were completed for twenty-four Down's syndrome children and adolescents by teachers or classroom assistants, for seventeen children with specific language impairment by teachers or speech and language therapists and for thirty-two typically developing children by parents or teachers. Only the WS subjects achieved a pragmatic composite score below the 132 cut-off indicative of impairment (mean score = 123.7). Eleven of the nineteen WS subjects scored less than 122, which is two standard deviations below the mean score achieved by the children with typical SLI in Bishop's (1998) study. The WS subjects obtained significantly lower scores than controls on all five subscales of the composite – inappropriate initiation, coherence, stereotyped conversation, use of context and rapport. In two of these subscales – inappropriate initiation of conversation and the use of stereotyped conversation – WS subjects achieved a significantly poorer score than either subjects with Down's syndrome or specific language impairment. WS subjects produced less coherent narratives and conversations than normal controls, even though they had similar levels of syntactic ability to these typically developing children. The WS subjects' ratings in these areas were comparable to those of DS and SLI subjects. Depressed performance in these latter subjects was related to poor syntactic skills.

The picture of extensive pragmatic impairment in Williams syndrome that is generated by Laws and Bishop's study is confirmed by other investigations. Sullivan *et al.* (2003) found that adolescents with Williams syndrome were unable to classify ironic jokes correctly at the end of stories. Like the adolescents with Prader-Willi syndrome and nonspecific mental retardation in the study, WS subjects judged ironic jokes to be lies, because they did not correspond to reality. In other studies, competence in pragmatics has been found to compensate for linguistic and cognitive deficits in Williams syndrome. Tarling *et al.* (2006) report considerable conversational ability in a twelve-year-old boy with Williams syndrome. This boy, called Brendan, was able to monitor comprehension in his interlocutor and reformulate his message when misunderstandings or requests for clarification occurred. He was able to foreground words prosodically that were integral to his interlocutor's understanding of his message. Brendan was also able to assess his interlocutor's apparent affective state during conversation and use this knowledge to adjust his persona within a developing narrative. An ability to engage in repair, usually jointly with his interlocutor over two or more turns, and to fulfill question-answer adjacency pairs was also in evidence. Tarling *et al.* (2006) state that 'it appears that Brendan is *communicatively* able notwithstanding considerable linguistic and cognitive limitations' (589; italics in original). The findings of this investigation may help to explain the impression of linguistic proficiency in WS individuals, notwithstanding their poor performance on standardised language tests.[51] The use of conversational strategies to compensate poor language and cognitive skills may also occur in other syndromes with mental retardation.[52]

There is now considerable evidence that the pragmatic language skills of males with fragile X syndrome are impaired. Sudhalter and Belser (2001) examined conversations between a researcher and individuals with fragile X syndrome, mental retardation due to other causes and autistic disorder. Males with fragile X produced significantly more tangential language than either mentally retarded or autistic subjects. Moreover, their production of tangential language was affected by conversational-pragmatic context, with significantly more tangential language produced within comments and questions than within responses.[53] Sudhalter and Belser state that 'because of their hyper-arousal and related social anxiety, males with fragile X syndrome are more strongly affected by the social demands of conversation than are members of other groups … this added stress exacerbates the effects of their already impaired inhibitory control system, resulting in the production of increased amounts of tangential language' (2001: 396). Abbeduto *et al.* (2007) state that 'perhaps the most studied aspect of pragmatics in FXS has been perseveration' (41). Verbal perseveration can lead to marked topic repetition in the conversation of individuals with fragile X syndrome. Murphy and Abbeduto (2007) found more topic repetition during conversation than narration in both male and female subjects with fragile X. Sheldon and Turk (2000) report the cases of ten-year-old monozygotic twin boys with fragile X. Twin A was more perseverative than twin B and responded to a request being denied by keeping making the same request. Referential communication is also problematic for fragile X subjects. Abbeduto *et al.* (2006) found that the fragile X subjects in their study were less likely than typically developing children to use unique descriptions for shapes and consistent descriptions for recurring referents. The latter finding was judged to be surprising, given the typical characterisation of verbal perseveration in these individuals.[54] Pragmatic deficits have also been reported in nonretarded subjects with fragile X. Simon *et al.* (2001) found a coherence deficit in nonretarded, full mutation women with fragile X. These women displayed a dramatic deficit in selecting appropriate endings to jokes relative to stories.

Laws and Bishop's (2004) study provides us with information about the pragmatic abilities of another group of subjects with mental retardation, individuals with Down's syndrome.[55] Twelve subjects (50 per cent) with Down's syndrome in this study scored 132 or less on the pragmatic composite of the Children's Communication Checklist. Only four DS subjects (17 per cent) scored within range of typically developing controls. Other findings suggest that the pragmatic language skills of the DS group may not be as impaired as these results indicate. The mean score for the DS subjects on the pragmatic composite was 132.6, a level just above the cut-off point for pragmatic language impairment. Also, examination of individual subscales showed that pragmatic problems were more closely associated with the coherence of narratives and conversations rather than with other scales on the checklist and that coherence was a function of the speech production and syntactic skills of DS subjects.[56] Abbeduto *et al.* (2006) reported impairments of referential communication (specifically, in the use of unique descriptions and referential frames) in the DS subjects in their study. Johnston and Stansfield (1997) found a normal range of pragmatic skills and communicative intentions in their study of six preschool children with Down's syndrome. In five of these children, pragmatic skills were equivalent or slightly superior to those of six comprehension-matched children without cognitive impairment in each of the areas examined by the Pragmatics Profile of Early Communication Skills (Dewart and Summers 1988). Papagno and Vallar (2001) found evidence of dissociation between literal and non-literal aspects of language in a single female subject with Down's syndrome. This subject displayed impaired comprehension of metaphors and idioms, while phonological, syntactic and lexical-semantic skills were largely preserved. Clearly, not all pragmatic impairments in subjects with Down's syndrome can be related to poor structural language skills in these individuals (cf. Laws and Bishop 2004).[57] With studies representing different aspects of pragmatics in Down's syndrome as impaired and relatively intact in roughly equal measure, it is difficult to discern a general pattern in the pragmatic skills of this clinical group.[58]

Although general intellectual functioning is significantly subaverage in mental retardation, studies have begun to examine the relationship between specific cognitive deficits and language and pragmatic skills in subjects with mental retardation. Several studies have examined the role of verbal, auditory or phonological short-term memory in the language deficits of mentally retarded subjects. In a study of thirty-one individuals with Down's syndrome, Chapman et al. (2002) found that auditory short-term memory, along with age at the start of the study and visual short-term memory, best predicted syntax comprehension in the DS subjects over the six-year period of the study. Laws (2004) confirmed the much reported presence of a specific deficit in verbal short-term memory (phonological memory) in a study of thirty children and adolescents with Down's syndrome. Laws also found that nonword repetition contributed about 50 per cent of the variance in MLU and sentence recall scores. This level of variance constituted a significant correlation between phonological memory and expressive language abilities in these Down's syndrome subjects. Rowe et al. (2006) found that DS adults performed at a significantly lower level than learning disabled subjects without Down's syndrome on a number of tests of executive function. Other studies of executive function have reported deficits in cognitive flexibility and planning in boys with FG syndrome (Ozonoff et al. 2000), working memory deficits in adults with idiopathic intellectual disability and in males with fragile X syndrome (Munir et al. 2000a; Numminen et al. 2001; Cornish et al. 2001) and attention deficits in FXS males (Munir et al. 2000b; Cornish et al. 2001).[59] However, none of these studies have attempted to relate executive function deficits to the language or pragmatic skills of subjects. The implications of these deficits for the pragmatic impairments of individuals with mental retardation are thus difficult to assess.

Researchers have begun to enquire if an impaired theory of mind (ToM) is present in children and adults with mental retardation.[60] ToM deficits have been reported in mentally retarded persons with genetic syndromes, including boys with fragile X syndrome, individuals with Down's syndrome and children with Williams syndrome (Yirmiya *et al.* 1996; Garner *et al.* 1999; Sullivan and Tager-Flusberg 1999; Abbeduto *et al.* 2001; Cornish *et al.* 2005). Tager-Flusberg and Sullivan (2000) found evidence of dissociation in the social-perceptual and social-cognitive components[61] of theory of mind in Williams syndrome, with only the social-cognitive component impaired in young WS children. Sullivan and Tager-Flusberg (1999) report that WS children (mean CA = 11.58 years) performed at a comparable level to age, IQ and language-matched groups of children with Prader-Willi syndrome or nonspecific mental retardation on a task examining second-order belief attribution. Sullivan and Tager-Flusberg argue that when one considers that the majority of four- to six-year-old children in an earlier study were able to pass second-order belief tests, it is clear that the performance of these WS children does not amount to 'success' in the domain of theory of mind. The ToM performance of mentally retarded subjects has been found to be similar to that of autistic individuals in some studies. Yirmiya and Shulman (1996) found no differences between the autism individuals in their study and subjects with mental retardation on a false belief task. Yirmiya *et al.* (1996) found that subjects with mental retardation of unknown aetiology and individuals with Down's syndrome performed similarly to subjects with autism on false belief and deception tasks. Other studies indicate that the ToM performance of subjects with mental retardation is superior to that of individuals with autism (Yirmiya *et al.* 1998).[62] Further research is needed to establish the specific features of ToM performance in different clinical groups and in syndromes with mental retardation in particular.

Investigators have been concerned to examine the effect of factors such as mental age[63] and language skills on ToM performance in mentally retarded children and adults. Language in particular has been shown to have a significant effect on ToM performance in subjects with mental retardation. Abbeduto *et al.* (2004) found that limited narrative language skills in subjects with intellectual disability contributed substantially to the failure of these subjects on a false belief task. ToM performance has also been found to vary across subjects with different genetic syndromes, each of which presents a distinct profile of linguistic strengths and weaknesses. Lorusso *et al.* (2007) compared indicators of theory of mind in the narrative production of subjects with Down's syndrome, Cornelia de Lange syndrome (CdLS), Williams syndrome and typically developing children who were matched for mental age and sex. The CdLS subjects displayed a number of problems in the use of ToM indicators in narrative production – specifically, they omitted more personal pronouns[64] in obligatory contexts than other intellectually impaired individuals and used a higher number of incorrectly introduced shifts in point of view than either typically developing or WS individuals. Mean length of utterance, which was lower in the CdLS subjects than in all other subjects, was shown to correlate with both these ToM indicators. Subjects with Williams syndrome produced more verbs denoting overt expressions of emotions (e.g. cry, shout) than even typically developing subjects. They also used personal pronouns with no clear antecedent significantly more often than either typically developing subjects or subjects with CdLS. Lorusso *et al.* remark that these findings are 'well in line with studies describing [WS] language as particularly rich and colourful at the descriptive and emotional level ... although other indicators ... suggest that this apparent richness is often redundant and syntactic complexity is not very well mastered at a finer pragmatic-communicational level' (2007: 49).

Clearly, these studies lend support to the view that language plays a role in ToM performance in subjects with mental retardation. However, they are noteworthy in a further respect that receives little or no discussion. The language domain that is central to the ToM investigations of Abbeduto *et al.* and Lorusso *et al.* is the pragmatic one of narrative. A speaker must be able to draw on a range of pragmatic language skills in order to produce a narrative. The key characters and events in a story must be appropriately foregrounded. Less significant information that the addressee may reasonably be expected to infer can be left implicit in the narrative. Events must be narrated in a way that will satisfy the addressee's expectations of relevance, manner, quantity, etc. For example, the addressee will expect to be told only about relevant events and for these events to be related in the order in which they occurred (compare with the conversational expectations that listeners have about the types of utterances that speakers should produce). These various pragmatic language skills are collectively aimed at addressing the informational needs of the addressee – the narrative will only be an acceptable one to the extent that the addressee knows the various characters and events in the story and how they are interrelated. Establishing the addressee's informational needs requires an imaginative capacity on the part of the narrator that is akin to a theory of mind – the narrator must be able to put himself in the addressee's mind in order to work out what type of information the addressee will want to be told. So the pragmatic language skills that enable us to construct coherent narratives are only possible to the extent that we have a theory of other minds. My point is not that we must first have a theory of other minds before pragmatic language skills can develop – pragmatic and ToM skills are more intimately intertwined, I believe, than this linear order of developmental events suggests. Rather, it is that researchers who examine the relationship between language and ToM appear to be at best uncertain, and at worst entirely neglectful, of the important role of pragmatics in this relationship. We will return to this issue in Chapter 4.

NOTES

1 These comments echo similar sentiments expressed by Bara *et al.* (1999). These investigators remark that 'currently, no single theory covers systematically the emergence of pragmatic capacity. We do not have a unitary account of the major

phenomena, viz. direct, indirect, ironic, and deceitful speech acts. Nor do we have a protocol by which to assess the normal stages at which a child is expected to produce and comprehend the different kinds of speech acts. Important as they could be, it is simply not possible to study deficits in communication without a comparable basis in normal development' (1999: 522).

2 The least restrictive diagnostic criteria were employed by Schodorf and Edwards (1983), who only required that the children in their study had normal hearing and intelligence. Rom and Bliss (1983) extended these criteria. In addition to having average IQ and normal hearing sensitivity, the children with developmental language disorder in their study had to satisfy a further negative criterion: an absence of orofacial or other medical problems. The most extensive exclusionary criteria were adopted by Prinz (1982) who required that children with known organic, intellectual, sensorial, learning and emotional problems were excluded from the study. Prinz's criteria are closest to those currently employed in diagnosing specific language impairment (see main text).

3 Craig (1991) states that 'children with Specific Language Impairment demonstrate poor expressive or poor receptive and expressive language skills in the absence of clinically significant neurological impairment, hearing loss, emotional problems, or sensory-motor defect, and their general intelligence appears to be within the normal range. The SLI diagnostic label is applied on the basis of well-accepted exclusion criteria' (166).

4 Not all studies have found deficits in the use of tense-marking morphemes in SLI children. Beverly and Williams (2004) found that eight boys with SLI (forty-two to fifty-eight months old) had a significantly higher percentage of 'be' use in obligatory contexts (46%) than younger controls matched for mean length of utterance (27%).

5 Notwithstanding these various syntactic impairments, SLI children have also been found to use a range of grammatical forms. Leonard (1995) examined the following functional categories in the spontaneous speech of ten children with SLI: determiner, inflection, complementiser. SLI children were able to use each of these functional categories. Examination of samples revealed the presence of three different types of determiners: articles (a, the), prenominal determiners (this, that) and pronominal possessive forms (e.g. my, his). Several examples of the inflection category were also in evidence: third-person singular or regular past verb inflection, some form of copula 'be', some form of auxiliary 'be', the modal forms 'can' and 'can't', the auxiliary form 'don't' and three different pronouns reflecting nominative case. The complementiser category was also represented in the SLI samples in the form of auxiliary inversion and an utterance-initial wh-phrase that could not be construed as the subject of the sentence (e.g. What is he making?). Although SLI children displayed evidence of these functional categories, Leonard found that these children used the grammatical elements associated with these categories to a more limited degree than controls matched for mean length of utterance.

6 Leonard (1998) captures this view as follows: 'given the criteria for SLI, it would be natural to assume that any pragmatic difficulties observed in these children were secondary to problems of linguistic form or content'. While Leonard acknowledges that 'some of the evidence of pragmatic difficulties in children with SLI is of this type', he also states that 'in other instances ... the basis of the problem is not so clear' (1998: 78).

7 One such study is conducted by Norbury and Bishop (2002). These investigators examined the story comprehension abilities of children with typical specific language impairment (SLI-T), children with pragmatic language impairments who were not autistic (PLI), high-functioning autism children and typically developing controls. During a story comprehension task, children were required to answer literal and inferential questions. Inferential questions required subjects to make text-connecting inferences and gap-filling inferences. Norbury and Bishop found that SLI and PLI children and children with high-functioning autism had more difficulty answering literal and inferential questions than age-matched controls. However, there was no significant difference between the clinical groups, SLI and PLI specifically included, on this inferencing task (although there was a trend for the high-functioning autism group to do more poorly than other clinical groups on questions requiring inferences, particularly gap-filling inferences). In an earlier study by Bishop and Adams (1992), school-age children with SLI performed a comprehension task in which they were asked questions about a story that was presented orally or in pictures. Half the questions were literal and half required subjects to draw inferences. Even taking into consideration their comprehension age, SLI children were impaired on this task. However, they did not have disproportionate difficulty with inferential questions. Children identified as having semantic-pragmatic disorder (an earlier term for pragmatic language impairment) attained lower scores than the other SLI children on this task, but again did not show disproportionate difficulty with inferential questions.

8 Several studies have revealed significant impairments in pragmatics or in skills essential to pragmatics in children with hydrocephalus. Dennis and Barnes (1993) examined oral discourse skills in fifty children who had experienced early-onset hydrocephalus. Admission to the study required either a verbal or performance IQ (or both) of above seventy. Four oral discourse tasks were investigated: establishing alternate meanings for ambiguous sentences; understanding figurative expressions; making bridging inferences; producing speech acts. Children with hydrocephalus performed more poorly than normally developing controls on all four tasks. Even hydrocephalus children with a higher-IQ (verbal IQ of eighty-five and above) performed more poorly than controls on these tasks (with the exception of figurative expressions). Barnes and Dennis (1998) examined inferencing and figurative language understanding during a narrative comprehension task in thirty children (mean age = 11.19 years) who had received a diagnosis of hydrocephalus in the first year of life. The mean verbal and performance IQ of these children was 103 and ninety-two, respectively. This group of hydrocephalus subjects had difficulty with coherence and elaborative inferences, even when prior knowledge was controlled. They also had difficulty interpreting novel (but not idiomatic) figurative expressions. In a later study, Barnes et al. (2004) found that children with hydrocephalus (mean age = 12.8 years) had difficulty suppressing contextually irrelevant meanings and in using an earlier read sentence to understand a new sentence, as the textual distance between these propositions increased. The verbal IQ of each of the twenty-eight hydrocephalus subjects in this study was above eighty. Huber-Okrainec et al. (2005) examined idiom comprehension in thirty-eight children with spina bifida meningomyelocele (SBM), each of whom was treated for hydrocephalus shortly after birth. Inclusion in the study required a verbal IQ score of seventy or above. The mean age of these subjects was 12.97 years. These investigators found that compared to age peers, SBM children were able to understand decomposable idioms (those that are processed like literal language) but not non-decomposable idioms (those that require contextual analyses for acquisition).

9 Although Bishop and Rosenbloom did not use the expression 'specific language impairment' in 1987, there are clear similarities between SLI and their account of the specific developmental language disorders of unknown origin to which semantic-pragmatic disorder belongs: 'Many children present with a language disorder for which there is no obvious explanation. Peripheral hearing is normal, non-verbal intelligence is good, the family home is perfectly adequate and there is no sign of physical or psychiatric abnormality. Little is known about the aetiology of these disorders. The vast majority of children have no detectable genetic or physical abnormality, even after detailed investigation' (Bishop and Rosenbloom 1987: 28).

10 Bishop (2000a) states that children with pragmatic language impairment are poor at inferencing, over-literal, neglectful of their listener's perspective and display a tendency to use socially inappropriate and/or stereotyped conversational responses.

11 Genetic factors appear to account for the similarity of these language impairments. Smith (2007) remarks of SLI that 'while there is co-morbidity of SLI with dyslexia, it appears that most of the common genetic effects may be with the language characteristics of autism spectrum disorders rather than with dyslexia and related disorders' (96).

12 This expression is taken from Newbury et al. (2005). These investigators review studies which suggest that 'a better understanding of the genetics of SLI might emerge if we move away from clinical criteria for diagnosis to look instead at a theoretically based quantitative and cognitive measure of the phenotype' (528). In the case of the studies reviewed by Newbury et al., that measure is a test of phonological short-term memory.

13 Botting (2005) states that 'increasing information about the presence of processing deficits in SLI have led some researchers to question the use of IQ criteria in clinical diagnosis' (317). In her own study of nonverbal cognitive development in eighty-two children with SLI, Botting (2005) recorded a significant fall in nonverbal IQ of over twenty points in these children between the ages of seven and fourteen years. Moreover, low nonverbal IQ has been found to be related to poor language skills in these children. Wetherell et al. (2007) found poorer narrative skills among adolescents with a history of SLI and poor cognitive levels (a mean nonverbal IQ of 78.4 in eight subjects) than in SLI adolescents with nonverbal IQ in the normal range (a mean nonverbal IQ of 96.6 in eleven subjects).

14 In a grammaticality judgement task, Hayiou-Thomas et al. (2004) found that normal language children can be induced to produce the verb morphology errors that occur in SLI by compressing the speech signal to 50 per cent of its original rate. This had the effect of simulating reduced speed of processing in SLI.

15 The infants in these studies had a positive family history of SLI. Their deficits in rapid auditory processing were found to predict later language skills – Choudhury et al. found that rapid auditory processing abilities predicted language scores at twelve and sixteen months, while Benasich and Tallal (2002) found that rapid auditory processing at 7.5 months was the single best predictor of language outcome at twenty-four months. Quite different results were obtained by van der Lely et al. (2004), who found 'no consistent evidence that a deficit in processing rapid acoustic information causes or maintains grammatical-SLI' (167).

16 In an earlier study, Montgomery (1995) examined the influence of phonological working memory on sentence comprehension in SLI children. SLI children and children with normal language participated in a nonsense word repetition task (an index of phonological working memory) and a comprehension task that used redundant

and nonredundant sentences. SLI children repeated significantly fewer three- and four-syllable nonsense words than normal language children and comprehended significantly fewer redundant (longer) sentences than nonredundant (shorter) sentences. Also, performance on nonsense word repetition and sentence comprehension tasks was positively correlated. Montgomery concludes that 'children with SLI have diminished phonological working memory capacity and that this capacity deficit compromises their sentence comprehension efforts' (1995: 187).

17 Other studies are less conclusive and suggest that SLI children may experience problems in visuospatial short-term memory after all. Archibald and Gathercole (2006a) found that 50 per cent of the SLI children in their study scored in the deficit range on a visuospatial short-term memory composite. Hick *et al.* (2005) reported that a visuospatial short-term memory task showed slower development over time in SLI children than in typically developing children.

18 Conti-Ramsden and Durkin (2007) examined the relationship of phonological short-term memory abilities to language and literacy skills over three years in eighty young adolescents with a history of SLI. Phonological short-term memory abilities were found to contribute significantly to later expressive language skills. Poor phonological short-term memory abilities were shown to be related to expressive-receptive profiles of SLI and to the presence of reading difficulties.

19 Sperber and Wilson (1995) state that 'we do maintain that inferential comprehension involves no specialised mechanisms. In particular, we will argue that the inferential tier of verbal comprehension involves the application of central, unspecialised inference processes to the output of specialised, non-inferential linguistic processes' (66). However, in more recent work Sperber and Wilson (2002) state that 'departing from our earlier views ... we will argue that pragmatic interpretation is not simply a matter of applying Fodorian central systems or general mind-reading abilities to a particular (communicative) domain' (5).

20 Schul *et al.* (2004) state that 'children with SLI present with a variety of perceptual, motor and cognitive processing problems that together share the common feature of performance slowness, or generalized slowness in processing' (661). To the extent that the slowness in SLI appears to affect a number of domains and modalities (i.e. it is not restricted to language or auditory stimuli, for example) and on the assumption that the inferential processes which are integral to pragmatic interpretation are part of cognition in general (i.e. they are not language-specific), it is reasonable to suggest that slowness may also be a feature of these processes.

21 Certain implicatures can be readily cancelled without creating an anomaly. If B responds to A's question 'Are you coming to the pub tonight?' by saying 'My parents are visiting this evening', A may take B's response to implicate that he won't be coming to the pub. However, this particular implicature can be cancelled if B goes on to say 'But I'll call in later on'. The inferential mechanism that is at work in utterance interpretation must be one that is capable of cancelling an implicature if upcoming linguistic or other information indicates the need for such cancellation.

22 If the reader thinks this is an unnecessarily negative stance on our current state of knowledge in this area, it is at least supported by prominent theorists. For example, in his 1983 book *The modularity of mind*, Jerry Fodor states that 'the reason why there is no serious psychology of central cognitive processes is the same as the reason why there is no serious philosophy of scientific confirmation. Both exemplify the significance of global factors in the fixation of belief, and nobody begins

to understand how such factors have their effects' (1983: 129). More recently, Levinson (2000) has remarked of utterance comprehension 'let us confess that we don't really have the faintest idea how it works' and 'books like those by Sperber and Wilson (1986) or Atlas (1989) or Horn (1989), or the present effort, which attempt to spell out some of the pragmatic processes involved, are pretty much stabs in the dark' (4). In his theory of generalised conversational implicature, Levinson (2000) argues that listeners use defaults to arrive at preferred interpretations of speakers' utterances. For an account of Sperber and Wilson's (1986, 1995) relevance theory, and a critical evaluation of this framework, the reader is referred to Chapter 4 of Cummings (2005).

23 The evolving nature of these classification systems can be seen in the inclusion of Asperger's syndrome for the first time in DSM-IV (American Psychiatric Association 1994). Following a large, international field trial involving over a thousand children and adults with autism and related disorders (Volkmar *et al.* 1994), it was decided that Asperger's disorder could be included in DSM-IV as a diagnostic category distinct from autism within the wider class of pervasive developmental disorders.

24 The ICD-10 (World Health Organisation 1993) includes the following PDD categories: childhood autism, atypical autism, Rett's syndrome, other childhood disintegrative disorder, overactive disorder associated with mental retardation and stereotyped movements, Asperger's syndrome, other pervasive developmental disorders and pervasive developmental disorder, unspecified.

25 Fombonne (2002) reviewed thirty-two epidemiological surveys of autism and PDDs and found four surveys that yielded estimates for childhood disintegrative disorder ranging from 1.1 to 6.4 cases per 100,000 subjects. Fombonne concluded that the prevalence rate for CDD is sixty times less than that for autistic disorder and that only one child out of 175 children with a PDD diagnosis meets criteria for CDD. Similarly low prevalence rates are reported for Rett's syndrome. Kozinetz *et al.* (1993) report a prevalence rate for Rett's syndrome of 0.44 cases per 10,000 females aged from two to eighteen years of age. Fombonne (2003) reports a prevalence rate of fifteen cases per 10,000 persons for PDD,NOS. This prevalence rate is higher than in other types of PDD. This may be related to over-diagnosis of this condition in the absence of specific diagnostic criteria for PDD, NOS.

26 Barton and Volkmar (1998) reviewed records on 211 subjects with autism and other developmental disorders. They found that the prevalence of medical conditions with suspected aetiological relationship with autism varied between 10% and 15%, depending on the system used to diagnose autism.

27 It should be emphasised that this only applies to autistic children who acquire verbal communication. The Yale Child Study Center states that speech (spoken language) is absent in about 50 per cent of autism cases.

28 The widely accepted clinical picture is one in which articulation skills are largely intact compared to other areas of language and communication. In a study of eighty-nine children with autism, for example, Kjelgaard and Tager-Flusberg (2001) concluded that 'among the children with autism there was significant heterogeneity in their language skills, [but] across all the children, articulation skills were spared' (287).

29 Noens and van Berckelaer-Onnes (2005) state that 'reviews suggest that the development of formal and semantic aspects is relatively spared, whereas pragmatic skills are considered to be specifically impaired' (123).

30 Rapin and Dunn (2003) state that many of the language deficits seen in autistic preschoolers parallel those of non-autistic preschoolers with developmental language disorders. Tanguay *et al.* (1998) argue that vocabulary and grammar deficiencies in autistic persons should be coded under developmental language disorder in DSM-IV.

31 In a study by Loveland *et al.* (1988), for example, behaviours as diverse as non-responses, gesture and vocalisation were classified as types of speech acts.

32 Studies have also failed to find evidence of a relationship between discourse skills and theory of mind in autism. Losh and Capps (2003) examined the narrative discourse abilities of twenty-eight high-functioning children with autism or Asperger's syndrome. These investigators found that the narrative abilities of these subjects were associated with performance on measures of emotional understanding, but not with theory of mind or verbal IQ.

33 This view of echolalia received support from early studies which purported to show a link between echolalia and poor receptive language skills in autism. In a study of ten autistic children, Roberts (1989) found that significantly more echolalic utterances were produced by children with poor receptive language skills than by children whose receptive language skills were age-appropriate.

34 In a study of immediate echolalia in eighteen autistic children, McEvoy *et al.* (1988) found that the validity of functional categories for echolalia was not strongly supported.

35 Oppositional defiant disorder (ODD) is an externalising problem. DSM-IV-TR states that 'the essential feature of oppositional defiant disorder is a recurrent pattern of negativistic, defiant, disobedient, and hostile behavior toward authority figures that persists for at least 6 months' (2000: 100). Gimpel and Holland (2003) remark that 'a substantial number of children with ODD eventually develop the more serious behavior disorder of CD. In fact, many researchers believe that ODD is a developmental precursor to CD, and the two disorders are often discussed together as "conduct problems"' (4).

36 It is perhaps a sign of how little research has been conducted in this area that the *Journal of Emotional and Behavioral Disorders* has only published two articles about language between 2002 and 2007 inclusive. This figure excludes papers on aspects of academic achievement such as reading and spelling. The findings of these two articles by Benner *et al.* (2002) and Nelson *et al.* (2006) are discussed in the main text.

37 Of course, children with language impairment can also be comorbid for emotional and behavioural problems. Benner *et al.* (2002) found that 57 per cent of children with diagnosed language deficits were also identified as having emotional and behavioural disorders. In a study of 581 second-grade children, Tomblin *et al.* (2000) found clinical levels of behaviour disorder in 29% of language-impaired children and in 19% of controls. Parent ratings for behaviour disorder were significantly correlated with spoken language scores (reading disability mediated the association between behaviour disorder and language impairment). Hummel and Prizant (1993) state that 'research clearly has established a 50–70 co-occurrence rate of speech, language, and communication disorders and emotional or behavioral disorders in children and adolescents in a variety of settings, including public schools, community speech and language clinics, and inpatient and day treatment psychiatric settings' (217).

38 The term 'elective mutism' was replaced by selective mutism in DSM-IV (American Psychiatric Association 1994). This change of terminology was intended 'to eliminate the implication that such children were electing not to speak due to underlying defiance' (Manassis *et al.* 2003: 154).

39 A question of some interest is whether the poor expressive language and speech skills of children with selective mutism may predispose them to developing this disorder – a child with these communication difficulties may actively avoid speaking in certain situations – or whether poor speech and language development is a consequence of the reduced practice in using communication skills in particular settings. Steinhausen and Juzi (1996) subscribe to the view that speech and language disorders may predispose a child to develop selective mutism. They state that 'these disorders may have acted as a preformation of speech avoidance that occurred primarily outside the home where, for instance, poor understanding of the child's speech may have resulted in harsh criticism by the social environment and may have consequently led to the child's withdrawal' (612). McInnes *et al.* (2004) argue that reduced communication experience in selective mutism may contribute to the development of poor language skills in this clinical group: 'Considering that these children have experienced temporary or extended periods of mutism in school and other settings, their reduced experience with age-appropriate social and didactic interactions may limit their overall development of higher level language skills' (311).

40 Grammatical intricacy describes the percentage of clause complexes used in a text. It is related to semantic complexity – the meaning of a text can be elaborated, extended or enhanced by combining simple clauses into clause complexes – but is independent of the length of a text (a long text with a large number of clauses can have a low rate of grammatical intricacy).

41 Heyer (1995) states that 'impulsivity ... leads to specific language-related deficits such as poor pragmatic skills, poor problem solving, an inability to maintain a topic or topic switch appropriately, and poor associative control' (280). Poor associative control, which describes an individual's inability to control the free flight of ideas, is 'frequently seen in ADHD children when they stray further and further from a topic by reacting to their random thought patterns. For example, an ADHD child is asked a simple question such as "Where do you live?" The child reacts to the word "live" and responds with "There is this stupid kid who lives next door to me and his brother plays on this baseball team and they never win any games but the Cleveland Indians are really winning a lot of baseball games this year. My dad takes me to games and I love peanuts but I can't buy them because I have braces and they get stuck"' (Heyer 1995: 280).

42 McInnes *et al.* (2003) state that 'a potential explanation for the ADHD group's poorer comprehension of inferences may be contextualized within Baddeley's model of working memory ... normal discourse comprehension processes ... and the particular task demands of the expository comprehension task in this study ... If the child showed an intact verbal span but weak ability to simultaneously recall and manipulate information from the passages, comprehension of inferences might therefore be limited' (438).

43 Although McInnes *et al.* (2004) do not account for these findings in terms of a theory of mind deficit, it is clear that a ToM deficit could have a role to play in explaining these results, particularly the difficulty of the children with selective mutism in

using story elements such as internal responses (a category that describes the emotional responses, goals, thoughts and desires of characters).

44 In the UK at least, changing social attitudes towards affected individuals have seen the label 'learning disability' replace the less acceptable terms 'mental handicap' and 'mental retardation' in many professional and everyday contexts (for example, in the UK the Department of Health uses the term 'learning disability'). The term 'mental retardation' is used extensively in the US and in medical and clinical literature. It is also a valid diagnostic term, as can be seen from its inclusion in DSM-IV-TR. For these reasons, and to avoid confusion caused by other uses of the term 'learning disability' (see note 38), the term 'mental retardation' will be used in the main text.

45 The term 'learning disability' is used extensively in the US to refer to individuals who have disorders such as dyslexia in the presence of normal intelligence. This usage is adopted by agencies such as the National Institute of Neurological Disorders and Stroke and the National Institute of Child Health and Human Development, two of the National Institutes of Health in the US.

46 Mental health clinicians have defined four degrees of severity of mental retardation or learning disability based on IQ score. These are mild mental retardation (IQ range 50–55 to about 70), moderate (IQ range 35–40 to 50–55), severe (IQ range 20–25 to 35–40), and profound (IQ level below 20–25). Mild mental retardation accounts for some 85% of cases. Approximately 10% of mental retardation cases have a moderate impairment. Severe and profound mental retardation accounts for 3–4% and 1–2% of cases, respectively.

47 'Learning disability includes the presence of a significantly reduced ability to understand new or complex information, to learn new skills (impaired intelligence), with a reduced ability to cope independently (impaired social functioning) which started before adulthood, with a lasting effect on development' (Department of Health 2001: 14).

48 This definition includes the three features of mental retardation listed in DSM-IV-TR: (1) significantly subaverage general intellectual functioning accompanied by (2) significant limitations in adaptive functioning (3) with onset before age eighteen years. Limitations in adaptive functioning must occur in at least two of the following skill areas: communication, self-care, home living, social/interpersonal skills, use of community resources, self-direction, functional academic skills, work, leisure, health and safety.

49 The last rubella epidemic to occur in the US prior to the introduction of a vaccine was in 1964–1965. In this epidemic, there were some 20,000 congenital rubella syndrome cases. Mental retardation occurred in 1,800 of these cases.

50 Notwithstanding their expressive difficulties with reference, mentally retarded subjects have been found to be adept at understanding referential expressions used by others. Abbeduto et al. (1998) found that school-age individuals with mental retardation are able to draw upon aspects of common ground (largely physical and linguistic co-presence but also community membership) to disambiguate referential expressions. Like typically developing children, these mentally retarded subjects requested confirmation of their referent choices most often when community membership formed the common ground. When common ground was not informative, these subjects were also able to signal a lack of comprehension.

51 This impression is most accurately conveyed in these remarks by Schultz et al. (2001): 'Upon meeting a person with WS for the first time, one might not immediately guess

that the person has developmental cognitive delays. They frequently show "cocktail party" verbal abilities – language abilities that are superficially quite intact, coupled with good adherence to social conventions and mores and a rather intense social interest' (607). There is now clear evidence that WS children and adults have considerable language deficits. The subject in Tarling *et al.*'s study had a significant deficit in his receptive and expressive language skills, as assessed on a range of standardised tests, and only a vocabulary score within normal limits. For further discussion of language deficits in Williams syndrome, the reader is referred to Cummings (2008).

52 Receptive and expressive language deficits have been found in individuals with foetal alcohol syndrome (Becker *et al.* 1990; Church *et al.* 1997). Subjects with FAS also have mental retardation which is in the mild to borderline range or 60–85 IQ points (Cone-Wesson 2005). Yet, these considerable language and cognitive deficits can be masked to some extent by the superior conversational skills of FAS children. Abkarian (1992) states that 'because of a superficial conversational talent, adults may wrongly surmise that children with FAS have better linguistic skills than they actually possess' (227).

53 Sudhalter and Belser (2001) explain these differences in the use of tangential language across responses, questions and comments as follows. Asking questions and producing comments rely 'less upon conditionalized language, and more upon the participant's own linguistic creativity' (2001: 396). Response type utterances, on the other hand, often involve answering well-rehearsed questions where 'semantic priming and associate responding would be expected to work to the speaker's advantage' (396). Also, in order to ask a question, one must make eye contact with and physically orientate oneself towards a conversational partner. This behaviour can be very arousing for individuals with fragile X. Sudhalter and Belser remark that 'the arousal experienced under these circumstances exacerbates the expression of their inhibitory control deficits, rendering them less able to block the production of questions and comments that are not pertinent to the ongoing conversation' (2001: 397).

54 Abbeduto *et al.* (2006) state that 'the fact that the youth with fragile X syndrome in this study were less perseverative (i.e., more inconsistent) suggests that there is a need for a more nuanced characterization of the language problems of this syndrome' (179).

55 Individuals with Down's syndrome experience elevated mortality due to dementia and Alzheimer's disease (Hill *et al.* 2003). Poor pragmatic language functioning has been reported in DS adults with Alzheimer's disease (Nelson *et al.* 2001). However, pragmatic deficits in these DS adults are likely to be caused by the neuropathological changes that attend Alzheimer's disease rather than by Down's syndrome per se.

56 Other studies have found that the narrative performance of Down's syndrome subjects exceeds what would be expected given their expressive syntactic and lexical limitations. Boudreau and Chapman (2000) found that compared to a group of typically developing children matched for expressive language, children and adolescents with Down's syndrome produced longer and more complex narratives. No differences were found in the event structure of the narratives produced by the DS subjects and subjects matched for expressive language. However, DS children and adolescents made poorer use of linguistic devices and cohesion than children

matched for mental age (but not children matched for expressive language). Despite expressive lexical and syntactic limitations, DS subjects were reported by Miles and Chapman (2002) to express more plot line and thematic content in their narratives of a wordless picture story and more misadventures of one of the protagonists in the story than controls matched for mean length of utterance.

57 Papagno and Vallar (2001) remark that 'what can be taken for certain is that the defective appreciation of metaphors and idioms cannot be interpreted in terms of impairments of the phonological, syntactic, and lexical-semantic aspects of language comprehension and production' (526).

58 Roberts et al. (2007b) state that 'in contrast to speech, vocabulary, and syntax skills, the pragmatic skills of children with Down syndrome appear to be a relative strength, although the findings in all areas of pragmatics are not consistent' (30).

59 Several studies have reported executive function deficits in nonretarded subjects who have syndromes in which mental retardation may occur. Kerns et al. (1997) found that nonretarded adults with foetal alcohol syndrome displayed clear deficits on neuropsychological measures sensitive to complex attention, verbal learning and executive function. Mattson et al. (1999) assessed executive function in alcohol-exposed children with and without a diagnosis of foetal alcohol syndrome. Alcohol-exposed children displayed specific impairments in the domains of planning and response inhibition, abstract thinking and flexibility. Kirk et al. (2005) found that nonretarded girls with fragile X or Turner syndrome exhibited executive dysfunction, as measured on the Contingency Naming Test. Other studies that have reported executive function deficits in nonretarded women with fragile X syndrome include Bennetto et al. (2001), Sobesky et al. (1994) and Mazzocco et al. (1993). Moore et al. (2004) reported significant impairments on tests of executive function in twenty adult male permutation carriers of fragile X who had an average full scale IQ of 113.

60 ToM performance in mentally retarded subjects is tested through the use of the same false belief tasks that are used to assess ToM deficits in autism. This raises the question of the reliability of these tasks for use with mentally retarded individuals. The reliability of theory of mind task performance by subjects with mental retardation has been examined by Charman and Campbell (1997). These investigators found that reliability was moderate across a series of three false belief tasks and two belief-desire reasoning tasks. Charman and Campbell state that 'given the important interpretations made regarding the representational skills of individuals on the basis of their responses in such experimental tasks, further work investigating the psychometric properties of the tasks is required with both typically and atypically developing individuals' (1997: 725).

61 Tager-Flusberg and Sullivan (2000) distinguish between social-perceptual and social-cognitive components of theory of mind. The social-perceptual component includes 'the capacity to distinguish between people and objects, and to make on-line rapid judgements about people's mental state from their facial and body expression' (2000: 62). The social-cognitive component of theory of mind 'entails the conceptual understanding of the mind as a representational system' (2000: 61).

62 Yirmiya et al. (1998) examined published data in journals and dissertations on ToM abilities of individuals with autism as compared to individuals with mental retardation and normally developing children. Publications up to and including 1997 were analysed. These investigators found a significant difference between the ToM

abilities of individuals with autism and those of subjects with mental retardation. Yirmiya *et al.* state that 'these data confirm that the deficit in ToM abilities characterizes individuals with autism but is not unique to autism because it is manifested by individuals with mental retardation as well. What may be unique to autism is the severity of the impairment rather than the impairment itself' (1998: 302).

63 It is generally held that the ToM performance of individuals with mental retardation, while delayed compared to normally developing children, is at least commensurate with the mental age of retarded subjects. This view receives support from studies such as that of Yirmiya and Shulman (1996), who found that performance on ToM tasks correlated with performance mental age in mentally retarded subjects. However, the findings of several studies suggest that ToM performance may not always be commensurate with the mental age of retarded individuals. Benson *et al.* (1993) found that mentally retarded adolescents performed worse than mental age-matched children without mental retardation on a task in which they were asked questions about the knowledge and beliefs of characters in stories. Zelazo *et al.* (1996) found that twelve low-functioning individuals with Down's syndrome performed worse than twelve mental age-matched, non-handicapped children on several ToM tasks.

64 Lorusso *et al.*'s study is not concerned with the syntax of pronouns, but rather with the way in which correct pronoun use requires skills that are as much representational (i.e. ToM related) as linguistic in nature: 'Pragmatically correct use of pronouns may ... be seen as the interface between different aspects of linguistic competence as well as between linguistic competence and representational (cognitive) skills' (2007: 48).

3 A survey of acquired pragmatic disorders

3.1 Introduction

For a significant number of children and adults, cerebral pathologies and injuries can result in the impairment of previously normal pragmatic language skills. This group of pragmatically impaired individuals includes the fifty-year-old man who has a right-sided cerebrovascular accident and the teenager who is involved in a road traffic accident and sustains a traumatic brain injury. It also includes the adult who develops a brain tumour in the language-dominant left cerebral hemisphere and the sixty-five-year-old woman with the onset of dementia related to Alzheimer's disease. In each of these cases, pragmatic disorder has a clear neurological aetiology – a focal cerebral lesion or a more diffuse pattern of cerebral degeneration is the cause of the individual's problems with the pragmatics of language. However, there is also a sizeable population of adults with schizophrenia in whom severe pragmatic disorder occurs in the absence of a clear aetiology, neurological or otherwise. In this chapter, I conduct a survey of pragmatic disorders in individuals where the onset of the disorder has occurred in adulthood or at least after the period when acquisition of most pragmatic skills has occurred.[1] Specifically, I will examine what is known about the nature and extent of pragmatic disorders in the following five clinical populations: individuals with (1) left-hemisphere damage; (2) right-hemisphere damage; (3) schizophrenia; (4) traumatic brain injury; and (5) neurodegenerative disorders (particularly Alzheimer's disease). This chapter will not be concerned with pragmatic disorders in adults with mental retardation or an autistic spectrum disorder, as these disorders first emerged in the developmental period. Pragmatic disorders in these adults thus fall within the discussion of Chapter 2.

Discussion of acquired pragmatic disorders in children and adults has largely been subordinated in the clinical literature to discussion of developmental pragmatic impairments, particularly in children.[2] Even within the literature on acquired pragmatic disorders, certain clinical groups have been discussed quite extensively (e.g. clients with right-hemisphere damage) while other groups have received little, if any, systematic investigation of their pragmatic impairments (e.g. clients with neurodegenerative disorders). This neglect of clinical populations is matched only by an equally widespread neglect of certain pragmatic phenomena. While studies of speech acts, implicatures, discourse and conversation are relatively common in the clinical literature, few studies have attempted to examine the use of pragmatic presuppositions and deictic forms by children and adults with acquired pragmatic disorder. The result has been that our body of knowledge of acquired pragmatic disorders finds some clinical groups and pragmatic phenomena disproportionately represented, often at the expense of other groups and phenomena. This chapter attempts to tease out what is known about pragmatic disorder in some of these less well investigated clinical populations and reports the findings of studies that have looked beyond certain standard pragmatic phenomena such as implicature.

Acquired pragmatic disorders are providing investigators with a valuable window onto the neurocognitive substrates of pragmatic impairment. The focal cerebral lesions that result from cerebrovascular accidents in the left and right hemispheres of the brain are allowing investigators to examine the neuroanatomical basis of pragmatic processing (e.g. Zaidel *et al.* 2002). Similarly, the degeneration of specific neural networks in certain neurodegenerative disorders and the cognitive deficits that attend this degeneration provide investigators with the opportunity to examine the relationship between pragmatics and cognition (e.g. Monetta and Pell 2007). Of course, research into the neurocognitive substrates of pragmatics can only proceed if cognitive models and brain imaging techniques such as functional magnetic resonance imaging (fMRI) are employed within studies of the pragmatics of language. There is now evidence that this is occurring – fMRI studies are beginning to examine the neural basis of pragmatic phenomena such as sarcasm in both pragmatically normal and disordered children and adults (Uchiyama *et al.* 2006; Wang *et al.* 2006). The findings of these studies will be reviewed in the sections below. The rather piecemeal results that are emerging from these studies do not permit any general statements to be made at this time about the neurocognitive substrates of pragmatics. However, they are an important first step on what will undoubtedly be a long road to determining the nature of those substrates.

Each of the clinical populations that will be examined below contains a significant number of heterogeneous individuals. For example, the population of individuals with neurodegenerative disorders includes a large proportion of adults with dementia related to Alzheimer's disease. However, there are other pathologies that can lead to dementia (e.g. Pick's disease, HIV infection, vascular disease). There are also a range of other conditions such as Parkinson's disease, multiple sclerosis and motor neurone disease that constitute the population of individuals with neurodegenerative disorders. The prevalence of these conditions varies, as do their clinical manifestations and implications for communication. To assist the reader's understanding of these complex populations, each section below will begin by introducing the diverse disorders and aetiologies that constitute these clinical populations. A general account of the language and communication impairments in each will be given before a more detailed discussion of pragmatic language disorders is presented.

3.2   Left-hemisphere damage

The left hemisphere of the brain can be damaged by a range of cerebral diseases and injuries. Cerebrovascular accidents and brain tumours can give rise to focal lesions in the left hemisphere, with other brain areas remaining relatively unaffected. The widespread degeneration that occurs in Alzheimer's disease or the multi-focal lesions that attend a traumatic brain injury can lead to damage of the left hemisphere alongside other brain areas. This section will address the pragmatic deficits that occur in individuals with a focal lesion of the left hemisphere to the exclusion of damage in other brain areas. Subsequent sections will examine pragmatic deficits in subjects for whom left-hemisphere damage is only one of many different lesion sites in a traumatic brain injury (section 3.5) or is part of a wider cerebral degeneration in a disorder such as Alzheimer's disease (section 3.6). Given the dominance of the brain's left hemisphere in language production and comprehension, it is to be expected that many of the studies that will be discussed in this section have been conducted into adults with aphasia. The reader should be aware, however, that non-aphasic adults may also fall within the population of persons with left-hemisphere damage and that several of the studies that will be examined below have such adults as their clinical subjects.

Cerebrovascular accidents or strokes are by far the most common cause of focal lesions in the left-hemisphere of the brain. A stroke may be caused by a blood clot that forms somewhere in the body (usually the heart) and travels to the brain (embolic stroke) or by a clot that forms in one or more of the arteries which supply the brain (thrombotic stroke). Alternatively, a blood vessel in the brain may rupture and bleed, leading to a haemorrhagic stroke. This may occur in a blood vessel within the brain (intracerebral haemorrhage) or in a large artery on or near the arachnoid membrane, the middle one of three membranes that cover the brain and spinal cord (subarachnoid haemorrhage). The American Heart Association reported in 2006 that 88% of strokes are ischaemic (blood-clot strokes), 9% are intracerebral haemorrhage and 3% are subarachnoid haemorrhage. Carroll et al. (2001) used data from the Fourth National Morbidity Survey to estimate the incidence of first ever and recurrent strokes in England and Wales. These investigators estimated that in 1999, 87,700 people had a first ever stroke and 53,700 had a recurrent stroke. Age-adjusted rates for first ever or recurrent strokes were 0.20% in males and 0.16% in females. Carroll et al. found that 81 per cent of the individuals in their study who suffered a first ever or recurrent stroke were over sixty-four years of age. Engelter *et al.* (2006) assessed the incidence of aphasia attributable to first ever ischaemic stroke (FEIS) in a geographically defined population of 188,015 inhabitants. These investigators report an overall incidence rate of aphasia attributable to FEIS of 43 per 100,000 inhabitants. They also found that the risk of aphasia attributable to FEIS increased by 4 per cent with each year of patient's age. Brain tumours can also cause focal lesions in the brain's left hemisphere. For further discussion of the causes of left-hemisphere damage, the reader is referred to Chapter 5 in Cummings (2008).

When language impairments occur as a result of left-hemisphere damage, it is usually in the form of aphasia. Although different classifications of aphasia exist, the currently dominant classification categorises aphasia into fluent and nonfluent types.[3] In fluent aphasia, language comprehension is often severely impaired in the presence of effortless, fluent speech. Fluent aphasics produce long, incoherent, well-articulated utterances that have the intonational and other suprasegmental features of normal speech (these features often give a listener the impression that the fluent aphasic has greater language competence than is actually the case). The lack of sense and incoherence of the fluent aphasic's language is related to his or her use of jargon (hence, the use of the term 'jargon aphasia' to describe this type of aphasia). In some types of jargon, English words are linked together to produce meaningless utterances (for example, the jargon speaker who described Interflora as 'A stage of firms that arrange the nation of children', or another jargon aphasic who described his/her daughter's holiday as 'She's got a rainbow, you know, three monthly rainbow going to Alaska').[4] In other types of jargon, new words are created ('neologisms'). For example, a jargon speaker, who was wanting to go for a walk in the park, uttered 'We have to go to the pargoney'. In still other forms of jargon, so many neologisms are used that utterances are entirely meaningless. For example, when asked what he had done during the week, one jargon speaker replied 'Oh I kegde treychoinge and cortlidge, oh erm partlie chulz, potiler crediss my children ringer'. The poor language comprehension of fluent aphasics makes it difficult for these subjects to monitor and correct their own incoherent output. Other features of fluent aphasia include echolalia, the use of circumlocution (talking around a target word that the subject can't produce), perseveration (continued use of a linguistic form beyond what is appropriate) and lexical retrieval problems.

In nonfluent aphasia, language production problems exist in the presence of relatively intact comprehension. Nonfluent aphasics struggle to produce utterances. Unlike their fluent counterparts, they are acutely aware of and frustrated by their often severe expressive difficulties. Articulation and suprasegmental features of speech are disrupted – intonation units are typically short. Syntax can be severely affected. Sentence structure is reduced and incomplete. The loss of function words (e.g. determiners, prepositions, pronouns) and verbs – two characteristics of Broca's spoken output – confers a telegrammatic quality on the expressive language of these subjects (hence, the use of the term 'agrammatic speech' in relation to nonfluent aphasics). For example, instead of saying 'I will take the dog for a walk', the nonfluent aphasic will struggle to utter 'Walk dog'. Stereotypical forms are often used to maintain interaction when problems of expression are particularly acute. There are considerable lexical-semantic disturbances in nonfluent aphasia. Subjects may mis-select vocabulary, with chosen and target lexemes often semantically related (e.g. use of 'eye' instead of 'ear'). These errors are called semantic paraphasias (a sound equivalent of these errors – phonemic (literal) paraphasias – occur in fluent aphasia, e.g. use of 'stowcan' instead of 'snowman').

The syntactic and lexical-semantic errors variously found in fluent and non-fluent aphasia have traditionally been assumed to reflect the role of the left hemisphere in the processing of rule-based aspects of language. Pragmatic aspects of language, it was argued, are essentially intact in adults with aphasia or, if present, are secondary to deficits of structural language. Recent studies of pragmatic skills in aphasic adults are beginning to reveal a more complicated picture of pragmatic impairment than is suggested by this traditional view. Specifically, studies show that pragmatic impairments in aphasic adults are not merely a consequence of deficits in structural language. In some cases, pragmatic language impairments have been shown to persist despite improvements in structural language (see Coelho and Flewellyn (2003) below). In other cases, pragmatic impairments have been demonstrated in the extralinguistic communication of subjects with left-hemisphere damage (see Cutica et al. (2006) below). In the paragraphs below, we examine these studies as part of a wider review of pragmatic impairment in adults with left-hemisphere damage.

Studies of discourse are a rich source of information for clinicians on the pragmatic language skills of adults with left-hemisphere damage. Borod et al. (2000) examined verbal pragmatic aspects of discourse production in sixteen subjects with left brain damage and sixteen subjects with right brain damage. To rate six pragmatic features for appropriateness, monologues were transcribed and analysed. The verbal pragmatic aspects examined were: conciseness, lexical selection, quantity, relevancy, specificity and topic maintenance. Both groups of brain-damaged subjects were impaired in pragmatic appropriateness relative to normal controls. Subjects with left brain damage were more impaired than subjects with right brain damage on each pragmatic feature, although differences were not significant. The pragmatic performance of LHD subjects was related to discourse content, with positive emotional content facilitating performance. Coelho and Flewellyn (2003) examined coherence in the story narratives of a subject with anomic aphasia over a twelve-month period. These researchers found that although microlinguistic skills improved over this period, local and global coherence failed to improve appreciably. Global coherence was more impaired than local coherence in this subject. Coelho and Flewellyn conclude that 'this pattern of impaired macrolinguistic abilities is consistent with that of individuals with Alzheimer's disease and closed head injuries, and suggests that difficulty with discourse organization may result from focal as well as diffuse brain pathology' (2003: 173).

Specific aspects of non-literal language have been shown to be impaired in aphasic and LHD adults. At least some of these impairments appear to be related to language disorder. For example, Chapman et al. (1997) examined the processing of proverbs in fluent aphasic patients. Subjects indicated their understanding of proverbs in two presentation conditions. In the spontaneous condition, subjects were required to express verbally their interpretation of proverbs that were presented in written and verbal form. In the multiple-choice condition, subjects were required to select from four proverb interpretations the one that most accurately reflected the proverb's meaning. Familiar and unfamiliar proverbs were presented in both conditions. Compared to normal controls, aphasic subjects had difficulty formulating an interpretation of both familiar and unfamiliar proverbs in the spontaneous condition. Aphasic subjects had little difficulty interpreting proverbs in the multiple-choice condition. The greater linguistic demands of the spontaneous condition, Chapman et al. argue, explain the poorer proverb performance of the aphasic subjects in this condition. Kasher et al. (1999) examined the processing of implicatures in thirty-one patients with LHD following a stroke. Implicatures of quantity, quality, relation and manner were examined by means of two-sentence conversational vignettes which were literally problematic. Famous paintings, which were also literally problematic, were used to examine nonverbal implicatures. Subjects were also administered a test of basic speech acts, which examined verbal and nonverbal assertions, questions, requests and commands. Subjects with LHD were significantly impaired relative to age-matched normal controls in implicature processing. Verbal and nonverbal implicatures intercorrelated highly in LHD subjects as did performance on most implicature subtests and most subtests of basic speech acts. On the basis of these results, Kasher et al. conclude that the left hemisphere includes a general 'implicatures processor'.

The finding that nonverbal implicatures were also impaired in the LHD subjects in Kasher et al.'s study suggests that not all pragmatic deficits are related to language impairments in this population. This view is further supported by the finding that only some implicatures in the LHD subjects in Kasher et al.'s study correlated significantly with only some language functions (particularly naming, reading and writing). A study of extralinguistic communication by Cutica et al. (2006) lends further support to the view that not all pragmatic impairments in LHD subjects can be accounted for by linguistic deficits. Subjects with LHD were presented with fifteen short videotaped fictions. In each fiction, an actor performs a gesture. After viewing each fiction, subjects are presented with a large photograph of the final frame. A white balloon above the actor's head must be filled by selecting from among four photographs the one that represents the actor's communicative intention. The performance of LHD subjects on fictions that contain non-standard acts – those involving simple deceits and simple ironies – was considerably poorer than in control subjects.

Conversation is an important arena for the use of pragmatic language skills. It is one of the most naturalistic means available to clinicians and researchers for examining deficits in these skills. Conversation also permits investigators to examine the interaction between pragmatics and other levels of language such as syntax and semantics. For example, the aphasic speaker may lack the requisite syntactic structures to produce certain speech acts or may make lexical selections that indicate a lack of awareness of social and politeness constraints in conversation. Given the many advantages of studying conversation, it is unremarkable that conversation analysis should have become one of the most extensively used techniques for examining pragmatic and linguistic functioning in aphasia. Conversation analysis has been used to examine collaborative repair in aphasic conversation (Perkins *et al.* 1999), hint-and-guess sequences in interactions involving a Norwegian aphasic speaker (Lind 2005), aphasic grammar within the context of turns at talk in conversation (Beeke 2003; Beeke *et al.* 2003a), word search strategies in aphasia (Oelschlaeger and Damico 2000) and the distribution of turns at talk in aphasic participants' conversations with a relative (Perkins 1995). The findings of these studies have often revealed considerable conversational skills on the part of aphasic subjects.[5] In this way, Damico *et al.* (2006) found that an individual with aphasia and dysarthria was able to collaboratively negotiate intelligibility with his clinician by using interactional strategies and knowledge resources. Motivated by an interactional need to produce unproblematic turns at talk, the agrammatic aphasic man studied by Beeke (2003) exhibited recurrent use of 'I suppose', when his production of subject-verb constructions was generally poor. Boles (1998) found that a woman with Broca's aphasia was able to engage in conversational self-repair and tripled her level of self-repair following therapy. For discussion of the application of conversation analysis to aphasia, the reader is referred to Beeke *et al.* (2007).

The neural correlates of pragmatic impairment are beginning to be examined by investigators. Zaidel *et al.* (2002) examined the relationship between the performance of thirty-one subjects with left brain damage on a Hebrew version of the Right Hemisphere Communication Battery (RHCB; Gardner and Brownell 1986) and the extent and location of lesions in different regions of the left hemisphere. The RHCB contains eleven subtests, many of which test aspects of language pragmatics. Zaidel *et al.* found a negative correlation between subtest scores on the Hebrew version of the RHCB and lesion extent in frontal and temporal perisylvian regions. In specific terms, verbal humour negatively correlated with the extent of lesion in the left inferior temporal gyrus; indirect requests negatively correlated with the extent of lesion in the middle and inferior frontal, superior temporal and supramarginal gyri; pictorial metaphors negatively correlated with the extent of lesion in the left superior temporal gyrus; verbal metaphors negatively correlated with the extent of lesion in the left middle temporal gyrus and in the junction of the superior temporal and supramarginal gyri; sarcasm negatively correlated with the extent of lesion in the left middle and inferior frontal gyri. On only one subtest was there any correlation with extent of lesion in subjects with right brain damage – narrative comprehension[6] negatively correlated with the extent of lesion in the junction area of the superior temporal and supramarginal gyri. These findings, Zaidel *et al.* conclude, fail to support the right prefrontal hypothesis of pragmatic deficit.[7] Other studies of the neuroanatomical correlates of pragmatic deficits include an investigation by Kasher *et al.* (1999) of the processing of conversational implicatures by subjects with left or right brain damage. In this study, both groups of subjects displayed weak correlations between performance on an implicatures battery and the extents of lesions in the left perisylvian language area or its right-hemisphere homologue.

Beyond linguistic impairments, cognitive deficits in aphasic and left-hemisphere damaged subjects have received relatively little direct investigation. Amongst those studies that have examined the cognitive skills of the LHD population are those that have investigated ToM skills in aphasic adults. It emerges that even in severely aphasic adults, these skills are largely intact. Varley and Siegal (2000) report the case of a severe agrammatic aphasic patient who was unable to process language propositions in any modality of language use. Notwithstanding his severe linguistic impairment, this patient exhibited ToM understanding and simple causal reasoning. Varley *et al.* (2001) report a second patient with severe aphasia and executive function deficits who retained the capacity to engage in ToM reasoning. These investigators concluded that 'these results reveal the functional autonomy of theory of mind from the capacity for propositional/grammatical language' (2001: 489). Similar preservation of ToM abilities was reported in a study by Stone *et al.* (1998). While patients with bilateral damage to the orbito-frontal cortex displayed similar ToM skills to individuals with Asperger's syndrome – they performed well on simpler ToM tests and displayed deficits on more advanced social reasoning tasks such as the recognition of faux pas – subjects with unilateral damage in the left dorsolateral prefrontal cortex exhibited no specific ToM deficits.

While ToM skills appear to be intact in aphasic and LHD subjects, there is clear evidence of executive function deficits in these same subjects. In a study of twenty-five aphasic individuals, Fridriksson *et al.* (2006) found that most subjects did not perform within normal limits on tests of executive function. Moreover, there was a clear relationship between executive functioning and functional communication in these subjects with decreased executive functioning ability occurring alongside decreased functional communication ability in aphasic subjects. Glosser and Goodglass (1990) found that aphasic patients with frontal lobe lesions were significantly more impaired on tasks of executive control than subjects with aphasia who had retrorolandic or mixed lesions in the left hemisphere. Nys *et al.* (2007) found that deficits in executive functioning, verbal memory and abstract reasoning were more prevalent and severe following left than right cortical stroke. Helm-Estabrooks (2002) examined aspects of nonlinguistic cognition in thirteen individuals with aphasia due to left-hemisphere stroke. A series of nonlinguistic tasks assessed visual attention, memory, executive functions and visuospatial skills. Ten aphasic subjects (77 per cent of sample) scored below the normal cut-off score on these four nonlinguistic areas. Moreover, no significant relationship was found between linguistic and nonlinguistic skills in these subjects. Rönnberg *et al.* (1996) examined verbal memory performance in nine subjects with mild aphasia as a result of subarachnoid haemorrhage. These investigators found impairments in the phonological loop and central executive of working memory. Impairments of long-term memory were also observed. Beeson *et al.* (1993) found that fourteen subjects with stroke-induced aphasia were impaired on tests of verbal memory relative to demographically matched controls. Subjects with anterior lesions displayed greater impairment of long-term memory while those with posterior lesions had greater impairment of short-term memory. Language ability and verbal memory performance did not correlate highly.

3.3   Right-hemisphere damage

The same cerebral pathologies and injuries that cause left-hemisphere damage can also compromise the brain's right hemisphere. Focal damage in the right hemisphere of the brain is most often caused by cerebrovascular accidents. Figures suggest that right-hemisphere strokes are less common, or perhaps less often diagnosed,[8] than left-hemisphere strokes. Amongst patients on a large hospital-based stroke registry in Germany, Foerch *et al.* (2005) found that 8,769 (44% of patients) had right-sided lesions and 11,328 (56% of patients) had left hemispheric events. Di Legge *et al.* (2005) examined 990 stroke patients in the Registry of the Canadian Stroke Network. Of these patients, 505 (51%) had a right-hemisphere stroke and 485 (49%) had a left-hemisphere stroke. Brain tumours, both primary and metastatic, can also cause focal damage in the right hemisphere. The Central Brain Tumor Registry of the United States reports that between 1998 and 2002, the state-specific incidence rates for malignant primary brain tumours among adults twenty years of age and older was 7.3

to 10.5 per 100,000 person-years (4.2 to 19.8 per 100,000 person-years for non-malignant tumours). The incidence for all brain tumours was highest among seventy-five- to eighty-four-year olds (50.3 per 100,000 person-years). The majority of tumours (32 per cent) in young adults aged twenty- to thirty-four-years were located in the frontal, temporal, parietal and occipital lobes of the brain. The most common histology in the twenty- to thirty-four-years age group was pituitary tumours with meningiomas most common in adults aged thirty-five years and above.

Although structural language deficits have been reported in clients with right-hemisphere damage,[9] it was clear from the earliest investigations of these clients that such deficits were not responsible for the inadequate communication skills observed in RHD patients. The publication in 1979 of a paper by Penelope Myers[10] was the first formal study to be undertaken of discourse-level communication disorders in adults with right-hemisphere damage. That paper arose out of the author's observation that RHD stroke patients who were receiving clinical treatment for dysarthria and who had intact language skills were nevertheless communicating inadequately. Specifically, these patients produced 'irrelevant and often excessive information' and seemed 'to miss the implication of [a] question and to respond in a most literal and concrete way' (38). When attempting to respond to open-ended questions, these patients 'wended their way through a maze of disassociated detail, seemingly incapable of filtering out unnecessary information' (38). The components of a narrative, although available to these patients, could not be assembled into a narrative. There was difficulty 'in extracting critical bits of information, in seeing the relationships among them, and in reaching conclusions or drawing inferences based on those relationships' (39). Although the detail provided by these patients was related to the general topic, its appearance seemed irrelevant because it had not been 'integrated into a whole' (39). Although Myers never used the term 'pragmatics' in relation to these communicative problems,[11] it is clear from today's pragmatically informed standpoint that these discourse and conversational impairments were part of a pragmatic disorder on the part of these RHD patients. Since Myers first described the features of communication in RHD patients, there has been considerable investigation of the right hemisphere's role in language processing and communication in general. Pragmatic aspects of language have come under particular scrutiny. In the rest of this section, we examine the findings of several studies in this area.

Non-literal language has been extensively investigated in the RHD population. Papagno et al. (2006) examined the comprehension of idioms in fifteen RHD subjects. Comprehension in these subjects was found to be severely impaired and was biased towards literal interpretation. The comprehension performance of these subjects was correlated with visuospatial abilities and was significantly affected by lesion site, particularly frontal lobe involvement.

Brundage (1996) examined the interpretation of proverbs in ten RHD subjects. Subjects were presented with a card, which had a proverb printed on it, and were asked to say what the proverb meant. Proverb familiarity and abstractness had a significant effect on interpretation. When explaining the meaning of proverbs high in abstractness, RHD subjects tended to produce literal explanations. Cheang and Pell (2006) administered tasks tapping humour appreciation[12] and pragmatic interpretation of non-literal language to ten subjects with RHD. Although the ability to interpret humour from jokes was relatively intact in these subjects, they had problems understanding communicative intentions. These findings, Cheang and Pell argue, 'imply that explicitly detailing communicative intentions in discourse facilitates RHD participants' comprehension of non-literal language' (2006: 447). McDonald (2000a) relates problems comprehending sarcasm in RHD patients to these subjects' difficulty processing information about the emotional state, intentions and beliefs of the speaker.

Discourse and conversation impairments are commonly reported in the RHD population. Lehman (2006) elicited discourse from eight RHD subjects. Discourse transcripts were rated by speech-language pathologists on content and quantity variables. RHD subjects produced discourse which was rated as more tangential and egocentric than that produced by healthy older controls. Extreme verbosity or paucity of speech also characterised the discourse of RHD subjects. Marini et al. (2005) examined stories generated during two picture description tasks in eleven RHD subjects, eleven LHD subjects and eleven neurologically intact controls. The performance of RHD subjects was poorer than that of controls in terms of information content and the coherent and cohesive aspects of narrative production.[13] Hird and Kirsner (2003) examined the ability of RHD subjects to take shared responsibility for the development of an intentional structure in conversation. Conversations between RHD subjects and normal speakers were audiotaped and analysed. Text-level discourse processing analyses and prosodic analyses were performed. Hird and Kirsner found that RHD speakers fail to use prosody to alert listeners to changes in discourse structure. Nor do they assume equal responsibility in conversation for the development and maintenance of discourse structure. Other features of right-hemisphere brain damage that compromise the conversational performance of affected subjects include an inability to respond to violations of Gricean maxims in conversation (Rehak et al. 1992), an inability to select appropriate terms of personal reference (Brownell et al. 1997), and reduced facial expressivity during conversation (Blonder et al. 1993).

The relationship between communication impairment in RHD and the ability to generate and manipulate inferences has been extensively investigated. Tompkins et al. (1999) examined the suppression of inferences in RHD and control subjects. The ability to suppress initial inferences in response to subsequent information was examined at two probe intervals (850 and 1200 ms). Both groups were unable to suppress initial inferences at these intervals. However, in RHD subjects suppression effectiveness was related to the comprehension of discourse stimuli that required inference revision.[14] Myers and Brookshire (1994) examined the effects of visual and inferential complexity on the picture descriptions of twenty-four RHD subjects. These investigators found that the communication impairments of RHD subjects on a picture description task were more strongly related to the inferential than to the visual complexity of the pictured stimuli. Purdy *et al.* (1992)[15] examined inferences based on text and those based on general world knowledge in fifteen RHD subjects and fifteen neurologically normal adults. Subjects watched a nine-minute film after which they were asked to answer a set of pre-recorded inference questions. Normal adults performed significantly better than RHD adults on both types of inference. Myers (1991) argues that RHD patients experience inference failure, that inference failure may occur at all levels of cognitive processing, that RHD can affect inference generation at early and late stages of cognitive processing and that inference failure may be a central deficit.[16]

As well as inferencing difficulties, RHD subjects have also been found to have theory of mind impairments, executive function deficits and problems with visuospatial processing. Griffin *et al.* (2006) found that RHD subjects have a functionally specific deficit in attributing intentional states, particularly those that involve second-order attributions. Happé *et al.* (1999) found that adults who had sustained a right-hemisphere stroke were significantly worse at understanding materials that required the attribution of mental states than they were at understanding non-mental control materials. Winner *et al.* (1998) found that RHD patients performed significantly worse than controls on a measure of second-order belief attribution. Moreover, the ability to distinguish lies from jokes correlated strongly with two measures of second-order belief attribution in these subjects.[17] In a case study of a patient with subcortical lesions of the right hemisphere, Rainville *et al.* (2003) found a severe executive function syndrome, as well as a memory deficit, neglect, anosognosia and impairments in spatial abilities. McDonald (2000b) reported that pragmatic performance in eighteen RHD patients was correlated to right-hemisphere visuospatial function, but not to executive function. Bartels-Tobin and Hinckley (2005) examined the relationship between discourse production and cognitive abilities in seven RHD subjects. Cognitive functioning was assessed in the following domains – attention, memory, executive functions, language and visuospatial skills. There were no statistically significant differences between the cognitive scores obtained by RHD subjects and those of neurologically intact control subjects (the investigators concede that this may be related to the small participant sample). Visuospatial skills, but not executive functions, were found to correlate to narrative discourse measures.

TOURO COLLEGE LIBRARY

Finally, investigators are beginning to examine the neuroanatomical correlates of right-hemisphere pragmatic and cognitive deficits. Shamay-Tsoory *et al.* (2005a) examined the neuroanatomical basis of sarcasm and its underlying social cognitive processes (i.e. ToM and emotion recognition) in subjects with right prefrontal and posterior damage. Subjects with prefrontal damage displayed impaired performance on a sarcasm task, with those with right ventromedial lesions exhibiting the greatest deficits understanding sarcasm. Right prefrontal damage was associated with ToM deficits and right-hemisphere damage was associated with deficits in emotion recognition. These investigators concluded that 'the right frontal lobe mediates understanding of sarcasm by integrating affective processing with perspective taking' (2005a: 288). Soroker *et al.* (2005) examined the neuroanatomical basis of the processing of basic speech acts (question, assertion, request, command) by RHD and LHD subjects. These investigators found no correlation between the location and extent of lesion in the perisylvian cortex of RHD subjects and performance on these speech acts. The neuroanatomical basis of visuospatial dysfunction was examined by Ricker and Millis (1996) in a study of patients with striatal, frontal white matter and posterior thalamic infarction of the right cerebral hemisphere. All three lesion groups, and particularly subjects with infarction of deep grey structures, were significantly impaired on tasks of visual synthesis and spatial analysis. In groups with striatal and frontal white matter lesions, performance on tasks of visual synthesis and spatial analysis correlated strongly with executive control performance.

3.4   Schizophrenia

Schizophrenia is a common mental illness. The Royal College of Psychiatrists in the UK reports that one person in 100 develops schizophrenia at some time in their life. Wu *et al.* (2006) used several administrative claims databases to calculate the annual prevalence of diagnosed schizophrenia in the US. These investigators report that in 2002, the twelve-month prevalence of diagnosed schizophrenia was estimated at 5.1 per 1,000 lives. The incidence of schizophrenia is considerably higher in men than in women. McGrath (2006) reports a male to female ratio of 1.4. The incidence of schizophrenia is also higher in migrants and in those living in urban areas (McGrath 2006). The age at onset also varies between men and women, with men typically developing schizophrenia earlier than women. Gorwood *et al.* (1995) examined a population of 663 schizophrenic patients and found that the mean age at onset in males and females was 27.8 years and 31.5 years, respectively. Twin and familial studies have shown that genetic factors play a significant role in schizophrenia. Tsuang (2000) reviewed concordance rates for schizophrenia in studies of monozygotic and dizygotic twins. For monozygotic twins, the concordance rates in these studies ranged from 31% to 58%; for dizygotic twins, concordance rates ranged from 4% to 27%. The risk of schizophrenia in the relatives of schizophrenic probands also correlates with the degree of shared genes. In first-degree relatives such as parents (50% shared genes) and in second-degree relatives such as uncles and aunts (25% shared genes), the morbid risk for schizophrenia is 6% and 2%, respectively (Tsuang 2000). It is now well known that schizophrenic individuals can exhibit cerebral anomalies such as ventricular enlargement. However, the exact relationship between these anomalies and clinical presentation and outcome in schizophrenia is somewhat less well known (Osuji *et al.* 2007).

There is now evidence that all levels of language are disrupted in schizophrenia. These levels include phonology,[18] morphology, syntax, semantics and pragmatics. Morphemic disturbances in schizophrenia are evident in the loss of word endings, like *–ed* and *–ion* in the following utterance produced by a patient studied by Chaika: 'I am being help with the food and the medicate ...' (1990: 24).[19] Syntactic errors are relatively common in schizophrenia. Schizophrenic subjects have been observed to use incomplete prepositional phrases and verb phrases. Chaika describes how one subject omitted the object of the preposition *for* in 'he was blamed for and I didn't think that was fair ...' (1990: 221). Ribeiro's schizophrenic subject routinely omitted the direct object of the verb *have* as in 'No, only if you have. Do you have?' (1994: 263). Clauses are started but not completed. In response to the interviewer's question 'Why do you think people believe in God?', a schizophrenic patient replied 'Um, *because* making a do in life. Isn't none of that stuff about evolution guiding isn't true any more now ...' (Thomas 1997: 40). The first sentence consists of a subordinate clause without a main clause. DeLisi (2001) found that sentence complexity was reduced in schizophrenia. The subjects with chronic schizophrenia in this study displayed reduced conjoined and embedded clauses. Lexical semantics is disrupted in schizophrenia. Neologisms occur frequently in schizophrenic speech, for example, the use of *geshinker* in the following extract from Thomas: 'I got so angry I picked up a dish and threw it at the geshinker' (1997: 38). Bizarre lexical choices are common. For example, Chaika's schizophrenic subject used 'the cash register man handled the financial matters' (1990: 202) to refer to his ringing up money for an ice-cream cone. Sumiyoshi *et al.* (2001) used the ANIMAL category fluency test[20] to examine semantic structure in fifty-seven patients with schizophrenia. These investigators found that while normal controls demonstrated the domestic/size distinction in semantic structure, no such dimension was evident in the schizophrenic patients.

Pragmatic deficits in schizophrenia have been extensively investigated over many years. Behavioural evidence indicates that schizophrenic speakers perform poorly on tests of discourse planning and comprehension, understanding humour, sarcasm, metaphors and indirect requests, and the generation and comprehension of emotional prosody (Mitchell and Crow 2005). These pragmatic aspects of language 'are essential to an accurate understanding of someone's communicative intent, and the deficits displayed by patients with schizophrenia may make a significant contribution to their social interaction deficits' (Mitchell and Crow 2005: 963). Tényi *et al.* (2002) examined the ability of schizophrenic subjects to recognise the intended meaning behind violations of Gricean implicatures. Twenty-six paranoid schizophrenic subjects and twenty-six normal controls were presented with four question-and-answer vignettes in which the maxim of relevance was violated. Subjects had to identify the speaker's intended meaning in each case. Tényi *et al.* found that schizophrenic subjects made significantly more errors than controls in identifying the communicative intentions that lay behind violations of this maxim. Corcoran and Frith (1996) examined politeness and appreciation of the Gricean maxims of quantity, quality and relation in schizophrenic patients with different symptom profiles. Subjects had to select an appropriate final piece of speech for one of the characters in a series of stories. One piece of speech adhered to the rule under question, while the other flouted the rule. Control subjects, schizophrenic subjects with paranoid delusions and schizophrenic subjects with negative symptoms adhered to the maxim of relation. However, all other maxims were flouted by subjects with negative symptoms. Subjects with paranoid delusions often failed to respond in a polite fashion, but performed at a similar level to controls on stories involving the Gricean maxims.

Meilijson *et al.* (2004) examined the pragmatic skills of forty-three subjects with chronic schizophrenia. To attain a general profile of pragmatic abilities in these subjects, Meilijson *et al.* used Prutting and Kirchner's (1987) pragmatic protocol. Schizophrenic subjects displayed a high degree of inappropriate pragmatic abilities relative to a psychiatric control group (individuals with mixed anxiety-depression) and to subjects with hemispheric brain damage (data from Prutting and Kirchner 1987). Pragmatic parameters that were more than 50 per cent inappropriate included topic selection, introduction, maintenance and change, lexical specificity/accuracy, prosody, turn-taking quantity/conciseness and facial expressions. Much of the incoherence of schizophrenic language can be related to failures of reference, particularly reference to earlier parts of spoken discourse. Docherty *et al.* (2003) examined disturbances of referential communication in forty-eight schizophrenic patients. These patients scored significantly higher (more disordered) than controls on each of six types of referential disturbance. Five types of referential disturbance were stable over time in these subjects (confused reference, missing information reference, ambiguous word meaning, wrong word reference and structural unclarity). A sixth type of reference – vague reference – was not stable over time. Referential disturbances showed little or no association with the severity of positive or negative symptoms in these patients.

Experimental studies have repeatedly shown that schizophrenic subjects are unable to process aspects of linguistic context. Bazin *et al.* (2000) conducted an experiment in which thirty schizophrenic subjects and thirty control subjects were required to complete sentences using the first word(s) that came to mind. Each sentence contained an ambiguous word, the less frequent meaning of which was primed by a preceding sentence. Results showed that only control subjects were able to use the linguistic context provided by the preceding sentence to prime the less frequent meaning of the ambiguous word. Schizophrenic subjects, particularly those with thought disorder, used the most common meaning of the ambiguous word more frequently than controls. Sitnikova *et al.* (2002) used event-related potentials to examine deficits in language comprehension in schizophrenia. Sentences that contained two clauses were read by schizophrenic and control subjects. These investigators hypothesised that the processing of target words in the second clause would be influenced by preceding linguistic context in the control subjects only. Schizophrenic subjects, by contrast, were expected to be inappropriately affected by the dominant meaning of homographs in the first clause (e.g. the 'structure' meaning of 'bridge' in the sentence *The guests played bridge because the river had rocks in it*). This hypothesis was confirmed.

Pragmatic impairments have been linked to cognitive deficits in schizophrenia. Linscott (2005) examined the relationship between pragmatic language impairment (PLI), thought disorder and generalised cognitive decline in twenty schizophrenic subjects. The Profile of Pragmatic Impairment in Communication (Hays *et al.* 2004; Linscott 1996) was used to score subjects for PLI. Significant PLI and generalised cognitive decline were found in the schizophrenic subjects. Furthermore, generalised cognitive decline predicted PLI. Linscott remarks that PLI in schizophrenia is secondary to generalised cognitive decline. Brüne and Bodenstein (2005) investigated the relation of proverb understanding in schizophrenia to the cognitive ability to engage in mindreading ('theory of mind'). Thirty-one schizophrenic patients completed a proverb test, a ToM test battery and a variety of executive functioning and verbal intelligence tests. These patients' psychopathology was also assessed. ToM performance, intelligence and executive functioning correlated strongly with the patients' ability to interpret proverbs correctly. Approximately 39 per cent of the variance of proverb comprehension in the schizophrenic patients was predicted by ToM performance. Brüne and Bodenstein conclude that 'the ability to interpret such metaphorical speech that is typical of many proverbs crucially depends on schizophrenic patients' ability to infer mental states' (2005: 233).[21] Champagne-Lavau *et al.* (2006) reviewed evidence which suggests that the co-occurrence of deficits in non-literal language understanding and theory of mind in schizophrenia may be explained by a context processing impairment that is associated with a lack of flexibility. Kiang *et al.* (2007)

found that proverb interpretation difficulties in eighteen schizophrenic patients were significantly correlated with working memory deficits in these patients, as well as with impairments in executive function, sensory-memory encoding and social/occupational function. In a study of thirty-nine subjects with schizophrenia, Corcoran (2003) found a substantial correlation between performance on an inductive reasoning task and a pragmatic language task that required subjects to infer a speaker's intentions.

Few studies have examined the neural correlates of pragmatic processing in schizophrenia. A notable exception is a study by Kircher *et al.* (2007) who examined processing of metaphoric sentences by twelve schizophrenic patients using functional magnetic resonance imaging. In the twelve control subjects in this study, reading metaphors as opposed to literal sentences produced signal changes in the left inferior frontal gyrus. In the schizophrenic subjects, an area 3 cm dorsal to the left inferior frontal gyrus was activated by the same metaphor activity. The severity of concretism was also found to negatively correlate with the response in the inferior frontal gyrus. Comparisons of the metaphor versus baseline conditions in control and patient groups revealed stronger signal changes in the right superior/middle temporal gyrus in the control subjects and in the left inferior frontal gyrus in the patients. Kircher *et al.* conclude that 'the inferior frontal and superior temporal gyri are key regions in the neuropathology of schizophrenia. Their dysfunction seems to underlie the clinical symptom of concretism, reflected in the impaired understanding of non-literal, semantically complex language structures' (2007: 287). In an earlier study, Kircher *et al.* (2001) examined the neural correlates of the processing of linguistic context in six schizophrenic patients with formal thought disorder (FTD). fMRI was used to measure cerebral activation during a task in which subjects read sentence stems and completed them orally. These investigators found an attenuated engagement of the right temporal cortex in FTD patients compared to schizophrenic patients without FTD and controls matched for cognitive and demographic variables.

3.5   Traumatic brain injury

Traumatic brain injury is a significant cause of hospitalisation and disability in both children and adults. The Centers for Disease Control and Prevention (2007) report that in 2003, 28,819 persons in nine US states (87.9 per 100,000 population) were hospitalised with a TBI-related diagnosis. There are two types of traumatic brain injury. In a closed head injury, the brain sustains damage in the absence of a fracture of the skull. In an open or penetrating head injury, a foreign object (e.g. a bullet) penetrates the skull and enters the brain. Traumatic brain injury can be the result of a road traffic accident (a common cause of head injury in young males), trips and falls (particularly in young children and elderly people[22]), a sports injury (boxing, skiing, etc.), violent crime (again, more common in young males) and child abuse.[23] The immediate effects on the brain of a severe blow to the head – called primary brain damage – are variable and include a skull fracture, contusion or bruising (usually immediately below the point of impact or where the brain has been driven against one of the bony ridges on the inside of the skull), haematomas or blood clots (either in the brain or between the brain and the skull), lacerations (tearing of the brain's lobes and blood vessels against the skull's bony ridges) and diffuse axonal injury (damage to nerve cells in the brain's connecting nerve fibres). These primary brain injuries are usually followed, after a period of hours or days, by secondary brain injuries. Examples of such injuries include brain swelling (oedema), increased pressure inside the skull (intracranial pressure), epilepsy and intracranial infection. While most traumatic brain injuries are mild (the ratio of mild to moderate to severe brain injuries is 8:1:1),[24] many sufferers are left with lifelong physical, cognitive and emotional problems that affect their ability to live independently, work and achieve normal social integration.[25]

Language impairments are a common consequence of traumatic brain injury. Demir *et al.* (2006) examined 103 patients with traumatic brain injury, fifty-one of whom had aphasia. These investigators report that the most frequent type of aphasia in these patients was Broca's aphasia (26.49%), followed by anomic aphasia (19.6%) and transcortical motor aphasia (15.6%). Gil *et al.* (1996) found aphasia in thirty-nine of 351 patients (11.1%) with severe traumatic brain injury. The most common forms of aphasia in these patients were amnestic (56%), expressive (10.3%) and receptive (10.5%). Whelan *et al.* (2007) examined the language skills of a nineteen-year-old woman twenty-two months after sustaining mild traumatic brain injury. A number of general language and high-level linguistic abilities were assessed. This woman displayed performance greater than 1.5 SD below the mean of a normal control group on 20/59 (34 per cent) of linguistic and cognitive variables assessed. She displayed below normal performance on tactile naming and digit span reversal, as well as on test items that involve complex lexical semantic operations. On a lexical decision task, this woman displayed prolonged reaction times to all word types and higher error rates on words with few meanings and low relatedness between meanings, as well as on legal nonwords. It was hypothesised that weakened coherence mechanisms may be responsible for prolonged responses on lexical decision tasks.

Pragmatic language deficits are increasingly being documented in the TBI population. MacLennan *et al.* (2002) studied pragmatic impairments in 144 TBI patients, who ranged in age from eighteen to seventy-one years (average age: 32.8 years). The mean time post-onset was 36.2 days. These patients were assessed using a pragmatic rating scale that was developed for the Defense and Veterans Brain Injury Center in Minneapolis. This scale measures nonverbal,

verbal and interactional aspects of communication. Ratings were based upon conversation, narrative discourse and procedural discourse. Pragmatic impairments were found in 86 per cent of patients. Cohesion, repair, elaboration, initiation and relevance were the five scales with the highest frequency of impairment. Impairments were evident in over 75 per cent of the pragmatic behaviours examined in fourteen subjects (10 per cent of the sample). MacLennan *et al.* conclude that pragmatic impairments are highly prevalent in the acute phase of TBI and that most impairments occur within propositional aspects of the message relating to the relevance, formulation and clarity of the message. Turkstra *et al.* (1995) examined pragmatic communication skills in three brain-injured adolescents aged 17.7, 18.3 and 16.8 years. One of these subjects, B.W., was unable to generate an alternative strategy to make a request when his first attempt failed. B.W. was also unable to produce a single indirect request, instead producing polite, direct requests. On a measure of accuracy and listener burden, B.W. obtained low scores as he was only able to give one procedural step out of a possible ten during the explanation of a simple board game to a listener. A second subject, J.H., obtained low scores on subtests examining the use of hints and the negotiation of requests. J.H.'s responses during his description of a board game tended to be concrete – he would describe the sequence of events that had just occurred rather than abstract the rules of the game. The third subject, P.W., had least pragmatic impairment of all subjects. However, he did have difficulty on a sarcasm task in which conversational dyads were verbally ambiguous and in which there weren't many contextual cues to aid interpretation. In all subjects, pragmatic performance was consistent with the results of neuropsychological testing.

Conversational discourse has also been found to be impaired in TBI subjects. Coelho *et al.* (2002) report that impairments include difficulties with topic management[26] and expressing information in a logical manner. The conversations of TBI subjects have also been found to be less interesting, less appropriate and more effortful. Coelho *et al.* examined response appropriateness and topic initiation in the conversations of thirty-two CHI subjects. These investigators found that head injured subjects depended on their conversational partner (the examiner) to maintain the flow of the conversation and that they often contributed information that did not facilitate the interaction. To compensate for these conversational impairments, the examiner asked more questions and introduced more topics than he did in conversations with non-brain-injured subjects. Togher and Hand (1998) examined the use of politeness markers during the telephone interactions of five TBI subjects with four different interlocutors. These interlocutors – a bus service employee, the police, a therapist, and the client's mother – varied according to relationships of power, status and contact with the TBI subject. The five politeness markers examined were finite modal verbs (e.g. could), modal adjuncts (e.g. possibly), comment adjuncts (e.g. I think), yes/no tags and incongruent realisations of the interrogative form (e.g. You don't know what time they go or anything?). In the therapist, bus and police interactions, TBI subjects used significantly less politeness markers per clause than control subjects (TBI subjects also used less politeness than controls in the mother interaction, although this only approached significance). Unlike controls, TBI subjects were unable to vary the number of politeness markers used according to the tenor of the social relationship in each interaction.[27]

Cognitive deficits such as executive function impairments are a common feature of individuals who have sustained a traumatic brain injury. McDonald (1992) takes the view that certain pragmatic impairments in head injured subjects can be related to frontal lobe cognitive deficits. Subjects with closed head injury (CHI) and matched control subjects were asked to perform a number of tasks that were designed to assess their expressive and receptive pragmatic skills. Tasks in which subjects had to issue requests in the form of hints and adhere to the conversational maxim of manner were used to test expressive pragmatic skills. Receptive pragmatic skills were assessed by asking subjects to perform a task that required them to understand indirect language. CHI subjects displayed various cognitive deficits related to frontal lobe pathology. Results revealed that CHI subjects had depressed performance compared to control subjects on all pragmatic skills. Within a more thorough analysis of the performance of these subjects, McDonald relates the impaired pragmatic skills of CHI subjects to their underlying cognitive skills. Specifically, a CHI subject who failed to adhere to Grice's maxim of manner[28] in his instructions to a blindfolded listener on how to play a novel game exhibited frontal lobe cognitive deficits like rigidity, perseveration and poor planning and problem-solving skills. Also, two CHI subjects who were unable to use indirect means (e.g. hints) of making requests exhibited considerable frontal lobe pathology. One subject was particularly concrete and perseverative. The other subject had less impaired abstraction skills but exhibited severe problems of impulse control. McDonald's findings would seem to provide at least tentative support for the view that pragmatic impairments in head injury are related to the underlying cognitive deficits of head injured subjects.

Investigators are also examining theory of mind (ToM) deficits in the TBI population. Milders et al. (2006) found ToM impairments in thirty-six TBI adults relative to thirty-four orthopaedic controls shortly after injury and at one-year follow-up (these adults also had executive function deficits). Henry et al. (2006) found that the capacity for mental state attribution in sixteen TBI adults was significantly reduced relative to controls and correlated substantially with phonemic fluency (a measure of executive functioning). Havet-Thomassin et al. (2006) found no relationship between the ToM impairments and executive function deficits of seventeen patients with severe TBI. ToM deficits have also been reported in adolescents with TBI (Turkstra et al. 2004). McDonald and Flanagan (2004) found that adults with TBI were able to recognise speaker beliefs in videotaped conversational exchanges only when this information was explicitly given. Second-order ToM judgements were related to the ability to understand conversational inference. In a study by Bibby and McDonald (2005), severe TBI subjects and healthy controls performed a range of verbal and nonverbal ToM tasks and verbal and nonverbal tasks that required them to draw general (non-mental) inferences. The TBI group performed more poorly than healthy subjects on ToM and general inference tasks. Further analysis suggested that TBI subjects have a general deficit in inferencing which, when combined with working memory and language impairments, adversely affects their performance on nonverbal and second-order ToM tasks. However, they may also have a specific ToM deficit which may impair their performance on verbal first-order ToM tasks. The exact relationship of these ToM impairments to the pragmatic deficits of TBI subjects requires further investigation.[29]

While numerous studies have examined the neuroanatomical correlates of cognitive impairments in TBI, few studies have sought to investigate the neuro-anatomical basis of pragmatic impairments in this clinical population. Two notable exceptions are investigations by Shamay-Tsoory et al. (2005a, 2005b). As discussed in section 3.3, Shamay-Tsoory et al. (2005a) found that subjects with prefrontal damage, and particularly those with right ventromedial lesions, exhibited deficits understanding sarcasm. Forty-one adults were included in this study, thirty of whom had brain contusions and haematomas following TBI. Shamay-Tsoory et al. (2005b) report that patients with ventromedial prefrontal lesions were significantly impaired in understanding ironic utterances and in identifying social faux pas compared to patients with posterior lesions and normal control subjects. These investigators relate the difficulties of these patients with irony and faux pas to underlying ToM deficits. The most severe ToM deficit was associated with lesions in the right ventromedial area. The neuroanatomical basis of executive function deficits in TBI has been extensively investigated. McDonald et al. (2002) state that impairments of executive function 'are generally attributed to frontal systems dysfunction, due either to direct insult to the frontal lobes or to disruption of their connections to other brain regions' (333). Lewine et al. (2007) found a significant association between frontal lobe dipolar slow wave activity (DSWA) on magnetoencephalography (MEG) and problems in executive function in patients with mild head trauma. Significant associations were also revealed on MEG between temporal lobe DSWA and memory problems, and parietal lobe DSWA and attention problems.

3.6   Neurodegenerative disorders

The group of neurodegenerative disorders is extensive and includes, amongst other conditions,[30] Alzheimer's disease, Parkinson's disease, motor neurone

disease and multiple sclerosis. Each of these disorders has a distinct neuropathology, epidemiology and prognosis (for detailed discussion, see Cummings
2008). Alzheimer's disease (AD) is by far the most prevalent of these disorders.[31]
It is also the most common cause of dementia, accounting for some 62 per cent
of all cases (Knapp and Prince 2007).[32] Alzheimer's disease can only be diagnosed definitively upon post-mortem examination, whereupon amyloid plaques
and neurofibrillary tangles are discovered in the brains of sufferers. The amy-
dala and hippocampus – part of the brain's limbic system – are particularly
susceptible to the degenerative changes that are associated with these plaques
and tangles. These histological aberrations are accompanied by biochemical
changes (e.g. deficiencies in neurotransmitters such as acetylcholine). In idiopathic Parkinson's disease (PD), there is a progressive loss of dopaminergic
neurones in the substantia nigra and nigrostriatal pathway of the midbrain.
When a diagnosis of Parkinson's disease is made, more than 60 per cent of
the dopaminergic cells in the substantia nigra may already have degenerated
(Berg 2006). Tremor, stiffness and slowness of movement (bradykinesia) are
symptomatic of the disorder. Motor neurone disease is not a single disorder,
but a group of progressive neurological disorders which includes amyotrophic
lateral sclerosis, progressive bulbar palsy, pseudobulbar palsy, primary lateral sclerosis and progressive muscular atrophy. In amyotrophic lateral sclerosis (ALS), the most common of these disorders, there is degeneration of the
anterior horn cells of the spinal cord and the motor cranial nuclei.[33] Multiple
sclerosis (MS) is a chronic, frequently progressive disease in which the body's
immune system attacks and breaks down the fatty insulating sheath (myelin)
that envelopes the axons of nerve cells. This process of demyelination can lead
to lesions in many different sites throughout the central nervous system. The
symptoms and course of the disorder vary according to its benign, relapsing/
remitting, primary progressive and secondary progressive subtypes.

The language disorder in Alzheimer's disease has been extensively described.[34]
In an early study of language in eighteen patients with Alzheimer's disease,
Murdoch et al. (1987) reported that syntax and phonology remained relatively
intact in these subjects, while semantic abilities were impaired. Subsequent
studies have confirmed marked lexical semantic deficits in AD patients and in
subjects with other forms of dementia. Laws et al. (2007) examined category
naming in patients with AD and in patients with Lewy body dementia (DLB).
Two tasks – picture naming and naming-to-description – were administered
to subjects. Both AD and DLB subjects showed significantly worse naming
on both tasks than healthy elderly matched controls, with the AD subjects
more impaired than the DLB subjects. Some AD and DLB subjects displayed
category-specific naming deficits, with all twenty-five significant category dissociations occurring for living things. Lexical semantic deficits have also been
documented during the course of Alzheimer's disease. Duong et al. (2006)

administered tasks of intentional lexical access (picture naming and semantic probes) and automatic access (lexical decision and priming) to sixty-one
subjects with mild cognitive impairment (a pre-AD stage) and thirty-nine
subjects with Alzheimer's disease. Subjects with mild cognitive impairment
were impaired on tasks of intentional access, while AD subjects were impaired
on both intentional and automatic access tasks. On the basis of these results,
Duong *et al.* conclude that 'intentional access to semantic memory is impaired
before automatic access' (2006: 1928). Adlam *et al.* (2006) also found evidence of semantic memory impairments early in the course of AD and specifically in patients with 'amnesic' mild cognitive impairment. Passafiume *et al.*
(2006) used a word-stem completion task to investigate semantic memory in
AD patients. AD subjects completed less stems than normal controls, indicating that there was 'a break down of the semantic network rather than a deficit
in the access to the semantic store' (2006: 460).

Alzheimer's disease is the only neurodegenerative disorder in which pragmatic impairments have been extensively examined.[35] There is evidence of substantial discourse impairments in AD subjects. Chapman *et al.* (1995) examined
the discourse coherence of picture-based stories produced by three groups of
subjects: individuals with early stage AD, normal old-elderly (OE) individuals
and normal control subjects. Significant differences were found between the AD
subjects and the OE and normal control subjects on content and form aspects of
discourse coherence. Specifically, AD subjects only supplied a typical frame of
interpretation 50 per cent of the time. Atypical frames were often applied or they
failed to interpret presented pictures within any frame. AD subjects also produced significantly fewer core and elaborative propositions and responses that
were organised according to a narrative structure than other groups. Cherney and
Canter (1992) elicited three types of discourse from patients with Alzheimer's
disease: descriptive, procedural and narrative. AD subjects produced more
irrelevancies, redundancies and incorrect utterances than either healthy, elderly
controls or subjects with right brain damage. They also produced less essential
utterances than either of these two groups and less elaborations than control
subjects. Carlomagno *et al.* (2005) examined the factors that underlie the lack
of reference and reduced informative content in the discourse of AD patients.
These subjects displayed reduced lexical encoding of information on both a referential communication task and a picture description task. AD subjects were
less efficient than aphasic subjects in establishing reference during the referential communication task as they presented more misunderstandings and needed
more explicit prompts from the listener. Also, the language used by AD subjects
during this task contained confounding and irrelevant information. The number
of these errors correlated negatively with the referring abilities of AD subjects.

Conversation is often an area of impairment in Alzheimer's disease. Mentis
et al. (1995) examined topic management during conversational interactions

between twelve subjects with Alzheimer's type dementia and a speech-language pathologist. Interactions between twelve normal elderly subjects and an SLP were also analysed. Normal elderly subjects and AD subjects differed significantly on parameters relating to topic introduction and maintenance. Specifically, AD subjects exhibited a reduced ability to change topic while maintaining the flow of discourse. They also had difficulty contributing to the propositional development of the topic and failed to consistently maintain a topic in a coherent and clear manner. Orange *et al.* (1996) examined conversational repair in five subjects with early stage dementia of the Alzheimer's type (EDAT) and in five subjects with middle stage DAT (MDAT). MDAT dyads spent a significantly higher percentage of conversation involved in repair than EDAT dyads; also, MDAT subjects created more discourse trouble sources than EDAT subjects. EDAT subjects produced more requests for repair than their conversational partners (a family member), but used less elaboration repairs than their partners. MDAT subjects created and repaired more conversational problems than their partners. Orange *et al.* state that 'despite the increase of conversational troubles with DAT onset and progression, the difficulties were repaired successfully the majority of the time' (1996: 881). Ripich *et al.* (1991) examined turn-taking and speech act patterns in the dyadic interactions between an examiner and eleven subjects with senile dementia of Alzheimer's type (SDAT). SDAT subjects spoke in shorter turns and used more nonverbal responses than normal elderly subjects. The examiner used shorter turns with SDAT subjects. More requestives and fewer assertives were used by SDAT subjects. Although there were significant discourse differences between SDAT and normal elderly subjects, SDAT subjects were still able to sustain conversation through their interaction patterns.

Studies have begun to examine the neurocognitive substrates of pragmatic deficits in subjects with neurodegenerative disorders. Cuerva *et al.* (2001) examined theory of mind and pragmatic abilities in thirty-four subjects with probable Alzheimer's disease. A test of indirect requests and conversational implications and a second-order false belief task were administered to these subjects and to a group of ten age-comparable healthy controls. AD subjects displayed significantly more severe pragmatic deficits than controls. Also, 65 per cent of these subjects did not pass the second-order false belief task. Cuerva *et al.* found a significant association between theory of mind and pragmatic deficits in the AD subjects in this study. McNamara and Durso (2003) examined the pragmatic communication abilities of twenty patients with Parkinson's disease. Prutting and Kirchner's (1987) pragmatic protocol was used to assess the pragmatic abilities of these patients. These investigators found that PD patients had significantly impaired pragmatic abilities, particularly in the areas of turn-taking, conversational appropriateness, prosodics and proxemics. Moreover, impaired pragmatic functioning was found to be significantly related to measures of frontal lobe function in these subjects. Monetta and Pell (2007) examined the comprehension of metaphorical language in seventeen subjects with Parkinson's disease. PD subjects who had impaired working memory on a measure of verbal working memory span were also impaired in the processing of metaphorical language. Monetta and Pell conclude that metaphor comprehension is dependent on fronto-striatal systems for working memory which are often compromised in the early course of Parkinson's disease.

NOTES

1 As the discussion of pragmatic development in Chapter 1 indicates, many pragmatic language skills are still being acquired during adolescence (e.g. complex speech acts such as persuasion). A head injury sustained by a fifteen-year-old is thus likely to disrupt both developmental and acquired aspects of pragmatics.

2 A search of Medline revealed that in the 6.5-year period between January 2000 and June 2007, fifty-four articles were published on developmental pragmatic disorders, while only twenty-four articles were published in the same period on acquired pragmatic disorders. These articles included reviews, experimental investigations and case studies. An assessment of these articles was made on the basis of their abstracts. If further information was needed to establish the age of subjects at the onset of pragmatic disorder, the articles themselves were examined. The fact that studies of developmental pragmatic disorder still outnumber investigations of acquired pragmatic disorder so heavily – by a ratio of 2.25:1, according to the figures above – was a central motivation for a recent issue of *Seminars in Speech and Language* entitled 'Pragmatics and adult language disorders' (Cummings 2007a).

3 The National Aphasia Association in the United States uses a system in which aphasia is broadly classified as fluent or nonfluent. In the Boston Diagnostic Aphasia Examination (Goodglass *et al.* 2001), subjects with aphasia are first classified as fluent or nonfluent. Subjects with fluent aphasia are subdivided into Wernicke's, anomic, conduction and transcortical sensory aphasia. Subjects with nonfluent aphasia are subdivided into Broca's, transcortical motor and global aphasia.

4 See Marshall *et al.* (2001). Also, see Marshall *et al.* (1996a and 1996b) for the source of 'A stage of firms …' The two examples of neologism in the main text are taken from Robson *et al.* (2003).

5 Studies of conversation have also revealed the use of linguistic forms that are not evident in language testing. For example, Beeke *et al.* (2003b) found that a speaker with nonfluent aphasia produced interactional grammatical phenomena during conversation that were not revealed using clinical assessments based on picture description and storytelling. Boles (1998) documented changes in the communication skills of a woman with Broca's aphasia using conversational discourse analysis that were not observable from test measures.

6 In other studies, impairments in narrative comprehension have been found in subjects with lesions of the left hemisphere. Channon and Crawford (2000) found that subjects with left anterior brain lesions were impaired relative to subjects with right anterior and right and left posterior lesions in story comprehension. These subjects commonly failed to make non-literal interpretations.

7 In an earlier study, Zaidel *et al.* (2000) found that verbal basic speech acts in subjects with left brain damage correlated with the extent of lesions in specific regions
   of the left perisylvian cortex. The speech acts in question were verbal assertions,
   questions, requests and commands. Zaidel *et al.* 'speculate that the classic localization of clinical language functions, such as auditory language comprehension or
   spontaneous speech, in left perisylvian cortex may be influenced by the localization
   of the basic speech acts used to assess those language functions in standard aphasia
   batteries' (2000: 443).
8 There is some evidence that right-hemisphere strokes are less readily diagnosed
   than strokes in the left hemisphere. Fink (2005) remarks of the findings of Foerch
   et al. in the main text: 'The conclusion that right-sided cerebral ischaemic events
   are under-recognised is hard to avoid. Foerch and colleagues' finding cannot be
   attributed to chance alone' (349).
9 Wacker *et al.* (2002) found aphasic symptoms in 36 per cent of patients with right-
   sided brain tumours using the Aachen Aphasia Test. Thomson *et al.* (1998) used the
   Western Aphasia Battery (WAB) and the Boston Naming Test (BNT) to examine
   language and communication function in patients with right-sided supratentorial
   intracranial tumours. Scores on the WAB showed that 21% were dysphasic, while
   35% obtained an abnormal language quotient. According to the BNT, 21 per cent
   of 47 patients were anomic. Lessa Mansur *et al.* (2006) describe the case of a right-
   handed patient who developed Wernicke's aphasia following a cerebrovascular accident in the right hemisphere. Bartha *et al.* (2004) describe the presence of linguistic
   deficits typical of conduction aphasia in three right-handed subjects with a lesion in
   the right hemisphere.
10 Myers presented her paper in May 1979 at the Clinical Aphasiology Conference
   (CAC) held in Phoenix, Arizona. It is a sign of the significance of this paper that
   it was published again in 2005 as a CAC classic in the journal Aphasiology. The
   reader is referred to Myers (2005).
11 Myers (1979) accounted for the 'inappropriate verbal output' of her RHD patients
   in terms of a 'deficit in integrating information on a higher level'. She remarks that
   'these results lend support to the hypothesis that RH patients have difficulty integrating information both on a perceptual and on a more formal level and that this
   deficit is reflected in their verbal output' (1979: 43).
12 Heath and Blonder (2005) found that eleven RHD patients and their spouses reported
   a statistically significant decrease in humour in these patients post-stroke. These
   investigators also found a significant positive association between RHD patients'
   self-reported orientation to humour post-stroke and their ability to decode prosody.
   Shammi and Stuss (1999) found that a specific brain region, the right frontal lobe,
   most disrupts the ability to appreciate humour.
13 Tompkins *et al.* (1992) take a different view of discourse impairments in RHD.
   These investigators analysed connected speech samples elicited from twenty-six
   RHD subjects. Samples were scored for literal and interpretive content units, among
   other features. It was found that many of the communicative behaviours routinely
   attributed to RHD subjects, such as high proportions of literal concepts, overper-
   sonalisation and excessive detail, failed to distinguish these subjects from either
   normally ageing controls or subjects with left-hemisphere damage. Tompkins *et al.*
   argue that studies demonstrating RHD communication impairments have been
   based on the most severely impaired RHD patients (e.g. those in treatment, in an

acute post-CVA stage, or with marked contralateral neglect) and that generalisation from these patients to the entire RHD population is not warranted.

14 In an earlier study, Tompkins *et al.* (1997) found that only RHD subjects had diffi-culty suppressing contextually inappropriate meanings of sentences at 1000 ms after sentence offset. Once again, the discourse comprehension performance of RHD subjects was correlated with suppression. Tompkins *et al.* (2004) found that RHD subjects were able to generate the lexical-semantic foundations of bridging infer-ences that were required to integrate text-final sentences in narratives. Activation of contextually incompatible interpretations of text-final sentences was associated with poor discourse comprehension performance in these subjects.

15 Purdy *et al.* (1992) were concerned to examine the use of context in inferencing by RHD subjects. Schmitzer *et al.* (1997) examined the influence of context on the interpretation of denotative and connotative meanings of homographs in RHD sub-jects. These investigators found that RHD subjects had a reduced ability to process connotative word meanings. Moreover, they were not assisted by the presence of semantically supportive linguistic information.

16 Other studies have failed to find evidence of inference failure in RHD subjects. Bisset and Novak (1995) found no difference in the ability of RHD subjects, aphasic subjects and normal controls to draw inferences from the feeling or sense of affect conveyed in videotaped vignettes.

17 Where most studies seek to relate the performance of RHD subjects on false belief tasks to an underlying conceptual deficit (i.e. a deficit in theory of mind), the focus of explanation of false belief test performance in a study by Siegal *et al.* (1996) is quite definitely not on such a deficit. These investigators relate the difficulties of RHD subjects on false belief tasks to problems in pragmatic understanding: 'the RHD patients' difficulties in making false belief predictions may be considered as due to pragmatic language deficits' (1996: 46). In a later study, Surian and Siegal (2001) found that RHD subjects had difficulties with ToM tasks when these were presented verbally, but performed as well as LHD subjects when these tasks were presented with visual aids. Moreover, RHD subjects exhibited reduced sensitivity to violations of Gricean maxims in conversation. Surian and Siegal explain these find-ings in terms of deficits in visuospatial representation and working memory, both of which are subservient to our pragmatic competence: 'their difficulties on tasks devised to test ToM understanding may stem from impaired visuospatial buffers and working memory processes required for pragmatic competence rather than a funda-mental representational deficit' (2001: 229–30).

18 The standard view is that phonology is intact in schizophrenia. Covington *et al.* (2005) state that 'according to all reports, segmental phonology in schizophrenia is obstinately normal' (90). However, findings such as those of Walder *et al.* (2006) suggest that this view may be in need of some revision. Walder *et al.* examined phonology, semantics and grammar in thirty-one schizophrenic outpatients and twenty-seven healthy controls. Male schizophrenic patients performed significantly worse than their healthy counterparts on all three language domains. While phon-ology was the least affected language domain in male patients, it was the most affected domain in female schizophrenic patients in the same study.

19 Covington *et al.* (2005) argue that what appear to be morphemic errors in schizo-phrenia might equally be related to disruptions of syntax or lexical retrieval. In this way, the schizophrenic patient studied by Chaika may have committed a syntactic

error by selecting the wrong part of speech (the infinitive form *help* rather than the past participle *helped*) or a lexical retrieval error by selecting a word with the correct semantic meaning but from the wrong syntactic category (the verb *medicate* as opposed to the noun *medication*). In any event, Covington *et al.* state that 'abnormal morphology in schizophrenia is quite rare' (2005: 90).

20 In the ANIMAL category fluency test, subjects are required to produce as many exemplars of the category ANIMAL as they can within a certain time limit, typically sixty seconds.

21 In a study of twenty-five patients with a diagnosis of schizophrenia or a related disorder, Langdon *et al.* (2002) obtained results that 'clearly support the view that there exists a domain-specific mind-reading capacity that is impaired in some patients with schizophrenia' (93). However, for some of these patients at least, poor mind-reading was caused by 'a more generalised problem with suppressing prepotent but inappropriate information' (94). Langdon *et al.* also found that the schizophrenic patients in this study were significantly impaired in their ability to recognise three types of non-literal speech – banter, sarcasm and metaphorical speech (banter was defined as an ironical utterance in which there was no intention to harm or to criticise). At least some of these patients' difficulty with the recognition of appropriate uses of ironical and metaphorical speech was related to problems suppressing prepotent inappropriate information. In addition, the general mind-reading capacity of these patients, as measured by false belief picture-sequencing scores, predicted understanding of ironical, but not metaphorical, speech. Langdon *et al.* conclude that 'the findings of this schizophrenia study suggest that not just a basic ability to attribute mental states but the more sophisticated mind-reading abilities of the kind needed to pass typical theory-of-mind tasks are critical for understanding ironical speech. In contrast, understanding of metaphorical speech may require only a very basic ability to represent mental states; this we know is intact in patients with schizophrenia' (2002: 97). A similar conclusion is drawn by Fine *et al.* (2001) who found a marked impairment on the comprehension of sarcasm in their patient B.M., a schizophrenic adult with congenital left amygdala damage who had also received a diagnosis of Asperger's syndrome. While the comprehension of sarcasm was impaired, B.M.'s performance on a metaphor comprehension task was normal. Fine *et al.* remark that 'B.M. may have performed normally on the metaphor task because, unlike sarcasm comprehension, the understanding of metaphor does not require the listener to take into account the thoughts of the speaker in order to reject the nonsensical literal meaning' (2001: 292).

22 Flaada *et al.* (2007) studied 1,433 confirmed incident cases of TBI sustained between 1985 and 1999 amongst a random sample of 7,800 residents of Olmsted County, Minnesota with a diagnosis suggestive of TBI. These investigators reported that 35% of these cases were paediatric (under sixteen years), 55% were adult (sixteen–sixty-five years) and 9% were elderly (over sixty-five years).

23 Sosin *et al.* (1996) estimate that road traffic accidents account for 28% of TBIs, sports injuries for 20% of TBIs and assaults and 'other causes' for a further 9% and 43%, respectively. Of those head injuries severe enough to require hospitalisation, almost half (49%) were caused by road traffic accidents. The two leading causes of TBI-related hospitalisation among the subjects recorded by the Centers for Disease Control and Prevention (2007) were unintentional motor vehicle traffic incidents and unintentional falls.

24 The source of this statistic is Kraus and McArthur (1996). In their study of TBI patients in Olmsted County in Minnesota, Flaada *et al.* (2007) report that moderate/severe injuries were found in 11.4% of paediatric cases, 8.5% of adult cases and 26.7% of elderly cases. Amongst moderate/severe injuries, 10.3% of paediatric cases, 40.3% of adult cases and 50.0% of elderly cases died within six months; in mild injuries, 0% of children, 0% of adults and 9.1% of elderly died within six months.

25 In a national survey in Canada, Dawson and Chipman (1995) described how 66% of TBI survivors living in the community reported an ongoing need for assistance with some activities of daily living. Some 75% of survivors were not working and as many as 90% reported problems with social integration.

26 Body and Parker (2005) argue that topic repetitiveness is a source of pragmatic impairment in TBI subjects and a cause of social exclusion in these subjects.

27 The recovery of conversational skills in TBI is by no means guaranteed. Snow *et al.* (1998) examined the conversational skills of twenty-four severely injured TBI speakers, first between three and six months post-injury and then at a minimum of two years post-injury. Conversational abilities did not improve in TBI speakers as a group over time. In a subgroup of eight patients who did improve over time, improvement was related to a significantly longer period of speech-language pathology intervention and to a greater initial severity of injury.

28 Another study that has revealed deficits in the adherence of TBI subjects to Gricean maxims was conducted by Douglas and Bracy (2006). These investigators examined forty-three dyads, each consisting of an adult with severe TBI and a close relative, at a minimum of two years post-injury. The La Trobe Communication Questionnaire (Douglas *et al.* 2000) was administered to all TBI adults and their relatives. These investigators found that fourteen behaviours were particularly problematic in the TBI adults and occurred significantly more frequently in TBI patients than in matched controls. These behaviours involved violations in the quantity, relation and manner domains of Grice's cooperative principle. Also, they reflected the impact on social discourse of impaired executive functions (namely, inhibitory control, fluency, attentional control and task management).

29 Martin and McDonald (2003) state that 'although there is good evidence for ToM deficits associated with communication difficulties in Autism and RHD, and potentially a similar link in TBI, the direction of this relationship is unclear' (455). Other investigators have failed to find a role for ToM deficits in the pragmatic language difficulties of TBI subjects (see Bara *et al.* 1997).

30 Some of these other conditions are Huntington's disease, Guillain-Barré syndrome and myasthenia gravis. These disorders are considerably less prevalent than those examined in the main text. For example, Naarding *et al.* (2001) report that the prevalence of Huntington's disease in Western Europe and Northern America is 5–10 per 100,000 persons.

31 Hirtz *et al.* (2007) estimate that among the elderly ($\geq$ 65 years) in the United States, the prevalence rate of Alzheimer's disease is 67 per 1,000 (or 6,700 per 100,000). Clough *et al.* (2003) state that a widely accepted figure for the prevalence of Parkinson's disease is 200 per 100,000 persons. Although epidemiological studies of multiple sclerosis in England and Wales have produced different prevalence estimates, the average prevalence is estimated to be 110 MS individuals per 100,000 population (Richards *et al.* 2002). Svenson et al. (1999) estimated the prevalence of motor neurone disease for the province of Alberta, Canada to be 7.38 per 100,000 population.

32 Many other diseases may also cause dementia. Problems with the blood supply to the brain may lead to vascular dementia. Some people with vascular dementia may also have Alzheimer's disease (so-called mixed dementia). Vascular and mixed dementia account for some 27 per cent of all dementia cases (Knapp and Prince 2007). Dementia with Lewy bodies and frontotemporal dementia (originally called Pick's disease) are less common forms of dementia. Rarer causes of dementia include HIV infection, Creutzfeldt-Jakob disease and Korsakoff's syndrome (alcohol-related dementia). It should also be noted that people with multiple sclerosis, motor neurone disease, Parkinson's disease and Huntington's disease can also develop dementia.

33 Average age of onset of ALS is fifty-six years, although patients may develop the disorder between forty and sixty years (Clem and Morgenlander 2006). Median survival is between three and five years, but it is not uncommon for individuals to survive longer than five years (30% of patients are still alive five years after diagnosis and 10–20% survive for more than ten years). Respiratory muscle weakness leads to death, with aspiration pneumonia and problems associated with immobility contributing to morbidity.

34 Few studies have examined language in patients with other neurodegenerative disorders. This is because of the widespread belief that dysarthria is the only communication disorder in clients with conditions such as multiple sclerosis and motor neurone disease. To the extent that language problems do occur, it is argued that they do so rarely: 'language disturbances such as aphasia, auditory agnosia, anomia, dysgraphia, and dyslexia are very rare in MS' (Merson and Rolnick 1998: 631). However, a study by Klugman and Ross (2002) of thirty persons with multiple sclerosis indicates that this may not be the case. These investigators found that more of their MS subjects reported language impairment than speech impairment (63.3% and 56.7%, respectively). Also, Rakowicz and Hodges (1998) found a language disorder in five of eighteen patients (28 per cent) with a new diagnosis of sporadic MND who presented consecutively to a regional neurology service over a three-year period. For discussion of language impairment in multiple sclerosis, motor neurone disease and Parkinson's disease, the reader is referred to Friend et al. (1999), Cobble (1998) and Berg et al. (2003), respectively.

35 Although most studies emphasise findings of pragmatic impairments in Alzheimer's disease, one study has demonstrated that some aspects of pragmatics are relatively intact in this disorder (at least in its early stages). Papagno (2001) examined metaphor and idiom comprehension in thirty-nine patients with probable early Alzheimer's disease. Only four patients (10.25 per cent) displayed an impairment of figurative language comprehension. A double dissociation between propositional and figurative language comprehension occurred in eleven patients (28.2 per cent). The more common dissociation was for propositional language to be impaired alongside preservation of figurative comprehension. Papagno concluded that 'the decline of figurative language is not an early symptom of dementia and can occur independently from the impairment of propositional language' (2001: 1450).

4 The contribution of pragmatics to cognitive theories of autism

4.1 Introduction

It is now widely acknowledged that a cognitive deficit underlies impairments in socialisation, communication and imagination in autism. Although many accounts of this cognitive deficit have been advanced, most clinicians and researchers have tended to coalesce behind one of three dominant theories in the field. These theories locate the core cognitive deficit of autism in an impaired *theory of mind*, in a cognitive processing style characterised by *weak central coherence* and in impairments of one or more cognitive processes referred to as *executive functions*. This multiplicity of cognitive deficits creates a primacy problem, in that only one of these impairments can be the core or primary deficit in autism while the others are secondary deficits. Deciding which, if any, of these impairments is more fundamental than the others is made all the more difficult by the fact that each cognitive deficit has received extensive experimental validation. Clearly, some non-empirical criterion needs to be found in order to address this question. In this chapter, I present *pragmatic adequacy* as just such a criterion. Motivated by the central role of pragmatic deficits in the communication impairment of autism, I argue that an acceptable cognitive theory of autism, particularly one that is foundational to other cognitive theories, must be pragmatically adequate. I assess the pragmatic adequacy of each of these cognitive theories in turn. It will be demonstrated that two of these theories – theory of mind and weak central coherence – can satisfy this criterion in principle. However, an examination of so-called 'pragmatics' research within each of these theoretical approaches reveals that neither theory can make a claim to pragmatic adequacy in practice. The third cognitive theory – executive function theory – cannot be assessed for pragmatic adequacy at this time due largely to the incomplete state of our knowledge of the cognitive and neurobiological substrates of pragmatic phenomena.

4.2 Cognitive theories of autism

In the absence of biological markers for autism,[1] clinicians have come to rely on behavioural criteria in their assessment and diagnosis of this disorder. These

118

criteria relate to the socialisation, communication and imagination impairments that have come to define autism since Dr Leo Kanner, a psychiatrist at Johns Hopkins University, first provided a clinical description of the condition in 1943. These criteria receive their most explicit formulation in two internationally accepted diagnostic systems, the fourth edition (text revision) of the *Diagnostic and statistical manual of mental disorders* (American Psychiatric Association 2000) and the tenth edition of the *International classification of diseases* (World Health Organisation 1993). These systems have undergone successive revisions as our knowledge of the behavioural features of autism has evolved. Moreover, even the current editions of these systems have not been exempt from criticism.[2] Notwithstanding these changes and criticisms, there is now considerable agreement amongst theorists and clinicians about the behavioural phenotype of autism and related disorders.

Clear behavioural impairments in autism have led theorists to consider if a core cognitive deficit might not explain some or all of these impairments. Motivated by the substantial growth that has occurred in recent years in the cognitive sciences, theorists have begun to advance several hypotheses concerning the nature and extent of this cognitive deficit. Chief amongst these hypotheses are explanations that locate the core cognitive deficit of autism in an impaired theory of mind. However, other equally significant, if somewhat less prominent, cognitive explanations of autism locate the core deficit in this disorder in a type of cognitive processing characterised by weak central coherence or in impaired executive functioning. In the rest of this section, we describe the main features of each of these cognitive theories and examine some of the experimental evidence that has been adduced in support of them. We then turn in the next section to discuss how these different cognitive theories are interrelated. As part of that discussion, we will consider what theorists mean when they claim that certain cognitive deficits are primary while other deficits are secondary.

4.2.1   Theory of mind (ToM) theory

Originally proposed by Simon Baron-Cohen and coworkers[3] in 1985, the theory of mind theory of autism posits that the core cognitive deficit in autism consists in a failure to attribute mental states both to one's own mind and to the minds of others:

By theory of mind we mean being able to infer the full range of mental states (beliefs, desires, intentions, imagination, emotions, etc.) that cause action. In brief, to be able to reflect on the contents of one's own and other's minds. (Baron-Cohen 2000: 3)

This deficit, it is argued, is responsible for the behavioural abnormalities seen in autism, particularly problems in socialisation and communication: 'It [ToM] seems to correlate with, on the one hand ... abnormal social behaviour and, on the other hand ... abnormal pragmatic competence in language. These correlations suggest that this cognitive deficit may indeed underlie these behavioural abnormalities' (Baron-Cohen 1991: 35). In order to test this ToM hypothesis, Baron-Cohen and his colleagues used an adaptation of a procedure developed by Wimmer and Perner (1983). This procedure was designed to assess children's understanding of false belief. It was hypothesised that if autistic children had a ToM deficit, they would fail tests of false belief (so-called Sally-Anne experiments[4]). This is because these children would be unable to conceive that people can have beliefs about a situation that differ from their own belief states. In their original 1985 study, Baron-Cohen *et al.* confirmed this hypothesis. These researchers found that while normal children and children with Down's syndrome passed the belief question on both trials of a false belief test (85% and 86%, respectively), 80% of the autistic children failed the belief question on these trials.

Since this early study, the theory of mind framework has been further elaborated. It has been shown, for example, that autistic children are not only delayed in their development of a theory of mind, but that this development may also be deviant. In a study conducted by Baron-Cohen (1991), it was found that the youngest autistic child to pass the belief test was almost ten years old. This represents a delay of almost six years compared to normal children: 'That this is almost 6 years later than the age at which normal children understand belief is evidence of substantial delay' (Baron-Cohen 1991: 46). It was also discovered that while normal subjects and mentally retarded subjects found pretence, perception and imagination equally easy to understand, subjects with autism had more difficulty representing pretence and imagination than perception: 'insofar as the group with autism progressed through a different *sequence* in understanding mental states to that seen even in the group with mental handicap, this is evidence of additional deviance in the development of their theory of mind' (Baron-Cohen 1991: 46; italics in original).

As part of their wider inability to understand and manipulate beliefs, autistic children have been found to fail tests of deception that are effortlessly executed by both normal and mentally retarded controls. Sodian and Frith (1992) found that autistic children performed significantly worse than normal and mentally retarded controls on an experimental task that required them to tell a lie (say that a box was locked). However, on a sabotage task, when the autistic children had a physical means of preventing a competitor from gaining access to a box (i.e. the children could use a padlock to secure the box), their performance was comparable to that of normal and mentally retarded controls (at least on the simple sabotage condition). This difference in autistic performance across deception and sabotage tasks shows that the crucial factor in the autistic children's failure on the deception task was their failure to manipulate the mental states of others. Specifically, they were unable to encourage a competitor to entertain a false belief. It was unsurprising, therefore, that the autistic children's performance on the deception tasks was shown to be predicted by their performance on a false belief attribution task.

4.2.2   Weak central coherence (WCC) theory

Uta Frith proposed the expression 'central coherence' to refer to 'the normal cognitive tendency to put a premium on the extraction of meaning, gist and gestalt in information processing' (Happé et al. 2001: 300). To the extent that autistic children display 'weak' central coherence, they exhibit a processing preference for parts over wholes. In the case of language processing, this preference leads the autistic child to neglect aspects of linguistic context. Jolliffe and Baron-Cohen (2000) found that subjects with autism and Asperger's syndrome were less able than normal controls to extract information from context and use it to make a global coherence inference about a character's action in a story. This processing preference also affects nonlinguistic domains. Jolliffe and Baron-Cohen (2001) investigated visuo-conceptual integration in normally intelligent adults with either autism or Asperger's syndrome. A modified version of the Hooper Visual Organisation Test (Hooper 1983) was used to test participants. Subjects were required to mentally (conceptually) integrate fragments in order to identify the object of which these pieces were a part. They were also required to identify an object from seeing just a single element or part of it. Both clinical groups were impaired in their ability to integrate fragments holistically but they were able to identify an object from a single part. Autistic subjects were more impaired than the group with Asperger's syndrome and the impairment applied to the majority of the autism group.

As well as leading to impaired performance, weak central coherence has also been linked to exceptionally good performance by autistic subjects on certain tasks. These are tasks that do not require subjects to perceive a gestalt. For example, Shah and Frith (1993) gave systematic variations of the block design task to autistic, normal and mentally retarded subjects. It was found that, regardless of age and ability, autistic subjects performed better than controls when presented with unsegmented designs. While autistic subjects were able to segment the gestalt in these designs with minimal processing effort, this was less easily achieved by control subjects. Clearly, the autistic cognitive tendency to process parts over wholes conferred processing benefits on the autistic subjects in Shah and Frith's study. The findings of this study and others like it have led Frith and coworkers not to present weak coherence as a cognitive impairment. Rather, while weak central coherence in combination with a specific deficit (e.g. in theory of mind) can lead to the impairments seen in autism, weak coherence by itself is more appropriately construed as a style of processing that has both benefits and disadvantages for autistic subjects: 'weak coherence plus an additional specific deficit (e.g. in theory of mind) may result in handicap (autism) while in the absence of such a deficit it may carry a balance of benefits and limitations and hence represent a cognitive *style* rather than an impairment' (Happé *et al.* 2001: 300; italics in original).

4.2.3   Executive function (EF) theory

The third cognitive theory of autism posits deficits in abilities that are mediated by the frontal cortex. These abilities, collectively termed 'executive functions', include cognitive processes such as planning, working memory, impulse control, inhibition and mental flexibility and the initiation and monitoring of action.[5] Bruce Pennington, a leading proponent of executive function theory, believes that a working memory deficit is responsible for executive dysfunction in autism: 'our executive dysfunction hypothesis is that in individuals with autism there is a severe, early disruption in the planning of complex behaviour, due to a severe deficit in working memory' (Pennington *et al.* 1997: 148). This deficit, Pennington *et al.* argue, can account for all the main behavioural symptoms of autism and for ToM impairments in autistic subjects.[6] We will return to this issue in the next section when we examine how cognitive theories are interrelated. In the meantime, we discuss the findings of some experimental studies that have revealed executive dysfunction in autism.

That autistic individuals display deficits in executive functions has been demonstrated in recent studies. Lopez *et al.* (2005) examined the relationship between executive functions and restricted, repetitive symptoms in adults with autistic disorder. These researchers found that several executive functions (i.e. cognitive flexibility, working memory and response inhibition) were highly related to restrictive, repetitive symptoms, while other executive functions (i.e. planning and fluency) displayed no such relationship to these symptoms. Kleinhans *et al.* (2005) found that high-functioning adolescents and adults with autistic disorder or Asperger's disorder performed significantly below average on a composite measure of executive functioning that was adjusted for baseline cognitive ability. The most consistent deficits were observed on complex verbal tasks such as a verbal fluency test that required cognitive switching and initiation of efficient lexical retrieval strategies. Cognitive inhibition was found to be intact in these subjects.

Ozonoff *et al.* (2004) examined the performance of autistic subjects and normal controls on two subtests of the Cambridge Neuropsychological Test Automated Battery. The two subtests – one a planning task and the other a measure of cognitive set shifting – produced significant performance differences between the groups. Moreover, these deficits were evident in both lower- and higher-IQ autistic subjects. Although impairment on these executive function subtests did not predict autism severity or specific autism symptoms, it was shown to correlate with adaptive behaviour. Joseph *et al.* (2005) examined the relationship between executive dysfunction and language ability in thirty-seven autistic children. Compared to normal controls, autistic children displayed deficits in three domains of executive function: working memory, inhibitory control and planning. Interestingly, executive function was only found to correlate positively with language ability in the control subjects. Joseph *et al.* conclude that 'executive dysfunction in autism is not directly related to language impairment per se but rather involves an executive failure to use language for self-regulation' (2005: 361).

4.3   The relationship between cognitive theories

By examining each cognitive theory in isolation, the reader may be left with the impression that these theories and the deficits they explain are essentially unrelated. It may seem, for example, that a ToM theorist cannot also see merits in a weak central coherence account of autism or that an executive function theorist cannot also accept the presence of ToM deficits in autism. However, the relationship between these theories is more complex than these simple characterisations suggest. In this section, we discuss the complex interconnections that exist between these cognitive theories. We will see, for example, how executive function theory includes a role for theory of mind deficits, if not ToM theory itself, within its cognitive account of autism. We then turn to examine the central question of the primacy of these theories. It will be argued that this question of primacy necessarily involves giving priority to one of these cognitive theories (after all, not *each* cognitive theory can be foundational to the other cognitive theories). This primacy question is currently being addressed through experimental studies that are testing the competing predictions of these theories. However, this experimental effort, it is argued, is misplaced because the primacy question is more conceptual than empirical in nature. In the next section, the case will be presented for using a communicative criterion, a criterion of pragmatic adequacy, in determining the primacy of cognitive theories of autism.

To understand the relationship between cognitive theories of autism, we first need to draw a distinction between theory of mind, central coherence and executive function *deficits* and the *theories* which purport to give an explanation of those deficits. One can subscribe to the claim that there are ToM *deficits* in autism – indeed, it would be difficult to deny this claim – without also subscribing to the ToM *theory* of autism. This distinction between 'deficits' and 'theories' has allowed researchers to reject opposing *theories* of autism while at the same time not appearing to deny the cognitive *deficits* that are explained by those theories. In this way, Russell (1997a) accepts the need to provide an account of ToM (mentalising) deficits within a cognitive theory of autism: 'my starting assumption will accordingly be that both executive and mentalizing impairments are fundamental components of autism and that a major task for cognitive theories of the disorder is to give an account of how the two are related' (256). However, such acceptance does not thereby commit Russell to subscribe to ToM theory itself. Russell's scepticism towards this theory is captured in a collection of essays that develop the executive function position. He remarks in relation to these essays:

Their common denominator is scepticism about a very particular and very ambitious theory, not about the existence of mentalizing deficits in autism. None of us is denying that persons with autism have such mentalizing impairments, and none of us would want to say that these difficulties can be, as it were, explained away in terms of executive deficits. (Russell 1997b: 1)

The relationship between cognitive theories of autism can thus best be characterised as follows. Clearly, the proponents of these theories acknowledge the need to give some account of the cognitive deficits explained by frameworks other than their own. Yet, this acknowledgement does not entail acceptance of the wider theoretical frameworks that explain those deficits. This plurality of cognitive deficits creates a problem of its own, however. For in order to achieve full integration of these deficits within a single theoretical account of autism, cognitive theorists argue, one of these deficits must have priority over the other deficits. This is tantamount to the claim that one cognitive deficit (e.g. executive dysfunction) is the proximal or primary cause of autism and that other deficits (e.g. ToM impairments and weak central coherence) can be explained in terms of this primary deficit. Just such a primacy claim is advanced by Pennington *et al.* (1997) when they present the following question as one of four validity tests of the executive dysfunction hypothesis of autism: can executive dysfunction theory be subsumed by central coherence theory? A similar primacy claim is implicit in Perner and Lang's statement that ToM is a 'prerequisite' for executive control (2000: 174). Also, when Plaisted states that 'it is a long-standing question whether the social deficits in autism are caused by what are often called "primary deficits" in perception, attention, and learning' (2000: 242), it is the primacy of 'asocial' theories of autism (i.e. EF and WCC theories) over ToM theory that she has in mind.

To address this question of the primacy of a specific cognitive deficit, researchers have typically adopted an experimental approach. In this way, Pennington *et al.* (1997) used modified versions of the block design task and a homograph ambiguity task to test the competing predictions of their working memory theory of autism and central coherence theory and to clarify the relationship between these two theories.[7] Plaisted (2000) turns to studies that have tested attention processes in very young autistic children in order to substantiate the primary role of these processes in the development of autism.[8] These investigators justify the use of an experimental approach by appealing to what they believe is the essentially empirical nature of the primacy question – experimental studies, they argue, will eventually reveal which of these cognitive theories captures the primary deficit in autism. This belief, it will be argued below, is mistaken, because the question of the primacy of a cognitive theory is one that is properly conceptual in nature. In addressing this question, investigators should first set themselves the task of listing those criteria that must be satisfied by a cognitive theory that is claiming primacy. As a start on this task, the criterion of pragmatic adequacy will be discussed at length in the next section. These criteria can then be used to test the primacy claims of competing cognitive theories.

4.4   The criterion of pragmatic adequacy

By starting with criteria that a cognitive theory of autism must satisfy, this conceptual approach reduces the contribution of experimental data in determining an answer to the question of primacy. This is advantageous in at least two respects. First, the results of many experiments are consistent with quite different theoretical accounts of the cognitive deficit in autism and are thus incapable of discriminating between competing cognitive theories.[9] Second, some experimental studies fail to assess the particular phenomena they are claiming to test (pragmatic phenomena, we will see subsequently, are a case in point). These studies are thus of questionable value in determining the primacy of cognitive theories of autism. The reduced significance of experimental data in a conceptual approach is matched only by the increased significance of criteria within this approach. These criteria are obtained by asking what type of cognitive theory could subsume other theories and provide an account of the primary cognitive deficit in autism. In considering the form that such a theory might take, it seems unproblematic to require that it should at a minimum be able to (1) account for a range of cognitive deficits in autism and not simply align itself with the deficits of a particular cognitive theory and (2) present an account of the main behavioural symptoms in autism. Although this enquiry is still in its initial stages, there is some early justification for claiming that a pragmatically adequate theory can accommodate (1) and (2). Such a theory can account for ToM and WCC deficits in autism. It can also account for the main communication deficits in autism and socialisation impairments where these are linked to communication failure. Both these points will be discussed in section 4.6. In the meantime, we can say that a theory that satisfies a criterion of pragmatic adequacy is a good place to begin the search for a foundational cognitive theory of autism.

To understand what a criterion of pragmatic adequacy involves, its main features can be explicated best by examining some of the communicative phenomena upon which it is based. Consider the following exchange between A and B:

A: Do you want to go into town?
B: I'm feeling really tired at the moment.

On hearing B's response, A will conclude that B does not want to go into town. In so forming this conclusion, A has established the implicature of B's utterance. Implicatures are just one type of implied meaning that speakers encounter during communication. However, their relevance in the present context is that they can be used to demonstrate the various cognitive processes that are integral to pragmatic interpretation in general. What appears to be, superficially at least, a relatively straightforward act of language understanding on A's part is, in fact, a complex inferential process that draws upon knowledge of conversational principles and much else besides. In order to recover the implicature of B's utterance, A must first view B as a sincere communicator who is attempting to make a relevant response to A's question. This assumption of conversational sincerity is the basis of Grice's cooperative principle. One of this principle's maxims, the maxim of relation, leads A to treat B's response as a relevant contribution to the conversational exchange. Using these conversational assumptions, A attempts to establish the relevance of B's utterance. On the basis of background knowledge, A knows that fatigue reduces one's desire to undertake physical activity and that going into town involves such activity. A also knows that B is fatigued (a fact introduced into the exchange by B's utterance). A concludes, therefore, that B does not want to go into town.

The inferential process outlined above is significant in at least two respects. The chain of reasoning that leads from an assumption of conversational cooperation to the implicature of B's utterance is none other than a series of inferences designed to establish B's communicative intention in producing that utterance. In recovering the implicature of any utterance, a listener must always go beyond the literal language used to determine what the speaker intended to communicate. This communicative intention is a mental state of the speaker in the same way that belief and knowledge are mental states. Establishing mental states is also integral to other forms of pragmatic interpretation. A speech act can only convey an illocutionary force beyond its literal meaning for the listener who is able to ascertain the communicative intention of the speaker who produces the act. For example, in order to understand that the utterance 'The dangerous dog is in the garden' is a warning to stay out of the garden, the listener must be able to establish that the speaker is intending to warn the listener rather than merely describe the dog's presence.

In addition to establishing the communicative intentions (mental states) of the speaker, the above inferential process is noteworthy in a further important respect. This process is a truly global cognitive operation which draws upon knowledge from a range of sources. Some of this knowledge may be perceptual in origin – for example, seeing a fatigued expression on B's face may serve to confirm B's statement that he or she is tired. Other knowledge may be retrieved from memory, from where it may go on to play a role in the recovery of implicatures. Still other knowledge may be obtained from earlier cognitive processes such as reasoning. As well as using knowledge from a range of sources, pragmatic interpretation must also draw upon a speaker's knowledge of conversational principles and facts. We saw above, for example, how Grice's cooperative principle and certain facts (e.g. that B was tired) were integral to the inferential process that led to the recovery of the implicature of B's utterance. In short, pragmatic interpretation can draw upon a potentially infinite range of knowledge, the source and nature of which cannot be fully circumscribed.

In summary, pragmatic interpretation proceeds by means of an inferential process that draws upon an indefinable range of knowledge and information. To the extent that we are basing the criterion of pragmatic adequacy upon this type of interpretation, this criterion must reflect the inferential, global nature of pragmatic interpretation. The criterion of pragmatic adequacy can thus be characterised as follows:

Pragmatic adequacy embodies the two features that are characteristic of any act of pragmatic interpretation. The first feature pertains to the inferential nature of pragmatic interpretation: establishing the implicature of an utterance or the illocutionary force of a speech act requires that a language user be able to engage in an inferential process that starts with a spoken utterance and concludes with the speaker's intention in producing that utterance. The second feature of this criterion captures the global nature of this inferential process: any item of information or knowledge, however remote, may be used in the inferential process by means of which a speaker's communicative intention is established.

A pragmatically adequate cognitive theory of autism must therefore be able to (1) explain the inferential process by means of which a speaker's communicative intentions are established and (2) account for the global nature of that process. In the next section, we examine how well each cognitive theory of autism is able to accommodate (1) and (2). We will see that, in principle, ToM theory can account for (1), while WCC theory can provide an account of (2). However, neither theory can satisfy both features of this criterion. Moreover, the studies that are used by ToM and WCC theorists to support (1) and (2), respectively, are problematic, in that they fail to capture the true nature of pragmatic interpretation. An assessment of the pragmatic adequacy of executive function theory is difficult at the present time, for reasons that will be outlined.

4.5   A pragmatic challenge to cognitive theories

The first of our three theories, ToM theory, has an understanding of (1) in the previous section, more broadly construed in terms of mental states, chief amongst its explanatory aims. Simon Baron-Cohen, the leading proponent of ToM theory, recognises the central role of ToM skills in pragmatic interpretation in a review[10] of ToM research in autism: 'Almost every aspect of pragmatics involves sensitivity to speaker and listener mental states, and hence mindreading' (2000: 13). Given the dependence of pragmatics on ToM skills, one might reasonably have expected ToM theorists to have extensively investigated this area of communicative function in autism. However, a review of the literature reveals that relatively few studies have used ToM concepts to examine pragmatic language skills in autism. This paucity of research is nowhere more evident than in the review by Baron-Cohen just mentioned. Although this review examines ToM research undertaken between 1985 and 2000, it has almost nothing to say about pragmatics beyond general comments about the type of skills that fall within this domain. Moreover, neither of the experimental studies included in this review succeeds in assessing the particular pragmatic phenomena that the authors of these studies are claiming to investigate. This last point is sufficiently important to warrant further examination.

The two experimental studies of pragmatics included in Baron-Cohen's review – Baron-Cohen *et al.* (1999) and Surian *et al.* (1996) – exemplify some of the weaknesses of ToM research in pragmatics. For this reason, we will examine each study in turn. Baron-Cohen *et al.* (1999) set out to investigate the recognition of faux pas by children with Asperger's syndrome (AS) or high-functioning autism (HFA). Twelve children with AS or HFA, and sixteen normal controls, were presented with ten short stories on audio cassette. In one of these stories, a man called Tim spills some coffee in a restaurant. He turns to a customer and, believing him to be a waiter, says 'I've spilt my coffee. Would you be able to mop it up?' Subjects were then asked a series of questions. One of these questions was designed to assess if subjects had detected the faux pas in the story ('In the story, did someone say something that they should not have said?'). A further question required subjects to identify the faux pas ('What did they say that they should not have said?'). A third question tested subjects' understanding of the language used in the story, while a fourth question aimed to assess if subjects were aware that the faux pas was a consequence of a false belief on the part of the speaker in the story.

There can be little doubt that this task is testing a range of language and cognitive skills in the autistic children in this study. It is far from clear, however, that the ability to recognise Tim's mistake in the above scenario is a form of *pragmatic* interpretation. The only thing that can be said about this scenario is that Tim has made a mistake – he has a false belief about a customer, a belief which leads him to ask the customer, inappropriately, to mop up his spilt coffee. In failing to detect this faux pas, autistic children are failing to detect Tim's false belief. But this particular failing is something quite different from the recognition of communicative intentions that is integral to pragmatic interpretation. Indeed, as Baron-Cohen *et al.* (1999) define faux pas, it is clear that no *intentional* communication is involved in either its production or recognition: 'A working definition of faux pas might be when a speaker says something *without considering* if it is something that the listener might not want to hear or know, and which typically has negative consequences that the speaker *never intended*' (408; italics added). Moreover, it is unsurprising that the autistic subjects in this study failed to detect instances of faux pas.[11] For the detection of faux pas is none other than the detection of false belief, and this particular ToM skill is known to be impaired in autism (see section 4.2.1 above).

The second study included in Baron-Cohen's review is equally problematic, but for different reasons. Surian *et al.* (1996) examined the ability of high-functioning children with autism to detect violations of Gricean maxims. The rationale for this study, as well as its predicted result, are captured as follows: 'If children with autism have deficits in ascribing mental states, and particularly ascribing intentions, then they should fail to recognise when such Gricean maxims are being violated' (1996: 58). One of the examples used in this study is the following violation of the quantity maxim:

A: How would you like your tea?
B: In a cup.

In this case, B's answer fails to provide a sufficiently informative response to A's question. However, this exchange is only pragmatically interesting to the extent that B's superficially uninformative response can be used by A to recover an implicature. In this way, it is reasonable to conclude that B is implicating that he wants his tea in a cup as opposed to a saucer (of course, to obtain this particular implicature, we are assuming that A is clumsy and tends to spill tea and that B is aware of this behaviour). The recognition that a response isn't maximally informative is an important step in the inferential process by means of which implicatures are recovered during pragmatic interpretation. However, it is only the first step in this process. Such interpretation is only fully achieved when a listener is able to use his recognition that a response isn't fully informative to derive a speaker's intended or implied meaning. Surian *et al.* found that while most children with autism performed at chance on this maxim task, all children with specific language impairment and all normal controls performed above chance. Yet, this finding lacks any real implications for our knowledge of pragmatic functioning in autism, given the failure of this maxim task to assess the processes that are integral to pragmatic interpretation.

Clearly, the ToM framework is compatible in principle with the emphasis on establishing communicative intentions (mental states) in pragmatic interpretation (the first feature of the criterion of pragmatic adequacy). However, in practice it emerges that this framework cannot yet claim pragmatic adequacy on the basis of the experimental studies of pragmatics that are currently being conducted within ToM theory. It remains to be seen if the central coherence proposals of Uta Frith and colleagues will fare any better in this regard. Once again, in principle, these proposals are compatible with one of the two features associated with the criterion of pragmatic adequacy, the global character of the inferential process by means of which a speaker's communicative intentions are established (the second feature of the criterion). Yet, upon further examination, it will be seen that the same experimental distortion of pragmatic phenomena that weakened ToM theory's claim to pragmatic adequacy also undermines the claim to pragmatic adequacy of WCC theory.

To appreciate this point, we need only consider the typical experimental methodology employed by studies within the WCC framework. Jolliffe and Baron-Cohen (1999) examined local coherence in normally intelligent adults with either autism or Asperger's syndrome. Local coherence was defined as 'the ability to make contextually meaningful connections between linguistic information in short-term or working memory' (1999: 149). Both clinical groups, and particularly the autism group, were impaired in achieving local coherence, as indicated by the following findings: (1) clinical subjects were less likely than normal controls to use sentence context spontaneously in order to obtain the context-appropriate pronunciation of a homograph (e.g. *bow*; *row*); (2) autism and AS subjects were less likely to choose a coherent bridging inference from among alternatives in order to link situations and outcomes in presented scenarios and (3) clinical subjects were less able to use context to interpret ambiguous sentences that were presented auditorily. Finding (1) was established through the use of the following experimental task. Subjects were asked to read aloud sentences that contained homographs. Each homograph had a frequent and rare pronunciation. An accompanying sentence or part of a sentence favoured one pronunciation over the other and appeared either before or after the homograph. Two of the test items for the homograph *row* are as follows:

Rare pronunciation, before context:
The man had a second row with his wife the day after.

Frequent pronunciation, after context:
Everyone who wanted to see the new film had to stand in a row.

Jolliffe and Baron-Cohen (1999) used an Ambiguous Sentence test to establish finding (3) above. Subjects were required to listen to pairs of sentences. The last sentence in each pair was either lexically or syntactically ambiguous. In each case, the ambiguity could be resolved by the preceding sentence that acted as a disambiguating context. Each ambiguous sentence was presented twice, with the preceding sentence biasing disambiguation towards either a rare or a common interpretation. Subjects were asked a question about the ambiguous sentence to which they had to choose one of three possible responses. These responses represent a context-appropriate interpretation, a context-inappropriate interpretation and an erroneous interpretation. One of the test items used in this study is given below:

Lexical ambiguity, rare interpretation:
Clare was robbed as she walked along by some water. The bank was the scene of the robbery.
Question: Where was the robbery?
Possible responses: (1) on a river bank; (2) in a bank; (3) in the village bank

A similar experimental task was employed by Hoy *et al.* (2004) in their study of coherence processing in autistic and normally developing children. These investigators used a visual illusions task and a verbal homophone task to test certain predictions of central coherence theory.[12] On the homophone task, children were asked to listen to a short story and then point to a picture that corresponded to a homophone in the story. One of the sentences in the story was intended to favour either a common or a rare interpretation of the homophone. For example, the ambiguous sentence 'The lady liked a long read/reed' would be followed by either 'She had lots of books' (common interpretation) or 'Especially the tall ones that grew by the river' (rare interpretation). Five pairs of homophones were used in this task, all of which had been checked for comprehension by four autistic subjects during a pilot study (none of these subjects were used in the main experiment).

The tasks described above are typical of the experimental methodology adopted by WCC theorists. In each task, subjects must draw upon linguistic context, usually an accompanying sentence, to achieve the disambiguation of a word or sentence or the correct pronunciation of a homograph. The assumption of studies that use these tasks is that language interpretation proceeds on the basis of a tightly circumscribed notion of context that is somehow determined in advance of interpretation. However, as the discussion of pragmatic interpretation in section 4.4 was intended to demonstrate, this assumption is mistaken for at least two reasons. First, context is a sprawling notion that evades all attempts to place limits on it. The potentially infinite range of factors that may be employed in the recovery of an implicature of an utterance is evidence enough of context's capacity to go beyond boundaries. It is in this respect that the inferential process involved in pragmatic interpretation is a truly global process. It is simply not possible to throw a net over those aspects of one's linguistic and other knowledge that may be deemed relevant to the interpretation of a word or sentence. Even less is it possible to represent these diverse aspects within a single sentence or part of a sentence, as the studies discussed above would appear to be claiming. Second, pragmatic interpretation is a dynamic process in which language users must *create* a context for the understanding of utterances. This context is not ready-made or somehow determined in advance of interpretation, as experimental tasks on the disambiguation of homophones would lead one to believe (recall that in Hoy *et al.*'s homophone task a disambiguating context in the form of a sentence is provided for subjects). Two prominent theorists of pragmatic interpretation, Dan Sperber and Deirdre Wilson, subscribe to the view of context as an essentially dynamic construct in their relevance theory. Cruse (2000) remarks of this theory that 'the proper context for the interpretation of an utterance is not given in advance; it is chosen by the hearer' (370). It emerges that in an effort to establish how autistic subjects process aspects of context, central coherence studies end up distorting the very notion of context that they are aiming to examine.

Central coherence theorists are motivated to explain the autistic tendency to engage in local over global processing. To this extent, it is reasonable to conclude that central coherence theory should be capable of accounting for the global character of the inferential process that is integral to pragmatic interpretation – this process, after all, is a type of global cognitive processing. However, we have just seen how the type of experimental investigation that is pursued by central coherence studies fails to deliver a viable account of the global nature of this process. Like ToM theory before it, central coherence theory can satisfy a key feature of the criterion of pragmatic adequacy in principle. But to the extent that neither theoretical approach has developed a suitable means of experimentally validating their respective claims, neither approach has thus far succeeded in producing a pragmatically adequate cognitive theory of autism in practice. The third cognitive theory of autism, executive function theory, must still be assessed against the criterion of pragmatic adequacy. While ToM and WCC theories could at least satisfy certain features of this criterion in principle, we are unable to make any assessment of the pragmatic adequacy of EF theory at the present time. However, we will see below that this is related more to our current lack of knowledge of what the neurobiological and cognitive substrates of pragmatic adequacy may be than to any feature of EF theory itself.

With improvements in neuroimaging and other investigative techniques, more is being discovered about the neurobiological basis of autism. It is becoming clear, for example, that many of the neurobiological processes implicated in autism underlie executive functioning itself. Russell (1997b) remarks that 'the neurobiology of autism has the sort of character one finds in the neurobiology of executive functioning' (8). Executive dysfunction in autism is believed to involve control processes that are widely distributed across brain systems. Robbins (1997) remarks that: 'It does not seem very likely that executive functioning is modular, probably representing instead a set of control processes that are widely distributed across neural systems, including the heterogeneous anatomical components of the prefrontal cortex and their connections with other brain structures' (21). Moreover, theorists also have a growing understanding of how neurobiological impairments in autism may relate to impairments at the cognitive and behavioural levels of the disorder. The three leading neurobiological theories of autism locate dysfunction in the following neural axes: the temporal lobe and limbic system, the frontal cortex and striatum ('frontostriatal' systems) and the cerebellum and brainstem. Russell relates each of these theories to cognitive and behavioural impairments as follows.[13]

These three are: frontostriatal (frontal lesions affect, at least, inhibition, working memory, the generation and monitoring of plans, and they cause stereotypies), medio-temporal (lesions affect aspects of the control of social behaviour, in addition to causing mnemonic and emotional deficits), and cerebellum (efference-copying and attention-shifting affected by lesions). (1997b: 8)

Clearly, much is now known about the neurobiological and cognitive correlates of executive dysfunction in autism. However, the same cannot be said of the criterion of pragmatic adequacy which lacks clear correlates at both neurobiological and cognitive levels. This criterion reflects a deeper lack of knowledge, that of the neurobiological and cognitive substrates of pragmatic interpretation itself. To date, we have a rather basic understanding of the cognitive substrates of pragmatic interpretation. Research in this area, in both normal and disordered subjects, has proceeded in a largely piecemeal fashion and few general statements are possible at this time (see Chapters 2 and 3). To this lack of knowledge of the cognitive substrates of pragmatic interpretation, we must add a further complicating factor. The very nature of the central inferential process that is involved in the recovery of implicatures still remains largely beyond our grasp (for further discussion, see Chapter 3 in Cummings, 2005). Even Grice was reluctant to speculate about the nature of this process beyond an oblique reference to deduction.[14] Wilson and Sperber (1991) capture the largely undeveloped state of our knowledge in this area as follows:

although the idea of conversational implicature has had enormous appeal and been used in an informal way to account for a wide range of pragmatic phenomena, little progress has been made in specifying the exact nature of the inference process by which conversational implicatures are 'worked out'. (378)

Even less is known about the neurobiological processes that are involved in pragmatic interpretation. Certainly, studies of pragmatic impairments in brain-damaged adults suggest some overlap between the neuroanatomical areas associated with these impairments and those identified in current neurobiological theories of autism.[15] In this way, McDonald (1992) takes the view that certain pragmatic impairments in head-injured subjects can be related to frontal lobe cognitive deficits in these subjects.[16] However, other studies have failed to link pragmatic impairments to specific neuroanatomical regions. Kasher *et al.* (1999) found that stroke patients with left brain damage and right brain damage were significantly impaired relative to age-matched normal controls on an implicatures battery. Yet, these investigators found only weak correlations of implicatures with extents of lesions in the left perisylvian language area or its right-hemisphere homologue. Still other studies have found evidence of pragmatic impairments in adults who have lesions in anatomical areas that do not so clearly overlap with the areas identified in the leading neurobiological theories of autism. For example, Bryan (1988) found that subjects with right-hemisphere damage performed less well on tests of metaphorical comprehension, the understanding of inferred meaning and humour than subjects with left-hemisphere damage and subjects with no impairment (for further discussion, see Chapter 9 in Cummings, 2005). In short, we can say almost nothing of a conclusive nature at the present time about the neurobiological substrates of pragmatic interpretation. By the same token, the criterion of pragmatic adequacy lacks any clear neurobiological correlates. Executive function theory may well be a pragmatically adequate cognitive theory of autism. However, on the basis of our current knowledge and, particularly, our lack of knowledge of the neurobiological and cognitive substrates of the criterion of pragmatic adequacy, we are unable to tell at this time if this is the case.

4.6   The validity of pragmatic adequacy

In section 4.4, we described how a foundational cognitive theory of autism should, at a minimum, be capable of satisfying two requirements. These requirements were that such a theory must be able to (1) account for a range of cognitive deficits in autism and not simply align itself with the deficits of a particular cognitive theory and (2) present an account of the main behavioural symptoms in autism. With the discussion of section 4.5 now complete, it should be clear that pragmatic adequacy can account for theory of mind and central coherence deficits in autism. Both ToM and WCC theories, it was argued, could accommodate features of the criterion of pragmatic adequacy in principle, even if the experimental methods currently used in these frameworks to examine aspects of pragmatics fail to satisfy this criterion in practice. With further elaboration of the neurobiological and cognitive substrates of pragmatic interpretation, it may well emerge to be the case that pragmatic adequacy can capture executive function deficits, in addition to ToM and WCC impairments. At this initial stage of enquiry, it seems reasonable to say that a pragmatically adequate cognitive theory of autism will be one that can subsume the full range of cognitive deficits in autism, not just the deficits of a single cognitive theory.

The criterion of pragmatic adequacy is based upon pragmatic processes such as those involved in the recovery of an implicature of an utterance. To this extent, pragmatic adequacy is first and foremost a communicative criterion. However, the scope of this criterion extends beyond communication to include other behavioural impairments in autism. Specifically, pragmatic adequacy can also account for some of the socialisation deficits in this disorder. An example of such a deficit is a failure to develop peer relationships appropriate to the child's developmental level. This deficit may occur as a primary disorder in autism (i.e. it may occur independently of other behavioural impairments). However, one can easily see how the autistic child with impoverished communication skills may also fail to develop age-appropriate peer relationships. Such a child is unlikely to participate in social interactions with peers, during which a wide range of social skills are practised and developed. Teasing is part of the normal social interaction that occurs between children and adolescents. The widely recognised difficulties that autistic children experience both in comprehending the teasing behaviour of others and in using teasing effectively in social interaction can be traced to the pragmatic language difficulties of these children.[17] Similarly, the autistic child with pragmatic language impairment will struggle to comprehend the non-literal communication used in humour and jokes during social interaction with peers.[18] Such a child is likely to find himself excluded from social activities with others. Here again, the child's communicative impairment, specifically his deficit in pragmatics, will lead to significant secondary social problems. It thus emerges that as well as accounting for the communicative impairment in autism, the criterion of pragmatic adequacy goes some way towards explaining the social deficits in this disorder also.

NOTES

1 In this chapter, the generic term 'autism' will be used to refer to all autistic spectrum disorders (ASDs) or pervasive developmental disorders (PDDs). The reader should be aware, however, that this term subsumes several distinct disorders. See section 2.3 in Chapter 2 of this book and Chapter 3 in Cummings (2008) for discussion of these disorders.

2 For example, the criterion in DSM-IV-TR requiring that there is no clinically significant delay in cognitive development in Asperger's disorder is now widely acknowledged to be mistaken: 'It is remarkable that DSM excludes, by definition, the use of this developmental diagnosis for individuals with mental retardation or intellectual disability; it is the only place in DSM where this occurs. However, clinicians and researchers are now aware that this is an error: Asperger's Syndrome occurs in individuals with (mild) mental retardation' (Baron-Cohen et al. 2000: x).

3 Baron-Cohen and his colleagues borrowed the phrase 'theory of mind' from Premack and Woodruff, two primatologists. Premack and Woodruff define theory of mind as follows: 'In saying that an individual has a theory of mind, we mean that the

individual imputes mental states to himself and others ... A system of inferences of this kind is properly viewed as a theory, first because such states are not directly observable, and second, because the system can be used to make predictions, specifically about the behaviour of other organisms' (1978: 515).

4 The expression 'Sally-Anne experiments' derives from the names of the two dolls in the false belief task used by Baron-Cohen *et al.* (1985). In this task, a doll called Sally places a marble into a basket and then leaves the scene. While Sally is gone, a second doll called Anne enters the scene, removes the marble from the basket and places it in her box. Sally returns to the scene, whereupon the experimenter asks the child the belief question 'Where will Sally look for her marble?' The child who points to the previous location of the marble passes this question. The child who points to the marble's current location fails this question, as he or she failed to consider Sally's false belief.

5 The phrase 'executive functions' is often given an inexact definition that usually involves a listing of cognitive processes (see definition in main text) along with some mention of the neurobiological correlates of these processes. The inexact nature of these definitions is remarked upon by Pennington *et al.* (1997): 'The term "executive functions" has been adopted as an umbrella term to refer to the cognitive processes involved in the planning and execution of complex behaviour, without necessarily specifying what those processes are more precisely. The term is also used even more broadly to refer to all behaviours disrupted by prefrontal lesions. Both uses lack theoretical precision' (147).

6 'Our executive dysfunction hypothesis could account for deficits in: (1) imitation; (2) joint attention; (3) theory of mind; and (4) symbolic play, which builds on both imitation and an understanding of goal-directed behaviour. It would also explain the motor stereotypies and behavioural rituals as practised, prepotent reactions that are not inhibited by a working memory representation of a more abstract goal for behaviour. Restricted and specialised interests would have a similar explanation. In addition, concreteness, inflexibility, and an impairment in discourse would all be readily explained by an executive dysfunction hypothesis. So, the executive dysfunction hypothesis has the potential to account for all the main symptoms of autism' (Pennington *et al.* 1997: 148).

7 These studies failed to establish any clear relationship between the working memory theory of autism and central coherence theory: 'The goal of this last validity test was to address the relationship between two currently separate cognitive theories of autism: namely, the central coherence theory and the working memory theory ... Taken together, these findings suggest that neither theory can currently be subsumed by the other' (Pennington *et al.* 1997: 166).

8 The view that Plaisted is discussing, if not directly espousing, assumes that early deficits in the primary processes of perception, attention and learning are the cause of later problems in the acquisition of a theory of mind. Plaisted states that 'this view makes the prediction that deficits in the primary processes are apparent from a very early age and possibly from birth' (2000: 243). Whilst acknowledging that this is a difficult prediction to *test* because autism cannot be diagnosed until at least eighteen months of age, Plaisted goes on to discuss the findings of several studies which have assessed 'the quality of attentional processing in social contexts exhibited by children with autism' (2000: 243). It is the impetus to engage in *testing* that is being challenged in the main text.

9 Plaisted (2000) notes that autistic children display abnormalities in their attention to faces but remarks that 'the question still remains, however, whether this abnormality results from deficits in processes specialised for face processing or from a more general abnormality in stimulus processing' (244). Plaisted is arguing here that the finding that autistic children are unable to attend to faces in the ways that normal children do is consistent with both a 'social' and an 'asocial' explanation of autism (deficits in specialised social processing systems or in general processes of perception, learning and attention, respectively).

10 In this review, Baron-Cohen (2000) uses the terms 'theory of mind' and 'mindreading' synonymously.

11 The performance of the AS/HFA subjects on this test was significantly impaired relative to the normal subjects. For subjects to pass the test, their score either had to be equal to or above eight out of ten. On the basis of this criterion, only 18% of the children with AS or HFA passed the test compared to 75% of the normal children. This difference in performance was highly significant.

12 These predictions were that autistic subjects would make more errors on the rare condition of the homophone task and fewer errors of judgement about the visual illusions than typically developing controls. This is because autistic children, according to central coherence theory, are less able than normal controls to use linguistic context to guide them towards a rare interpretation of a homophone and that they operate instead with the common interpretation of the homophone as a default position. Similarly, autistic children are better than normal children at ignoring or not seeing the inducing context of visual illusions. Hoy *et al.* (2004) found that the autistic and typically developing children performed equally well on the visual illusions task. Although autistic subjects made relatively more errors than controls on the rare condition of a homophone task, these differences were accounted for by variation in the verbal ability level of the autistic subjects rather than by the diagnostic status of these children. Hoy *et al.* conclude that 'if it is assumed that … these experimental tasks are effective measures of weak central coherence then none of the predictions made by the weak central coherence theory of autism is supported' (2004: 274).

13 Russell also remarks that 'it is interesting to note that each of the three main neurobiological theories of autism locates the core impairment in an area with a significant executive role' (1997b: 8).

14 The closest Grice comes to making a comment that is revealing of the nature of this inferential process is his use of the term 'derivation' (suggestive of a deductive process of reasoning) in the following quotation from 'Presupposition and conversational implicature': 'the final test for the presence of a conversational implicature had to be, as far as I could see, a *derivation* of it. One has to produce an account of how it could have arisen and why it is there. And I am very much opposed to any kind of sloppy use of this philosophical tool, in which one does not fulfill this condition' (1981: 187; italics added).

15 The differences between the neurological status of a subject (child or adult) with autism and a brain-damaged adult are considerable. These dissimilarities prevent us from drawing any firm conclusions about autism from studies of brain-damaged adults.

16 In this study, subjects with closed head injury (CHI) and matched control subjects were asked to perform a number of tasks that were designed to assess their expressive

and receptive pragmatic skills. Tasks in which subjects had to issue requests in the form of hints and adhere to the conversational maxim of manner were used to test expressive pragmatic skills. Receptive pragmatic skills were assessed by asking subjects to perform a task that required them to understand indirect language. CHI subjects displayed various cognitive deficits related to frontal lobe pathology. Results revealed that CHI subjects had depressed performance compared to control subjects on all pragmatic skills. Within a more thorough analysis of the performance of these subjects, McDonald relates the impaired pragmatic skills of CHI subjects to their underlying cognitive deficits. Specifically, a CHI subject who failed to adhere to Grice's maxim of manner in his instructions to a blindfolded listener on how to play a novel game exhibited frontal lobe cognitive deficits like rigidity, perseveration and poor planning and problem-solving skills. Also, two CHI subjects who were unable to use indirect means (e.g. hints) of making requests exhibited considerable frontal lobe pathology. One subject was particularly concrete and perseverative. The other subject had less impaired abstraction skills but exhibited severe problems of impulse control.

17 Heerey *et al.* (2005) remark that 'much of the playful content of a tease is nonliteral, seen in similes, prosodic variations … and grammatical devices … that indirectly render the provocation less hostile' (56).

18 Emerich *et al.* (2003) investigated the ability of adolescents with high-functioning autism or Asperger's syndrome to comprehend humorous material. Typical subjects and subjects with HFA or AS were required to choose funny endings for cartoons and jokes. For cartoon and joke tasks combined, adolescents with autism performed significantly more poorly than typical adolescents. Martin and McDonald (2004) found that individuals with Asperger's syndrome performed significantly more poorly than controls on tasks requiring the interpretation of ironic jokes. AS subjects were more likely to conclude that the protagonist in stories was lying than telling an ironic joke.

5   The cognitive substrates of acquired pragmatic disorders

5.1   Introduction

Explanations of acquired pragmatic disorders in adults are increasingly adopting some of the same theoretical constructs that have been used to account for developmental pragmatic disorders in children. As the discussion in Chapter 3 demonstrates, growing numbers of empirical studies are examining ToM impairments and executive dysfunction in a range of adult clinical subjects. Even more importantly for our present purposes, these studies are increasingly attempting to relate these cognitive deficits to various aspects of pragmatic language function (or dysfunction). The clinical rationale for these studies is clear enough. Developmental models have limited application to the study of acquired impairments of cognition and pragmatics in adults who have previously undergone normal development of these capacities. The autistic child who has failed to develop a theory of other minds, either in whole or in part, is certainly undertaking pragmatic language learning against a background of significant neurocognitive compromise. Yet, this child's neurocognitive status is likely to differ in marked ways from that of the adult who has acquired brain damage and who has extensive experience prior to the onset of injury or disease of the type of mental state attribution that is integral to pragmatic interpretation. Langdon *et al.* (2002) caution against the use of developmental models to understand acquired cognitive and pragmatic impairments in adults when they state that:

Evidence of a link between poor mind-reading and poor pragmatics in an early-onset neurodevelopmental disorder such as autism may potentially say more about the role that normal mind-reading ability plays in the *acquisition* of a normal understanding of pragmatic uses of language than it does about the role that normal mind-reading ability plays in the *on-line* processes that underpin pragmatic uses of language in developed adults ... it is important to find out whether the link between poor mind-reading and poor pragmatics that holds for autism also holds for an acquired neurological disorder, such as that following stroke damage, or a late-onset neurodevelopmental/ neurodegenerative disorder, such as schizophrenia. (75–6)

In this chapter, we examine what is known about the cognitive substrates of acquired pragmatic disorders. This area of clinical pragmatics is still very much a fledgling study. A number of factors are responsible for the largely undeveloped state of our knowledge of the cognitive substrates of pragmatic disorders in adults. First, the type of theoretical advances that are required to support progress in this area have been quite limited to date. One such advance is the development of what Carston *et al.* (2002) have described as 'a cognitively plausible pragmatic theory' (1). In a collection of papers to emanate from a workshop on Pragmatics and Cognitive Science held in September 2000, Carston *et al.* convey something of the extent of the problem when they remark that:

The aim of the workshop was to broaden the understanding of pragmatics in the cognitive science community and to encourage interdisciplinary research on verbal communication. Until quite recently, the study of verbal communication was approached primarily from a philosophical or sociological perspective, and there was little attempt to construct a cognitively plausible pragmatic theory. (2002: 1)

Until such time as cognitively plausible pragmatic theories are forthcoming,[1] it is difficult to see how any substantial progress can be made on questions relating to the cognitive substrates of pragmatic disorders.[2] Second, if pragmatic theories are not cognitively plausible, it is at least as true to say that cognitive theories are not pragmatically plausible. It is often the case that when theorists devise cognitive models to explain symptoms in disorders such as schizophrenia, for example, that impairments of pragmatics (or even communication in general) are overlooked or, at least, are not afforded the same explanatory emphasis as positive symptoms such as delusions and hallucinations.[3] However, cognitive impairments in schizophrenia such as mentalising (ToM) deficits are as likely to have implications for communication as for delusions, as the following extract from Langdon and Coltheart (1999) clearly demonstrates:

If patients cannot reflect on beliefs as representations of reality, then the distinction between subjectivity and objectivity collapses, leading to maintenance of delusions. If patients cannot mentalise about the unique subjective point of view of others, then they will make no allowance for others' knowledge when planning to communicate and they will fail to monitor for signs of listener confusion ... if patients cannot represent the intentional instigation of their own actions, as distinct from monitoring subsequent action in the world once those intentions have been realised, then actions will be experienced with no accompanying sense of self-generation, leading to delusions of alien control. (44–5)

If, as I am claiming, cognitive theories of neurodegenerative and other late-onset disorders are largely being developed in isolation from communicative and pragmatic concerns, then it is unsurprising that these theories should be so poorly equipped to explain the pragmatic impairments that are found in schizophrenic adults or in patients with right-hemisphere damage, for example. One consequence of cognitive theories being developed in a communicative vacuum was discussed in Chapter 4, where we examined how

experimental ToM studies had misrepresented the essential character of pragmatic phenomena such as implicatures. However, an altogether more pernicious consequence of the tendency of cognitive theorising to be conducted in
isolation from pragmatic concerns is that this theorising is unable to generate
the type of testable hypotheses that would advance our knowledge of the
cognitive substrates of acquired pragmatic disorders. Hypothesis testing in
cognitive science has produced considerable gains in our understanding of
several language disorders (e.g. aphasia and dyslexia). The widespread lack
of hypothesis testing on the question of the cognitive basis of pragmatic disorders is a real impediment to progress in this area that should be of genuine
concern to cognitive theorists.

Notwithstanding the lack of cognitive and pragmatic plausibility of pragmatic and cognitive theories, respectively, we will endeavour in this chapter
to examine what is known about the cognitive basis of acquired pragmatic
disorders in adults. We begin by considering the different theoretical positions
that have been suggested by findings of cognitive deficits in the adult clinical
populations that were examined in Chapter 3. Some of these positions have
greater initial plausibility than other positions in a causal explanation of pragmatic disorders in adults. For example, the cognitive ability to recognise and
manipulate mental states that is integral to theory-theory, or metarepresenta-
tion, accounts of mentalising is a more general case of the scenario that obtains
when a listener recovers a speaker's communicative intention in producing a
particular utterance (communicative intentions, after all, are simply another
type of mental state like belief and knowledge).[4] As such, it is relatively easy to
see a role for theory-theory accounts in an explanation of acquired pragmatic
disorders (even if the question of the exact nature of that role – a domain-
specific cognitive module or some non-modularised process – is altogether less
straightforward). For each cognitive theory that will be examined, we consider
its likely relevance to an explanation of pragmatic disorders in the adult clinical populations that were surveyed in Chapter 3. In the absence of specific
theoretical proposals about the form that such an explanation might take, or
even a substantial basis in empirical facts, some of these deliberations are of
necessity speculative in nature (at this initial stage of enquiry, we are still at a
loss to say with complete certainty exactly what are the acquired impairments
of pragmatics that we need to explain and whether cognitive deficits have a
direct, causal role in such an explanation or a more indirect role through their
influence on other factors that impact upon pragmatics). However, speculation
can still involve rational guesswork based upon our best knowledge in other
domains (pragmatic interpretation in normal subjects, cognitive deficits in neurodevelopmental disorders such as autism, etc.). It is hoped that these deliberations will be judged worthwhile by the reader as much for what they can tell
us about the direction that should be taken by future research in this area as for

the summary that they provide of the different theoretical possibilities that are currently on offer.

5.2   Pragmatic theory

A sensible place to begin an examination of the cognitive substrates of acquired pragmatic disorders is to consider the views of pragmatists on the different types of processes that are involved in utterance interpretation. In discussing their respective views, these pragmatists have made more or less explicit claims about the type of cognitive architecture upon which these processes are dependent. At least some of these pragmatists[5] subscribe to the dominant cognitive scientific view of the mind that is generally attributed to Jerry Fodor and his modularity thesis, or some version thereof.[6] Almost without exception, these pragmatists have based their claims on theoretical arguments about the nature of pragmatic concepts. So in an important respect, these claims lack essential validation in terms of the type of psychological processes that are involved in the interpretation of utterances by normal language users.[7] Even less have these pragmatic theories been used to account for the range of pragmatic disorders in adults that we described in Chapter 3. This general lack of empirical validation has implications for the type of discussion that can be conducted in this section. Rather than base claims about acquired pragmatic disorders on clinically validated pragmatic frameworks, we can at best discuss which (if any) of these frameworks offers the greatest possibility of an explanation of these disorders. In saying this, I am not subscribing to a sceptical view in which we must relinquish the ambition of describing what a clinically valid pragmatic theory might look like. Instead, my aim is to point researchers in the direction of where I believe such a clinically valid theory may lie.

Carston (2002: 141) describes three positions on the pragmatic systems that are believed to be involved in utterance interpretation:

[1] The various different pragmatic tasks are performed by processes that comprise a single system, which takes decoded linguistic meaning as its input and delivers the propositions communicated (explicatures and implicatures).

[2] There is a crucial split between the processes involved in deriving explicit utterance content, on the one hand, and the processes of implicature derivation, on the other, with the two sets of processes each belonging to a distinct cognitive system, the output of the first (explicature or 'what is said') being the input to the second.

[3] There are distinct processes for at least some of the (conceptually) distinct pragmatic tasks (disambiguation, indexical reference assignment, recovery

of unarticulated constituents, speech act assignment, etc.) and each of these distinct processes is performed by a distinct cognitive system.

These positions, Carston argues, are held by different pragmatists: position [1] by Sperber and Wilson; position [2] by, amongst others, Grice, Levinson and Recanati; and position [3] by Kasher. In Cummings (2005), I challenged Sperber and Wilson's relevance theory and Kasher's views on the modularity of pragmatics on independent philosophical grounds. Specifically, I argued that neither theoretical standpoint could adequately capture the true nature of pragmatic phenomena given their adherence to the dominant cognitive scientific (modular) view of our mental architecture. In the present context, I do not wish to revisit those arguments. Rather, I want to consider the particular features of positions [1] and [3] that are consistent with our current best knowledge of pragmatic disorders in adults in the hope that ultimately these accounts will be able to tell us as much about pragmatics in the disordered case as in the case of the normal language user. To this end, we begin with an examination of Sperber and Wilson's (1995) relevance theory.

5.2.1   Relevance theory

As Carston's characterisation under [1] indicates, relevance theory posits a single pragmatic comprehension system that is responsible for generating both the explicatures (explicitly communicated propositions) and implicatures of an utterance. This system is guided by an overarching principle of relevance which has both communicative and cognitive applications:

Relevance, as we see it, is a potential property of external stimuli (e.g. utterances, actions) or internal representations (e.g. thoughts, memories) which provide input to cognitive processes. (Sperber and Wilson 2002: 14)

This principle confers a certain legitimacy and order on an individual's processing of communicative stimuli (utterances) on the one hand and internal representations on the other hand. To the extent that speakers are aiming to produce maximally relevant utterances,[8] listeners are justified in arriving at an interpretation of these utterances that satisfies their expectations of relevance. The cognitive mechanisms that permit such interpretation would have poor survival value[9] for humans if they were not somehow geared up towards maximising the relevance of the information that they process. After all, a relevant interpretation is the interpretation that the speaker most likely intended his listener to understand, i.e. it is a *true* representation of what the speaker intended to convey. Yet, the maximisation of relevance must be balanced against the costs of achieving such relevance – a relevant interpretation or other representation that has been extremely costly to obtain will use valuable cognitive resources with little overall gain in a person's representation of the world. Relevance must therefore be constructed along cost–benefit lines:

The relevance of an input for an individual at a given time is a positive function of the cognitive benefits that he would gain from processing it, and a negative function of the processing effort needed to achieve these benefits. (Sperber and Wilson 2002: 14)

This relevance-guided comprehension procedure can be demonstrated as follows. Consider the following exchange in which Rob and Pete discuss the recent divorce of a mutual friend Bill:

ROB: Did Bill have an easy divorce?
PETE: He went through a minefield!

A number of attributes in Rob's concept of a minefield are activated by Pete's use of the word in his response to Rob. Some of these attributes will receive more activation than others based upon features of the context. For example, Rob's use of the word 'divorce' in his question to Pete has the effect of raising the accessibility of those attributes that describe emotional upset and turmoil. The different attributes that are activated in Rob's concept of a minefield give rise to possible implications of Pete's utterance:

(a) Bill has experienced considerable psychological distress.
(b) Bill has confronted protracted and difficult legal issues.
(c) Bill has incurred severe financial penalties.
(d) Bill has limited access to his children.
(e) Bill has been exposed to considerable danger during conflict.
(f) Bill is lucky to be alive and not seriously injured.
(g) Bill has shown considerable heroism in the face of grave danger.

Rob's relevance-theoretic comprehension procedure leads him to consider these implications, starting with (a) and terminating with (d), when presumably there are no further contextual effects to be gained from the continued relevance processing of Pete's utterance. Implications (a) to (d) are consistent with the metaphorical interpretation of Pete's utterance, the interpretation that Pete intended Rob to derive from his utterance. However, if the exchange between Rob and Pete took the following form:

ROB: Why did Bill receive a military honour?
PETE: He went through a minefield!

then Rob could be expected to access the above implications in an altogether different order. Specifically, (g) may be the most accessible implication, while implication (a) may be least accessible. Rob's relevance-theoretic comprehension procedure would lead him to process implications (e), (f) and (g) – implications that are consistent with a literal interpretation of Pete's utterance – at which point his expectations of relevance would be satisfied and further relevance processing ceases. The altogether less accessible implications (a) to (d) would not be processed, as to process these implications would incur cognitive costs in excess of any cognitive gains that could be achieved through contextual effects. In both cases, Rob has successfully established the intended meaning of Pete's utterance through the observance (admittedly subconscious) of the following two-step procedure:

(a) Follow a path of least effort in computing cognitive effects. In particular, test interpretive hypotheses (disambiguations, reference resolutions, implicatures, etc.) in order of accessibility.
(b) Stop when your expectations of relevance are satisfied (Sperber and Wilson 2002: 18).

The relevance-theoretic comprehension procedure just outlined is located, according to Sperber and Wilson, in a dedicated module that is a specialisation of a more general mindreading module.[10] The advantage of such a modular mechanism is that it can exploit certain regularities within its domain that are not afforded to a general inferential capacity such as Fodor's central system:

A general-purpose inferential mechanism can only derive conclusions based on the formal (logical or statistical) properties of the input information it processes. By contrast, a dedicated inferential mechanism or module can take advantage of regularities in its specific domain, and use inferential procedures which are justified by these regularities, but only in this domain. (Sperber and Wilson 2002: 9)

Sperber and Wilson explicitly set their proposals for a relevance-theoretic comprehension procedure against the two dominant theories of mindreading, the rationalisation (or 'theory-theory') account and simulation theory (to be examined in section 5.3.1.2): 'we want to argue that neither the rationalisation nor the simulation view of mind-reading adequately accounts for the hearer's ability to retrieve the speaker's meaning' (Sperber and Wilson 2002: 10). Their arguments against these cognitive theories, both of which will be examined in section 5.3, are beyond the scope of the current discussion. What we are concerned to consider now is whether certain features of relevance theory are able to account for what we know about pragmatic deficits in adults. Also, we want to discover if the theory is able to generate certain testable predictions that could be the basis of future experimental work in pragmatically impaired adults.

As we have seen, Sperber and Wilson's relevance-theoretic comprehension procedure makes two specific claims about the order in which hypotheses about the speaker's intended meaning should be processed. The first of these claims is that highly accessible interpretive hypotheses are first to be 'tested', while less accessible hypotheses will incur excessively large processing costs for any contextual effects that they may produce and are unlikely to undergo

relevance processing. The second claim is that this process of hypothesis testing should cease as soon as a listener's expectations of relevance are satisfied.
While this situation may reflect the position of the normal language user, it is
conceivable that it may be disrupted in one of several ways in the pragmatically impaired adult. Such an adult may lack the interpretive flexibility shown
by Rob in the above exchanges. Specifically, he may be unable to vary the
order in which he sets about testing interpretive hypotheses or even generate
certain hypotheses. In the latter case, the dominant (literal) meaning of a word
such as 'minefield' may make implications (e) to (g) accessible to the complete
exclusion of implications (a) to (d).[11] The literal interpretation of the utterance
'He went through a minefield!' would be understood by such an adult, even in
cases where the metaphorical interpretation is intended by the speaker. Such a
scenario appears to account for what we know about utterance interpretation
in the case of schizophrenic patients. There is now clear experimental evidence that schizophrenic adults are unable to use linguistic context to prime
non-dominant meanings of words (Bazin *et al.* 2000; Sitnikova *et al.* 2002).
One can imagine how these adults would be unable to use the word 'divorce'
in Rob's question to Pete to make the non-dominant (metaphorical) meaning
of 'minefield' more accessible than the dominant (literal) meaning of the same
word. If schizophrenic adults are unable to generate implications such as (a) to
(d) above, then it is unsurprising that they should fail to recover the intended
metaphorical interpretation of Pete's response and draw instead the unintended
literal interpretation of the same utterance.

As well as being unable to generate certain interpretive hypotheses, it
appears likely that some pragmatically impaired adults are also unable to
comply with the second aspect of Sperber and Wilson's relevance-theoretic
comprehension procedure: the requirement to stop testing interpretive hypotheses as soon as expectations of relevance are satisfied. For such an individual,
expectations of relevance would not be satisfied by any of the implications (a)
to (g) above. Indeed, as relevance processing proceeds, a series of ever more
implausible implications would be processed for their contextual effects. Not
only will this processing incur considerable costs for this individual for little
or no return in contextual effects, but it will take him or her steadily further
away from the speaker's intended meaning in producing a particular utterance. Such a scenario appears to characterise patients with the paranoid subtype of schizophrenia.[12] The paranoid schizophrenic patient, as Langdon *et
al.* (2002) emphasise, can certainly attribute intentions to other people. Such
an individual would have little difficulty, for example, in understanding that
a speaker can entertain thoughts and beliefs that are both different from his
or her own and that are the opposite of utterances that are expressed (e.g. the
speaker who produces the ironic utterance 'What a delightful child!' in the
presence of a disruptive five-year-old believes that the child is *not* delightful).

However, a pathological situation obtains when this possibility – the possibility that a speaker is entertaining thoughts and beliefs that differ from his expressed utterances – is pursued to an implausible and irrational extent (e.g. the speaker who believes that the person who utters 'What a delightful child!' is making some reference to the listener's own negative childhood experiences rather than merely producing an ironic utterance). Langdon *et al.* capture this situation as follows:

Schizophrenic patients who fail theory-of-mind tasks are not unable to represent people's mental states. These individuals know that people have beliefs and intentions and they are perfectly capable of representing that other people can believe things that differ from what they themselves believe. Indeed, they are often very adept at concealing their own beliefs from other people. If anything, these individuals can sometimes over-attribute intentions. A paranoid schizophrenic patient who believes that other people are harbouring hostile or persecutory thoughts about him or her (common in schizophrenia) can hardly be thought of as someone with an *inability* to represent the mental states of others. (84; italics in original)

Clearly, the over-attribution of intentions to others by the paranoid individual has special significance for a pragmatic theory of utterance interpretation. Indeed, Cram and Hedley (2005) have already characterised this behaviour in relevance-theoretic terms. The paranoid individual, these theorists argue, will not stop relevance processing[13] when an ironic interpretation of the above utterance has been obtained. Rather, this individual will continue to process the speaker's utterance with a view to establishing some other, ulterior intention on the part of the speaker. Cram and Hedley use the term 'praeter-relevance' to describe such cases of pragmatic overshoot:

What we would like to focus on ... is the polar complement to such cases of pragmatic deficit, namely cases of paranoid delusion (and more specifically, non-bizarre paranoid delusion), where an individual overshoots rather than undershoots in the interpretation of an utterance ... In cases of paranoid interpretation ... an individual will indeed first arrive at an intended ironic reading, but typically will not stop there: an ulterior intention will be suspected and a further level of implicated meaning will be constructed. We should like to propose the term 'praeter-relevance' as a linguistic (rather than a clinical) identifier for such cases of pragmatic overshoot, on the hypothesis that the overshoot is guided by the same pragmatic principles as apply to the interpretation of utterances elsewhere. (2005: 199)

We have considered how a specific component of Sperber and Wilson's relevance-theoretic comprehension procedure, when disrupted in a schizophrenic speaker, may lead to a failure in generating certain interpretive hypotheses (usually metaphorical, ironic and other non-literal hypotheses). When another component of the same procedure is disrupted, a schizophrenic speaker may exhibit an inability to cease the relevance processing of utterances. A relevance-theoretic explanation of pragmatic deficits in schizophrenic patients appears to receive some degree of validation from what we know about how schizophrenia presents in sufferers (these patients typically experience paranoia, for example) and from the results of experimental studies (e.g. Bazin *et al.* 2000). However, it is nevertheless the case that substantial empirical investigation is needed to validate the claims that have been made in this section. Langdon *et al.*'s (2002) study of the understanding of non-literal speech in schizophrenic patients is an excellent example of the type of study that is needed to expose pragmatic theory (in this case, relevance theory) to rigorous testing in clinical subjects.[14] These investigators base certain predictions about the understanding of metaphor and irony in schizophrenic patients on the relevance-theoretic distinction between metaphor as a descriptive use of language, and irony as an interpretive use of language. Specifically, they predict that schizophrenic patients will show greater impairment in the understanding of irony than in the understanding of metaphor because the interpretation of irony requires more complex mindreading skills (the ability to attribute second-order mental states) than those required for the interpretation of metaphor – the latter, Langdon *et al.* claim, 'requires some appreciation that the speaker is capable of having thoughts about the world, [but] it is far from clear that it requires the kinds of abilities that are assessed by typical theory-of-mind tasks' (83). These relevance-theoretic predictions were confirmed.[15] Moreover, metaphor and irony hit rates made highly significant and independent contributions to predicting the odds of being a patient, which indicated that impairment of different cognitive processes caused these patients' difficulties understanding metaphorical and ironical speech.

5.2.2   Modular pragmatics

In the concluding section of his paper 'Pragmatics and the modularity of mind', Kasher (1991a) proposes the following 'basic formula of the modular structure of pragmatics' (579):

Pragmatics in the mind = a pragmatic module
+ a pragmatic part of the centre
+ pragmatic interface

This tripartite formula derives from the examination of six pragmatic phenomena: deixis; lexical pragmatic presuppositions; forces (of speech acts); performatives; conversational implicatures; and politeness principles. Specifically, it is argued that speech acts indicate the need for a pragmatic module that is linguistic in nature; conversational implicatures and politeness principles suggest the presence of a pragmatic component in the mind's central system; and indexicals and lexical pragmatic presuppositions provide evidence for an interface between the pragmatic module and the pragmatic part of the central system. In this section, we examine the arguments that Kasher advances to support the involvement of different cognitive processes in these various pragmatic phenomena. We then consider what, if any, relevance Kasher's proposals hold for the study of pragmatic deficits in clinical subjects.

Kasher uses the case of speech acts in general, and indirect speech acts in particular, to argue for the existence of a pragmatic module in the mind. This module, he argues, is responsible for the syntactic and semantic processing of utterances, from which their literal force is obtained. However, to account for the frequently observed phenomenon that the intended force of many speech acts differs from the force that is encoded in language – for example, that the declaration 'It's warm in here' often has the force of an indirect request (possibly to have the heating turned down), as opposed to the force of an assertion – the literal forces of utterances go forward as presumptions to the central system.[16] In this system, they interact with beliefs about the speaker's communicative intentions, with the result that some presumptions survive – that is, the literal force of an utterance comes to stand as its intended force – other presumptions are rejected, and still other presumptions are used and then rejected:

The linguistic modules determine a literal force using the syntactic properties of the utterance under analysis and the semantic properties of lexical or other elements of the utterance ... these literal forces are taken by the related central device to presumably be the forces of the utterances under consideration ... many of the presumptions that the linguistic modules create for the central systems of understanding are left intact by it: the force of many declarative sentences, for example, is that of assertion. On other occasions these presumptions are not retained, because beliefs available to the central device are found to be incompatible with them ... On still other occasions, the input presumption with respect to the force of a given utterance is not discarded but rather used and dismissed. (Kasher 1991a: 576)

The operation of conversational implicatures and politeness principles, Kasher argues, suggests the presence of a quite different cognitive mechanism: not a pragmatic module as in speech acts, but a central cognitive system. Kasher places an often neglected Gricean point at the centre of his account of conversational implicatures. It is frequently overlooked in discussions of implicatures that Grice intended his cooperative principle and maxims to form the communicative subcase of a more general principle of rational action:

The philosophical foundations on which Grice's theory of conversational implicature rests is a general theory of rational action. (Kasher 1991a: 577)

Applied to the domain of action, rationality consists in a principle of effective means. This principle amounts to the claim that a rational agent chooses those actions that most effectively, and with minimal cost, achieve particular ends. It is impossible to circumscribe the range of factors that may play a part in an agent's choice of such an action. For this reason, Kasher locates this general rationality principle (and the conversational implicatures that rest on this principle) within the mind's central system:

> Obviously, our principles of general rationality and of effective means are not domain specific in any reasonable sense and hence, if they constitute the principles of operation of some mental device, then the latter must be a central cognitive system which employs the former principle in forming beliefs and in planning action, not only when language plays an overt role. (Kasher 1991a: 147)

The appropriate application of politeness principles, Kasher contends, demands knowledge of a range of factors within the context of utterance. Kasher cites Leech in this regard, who claims of these principles 'their relative weights will vary from one cultural, social, or linguistic milieu to another' (1983: 150). Such is the context-dependence of these principles that Kasher locates them within the operation of a central system:

> The information required by a speaker s for applying politeness maxims to s's own speech could not be considered encapsulated in any interesting sense. What regulates certain aspects of speech and understanding are, then, principles by which some central cognitive system operates on varied data. (1991a: 578–9)

According to Kasher, two pragmatic phenomena suggest the existence of interfaces in the mind. Indexical expressions, such as 'she' and 'here', reveal, he argues, a complex set of interface features between language and perception modules on the one hand and the central system on the other hand:

> Indexicals ... involve the output of a language module and its integration with some output of a perception module, where both serve as input for the same central cognitive device which produces the integrated understanding of what has been said in a given context of utterance. (1991a: 579)

In this way, the referent of 'she' in an utterance is not determined by the operation of some language module alone. Even if such a module did exist and contained the knowledge that 'she' refers to a human female – at least this much of the reference of 'she' is acquired when we master English – the identification of this individual depends on the operation of a central device which, importantly in this case, has access to information from a perception module. The cognitive specification of pragmatic presuppositions is revealing of Kasher's second pragmatic interface: 'Lexical pragmatical presuppositions involve another type of interface between a language module and ... central device' (1991a: 579). Specifically, the language module establishes the contribution to these presuppositions of certain lexical items within utterances:

> Though the output of such a cognitive module is an intermediate representation it might be of some theoretical significance, marking the analytical, lexical contribution to the specification of pragmatic presuppositions. (1991a: 575)

What an informationally encapsulated pragmatic module cannot explain, Kasher contends, is that range of beliefs that come ultimately to play a part in the defeasibility of presuppositions. This feature of presuppositions suggests the operation of a central device within a complete specification of the presuppositions that attend an utterance:

> Thus, the most a module can do in service of the process of specifying the lexical pragmatic presuppositions in a context of utterance and understanding is to provide input for some central cognitive device which is to use both this input and the classes of present beliefs, assumptions and the like, as grounds for establishing the current class of pragmatic presuppositions. (1991a: 575)

A number of testable hypotheses are readily suggested by Kasher's claims regarding the modularity of pragmatics. First, to the extent that certain pragmatic phenomena depend on the same cognitive processes, one could reasonably expect to find these phenomena jointly impaired in certain clinical subjects. If it was discovered, for example, that certain clinical subjects had marked deficits using and recovering conversational implicatures, but exhibited normal use of politeness principles, then Kasher's claim that both phenomena are mediated by a pragmatic component in the mind's central system would begin to look decidedly weak. The finding of a double dissociation[17] in these pragmatic abilities would be particularly devastating to Kasher's claims. Second, to the extent that certain pragmatic phenomena (e.g. indirect speech acts) are conventional in character and exhibit the type of linguistic regularities that can be handled by a domain-specific pragmatic module, we might expect to find impairments of these phenomena in subjects with language disorders (e.g. aphasia). This second hypothesis can be extended into a claim about the neuroanatomical location of a pragmatic module. For if a particular type of (modular) pragmatic impairment is more likely to be found in subjects with a language disorder such as aphasia, then we might reasonably conclude that the brain's left hemisphere (the location of the language centres that are damaged in aphasia) may also be the location of a pragmatic module. We will see below that these particular hypotheses receive considerable validation from recent experimental studies that have been conducted by Kasher and his coworkers. Third, to the extent that the output of a modular pragmatic capacity acts as input to a central pragmatic capacity, we might expect to find some correlation between modular and central pragmatic phenomena in clinical subjects. If the output of a pragmatic module (the input to the central system) is degraded in the presence of brain damage, for example, one might expect to find related impairments of central pragmatic functions. The absence of such a relationship would suggest a greater level of functional independence between modular and central pragmatic capacities than is suggested by Kasher's framework. We consider each of these hypotheses further below.

The type of empirical findings that are needed to address the first hypothesis above have been stubbornly slow to emerge from the clinical literature. Specifically, we need to be able to show that certain pragmatic impairments occur 'in clusters' in clinical subjects according to the modular or central processes that are believed to mediate these pragmatic abilities in the normal subject. By the same token, we need evidence that if certain areas of pragmatic functioning are preserved in clinical subjects, that these areas of preserved ability occur along the lines of the distinction between modular and central processes that is integral to Kasher's framework. However, such evidence is not readily forthcoming. If the ability to compute conversational implicatures and to observe politeness principles is truly mediated by central pragmatic processes, then some covariation in these abilities may be expected. In other words, the subject who struggles to recover the intended implicature of an utterance should also be expected to experience difficulty observing politeness constraints on the use of language. However, while a growing number of studies are testing the use and understanding of implicatures by clinical subjects, the same cannot be said of politeness principles. Experimental and qualitative studies have almost completely neglected to examine how adults with acquired pragmatic disorders negotiate considerations of politeness in a range of conversational interactions. The same can be said of other pragmatic phenomena (e.g. lexical pragmatic presuppositions) that are central to components within Kasher's framework (in the case of presuppositions, a pragmatic interface). Quite simply, in the absence of research on how these various pragmatic phenomena are used by a range of clinical subjects, it is difficult to make much progress on the first of the three hypotheses considered above.

Thus far, we have established that it is not yet possible to say if groups of pragmatic phenomena are disordered or preserved along the modular and central lines that are integral to Kasher's framework. If certain pragmatic phenomena are jointly mediated by a pragmatic module or by a pragmatic component of the mind's central system, then we would expect all modular phenomena and all central phenomena to be either disordered or preserved in clinical subjects. The finding that one central pragmatic concept (e.g. conversational implicature) was impaired while another central pragmatic concept (e.g. politeness) was preserved, we argued, would be damaging to Kasher's view of the modularity of pragmatics. If basic research on politeness, lexical pragmatic presuppositions and other pragmatic phenomena (e.g. indexicals) in a range of clinical subjects has not yet been conducted to the extent that is necessary to examine the types of pragmatic skills that are jointly impaired or preserved in these subjects, then maybe there is some other way in which the pragmatic phenomena that Kasher assigns to different pragmatic competences can be examined. For example, putting politeness principles aside, if it can be demonstrated that pragmatic phenomena such as conversational implicatures vary with other capacities of the mind's central system, specifically, its mind-reading capacity, then surely Kasher's framework receives some initial validation from this fact. The difficulty here is that few studies have attempted to relate in any direct way the ToM (mentalising, mindreading) abilities of clinical subjects with their performance on tasks involving the use and understanding of conversational implicatures, for example. In fact, of all the studies reported in Chapter 3 that attempted to examine ToM skills in adults, only five have in any way related those skills to pragmatic phenomena – Brüne and Bodenstein (2005) and Champagne-Lavau et al. (2006) in schizophrenic adults, McDonald and Flanagan (2004) in TBI adults, Cuerva et al. (2001) in adults with Alzheimer's disease and Winner et al. (1998) in RHD adults. Once again, there is an inadequate empirical basis for allocating some pragmatic phenomena to a pragmatic central system, while others are allocated to a pragmatic module (and even others to a pragmatic interface).

It might be instructive at this juncture to step back and ask why so few of the very large number of empirical studies of pragmatics that have been conducted in clinical subjects are unable to address the type of theoretical concerns that we have been addressing in this section. The answer is that these studies have been undertaken in a largely ad hoc fashion. It is not an exaggeration to say that in the last thirty years, few studies that have examined pragmatic impairments in adults (or indeed children) have had a clear theoretical rationale. The result has been a large collection of studies that report all sorts of pragmatic deficits without any explanation of how one pragmatic deficit relates to any other pragmatic deficit. For example, if certain pragmatic phenomena are all mediated by a pragmatic module or by a pragmatic central system, it would be virtually impossible to discern such a pattern across a set of studies that often don't even appear to be describing the same pragmatic behaviours. In fairness to investigators, there has been a noticeable lack of pragmatic theory with which to drive empirical studies. Theorists' frameworks have often been too abstract in nature to derive any testable predictions or have appeared to lack relevance to the study of clinical subjects. It is still often the case that we don't have clear theoretical models of the pragmatic phenomena that clinical researchers are attempting to investigate. Kasher has been quick to make this very point in relation to metaphor, sarcasm and humour:

In the absence of appropriate theories of metaphor, sarcasm and humor, for example, it is not clear what exactly is being tested. Moreover, without better understanding of each of these phenomena there seems to be no good reason for combining them to form a separate competence. (1991b: 393)

Some progress is undoubtedly being made in bridging this considerable theoretical–empirical gulf. Langdon et al. (2002) use relevance theory to make predictions about the understanding of irony and metaphor[18] in schizophrenic adults. However, such theoretically motivated studies are still a minority. It is not until such time as studies of this type become commonplace that we can expect to gain really significant insights into disordered pragmatics.

The second hypothesis introduced above has spawned a research agenda that has produced a number of interesting empirical findings. Kasher's argument in support of a pragmatic module rests on the supposition that certain pragmatic phenomena, such as speech acts, have a 'conventional' component that is mediated by the domain-specific linguistic processes of an input module. To the extent that this is the case, we may expect to find impairment of those phenomena in individuals with a language disorder such as aphasia. Also, if aphasic and other left-hemisphere damaged subjects display impairment of these conventional aspects of pragmatics, then it is at least reasonable to suppose that a pragmatic module is located in the brain's left hemisphere. This second hypothesis has received considerable confirmation from the findings of recent studies. Soroker *et al.* (2005) examined the processing of the basic speech acts of question, assertion, request and command in LHD and RHD patients. It is clear from how these investigators define these speech acts that they are the types of pragmatic phenomena that Kasher would locate within a modular pragmatic competence: 'Usually a [basic speech act] is performed by uttering a specific kind of sentence which is linguistically marked as appropriate for it' (2005: 215). In this study, a graded series of tasks was implemented in interactive situations to avoid the problem of creating an unnatural setting. These tasks assessed appreciation of the target speech acts, through comprehension of their meaning to the ability to produce them. Of the thirty-one LHD patients included in this study, twenty-nine had language problems of different kinds. Three findings from this study provide confirmatory evidence for our current hypothesis. First, an ANOVA of percent-correct responses that included group (LHD and RHD) and speech act (assertion, question, request, command) revealed a main effect of group, with LHD subjects displaying a significant disadvantage. Second, impairments of the four basic speech acts correlated significantly with the extent of damage in left perisylvian cortical regions. Third, for the LHD subjects, there were significant correlations between the four basic speech acts and almost all the components on the Hebrew version of the Western Aphasia Battery. Soroker *et al.* conclude that 'there is systematic localization of basic speech acts in the left hemisphere but not in the right hemisphere' (2005: 216).

The right hemisphere did not lack all involvement in the basic speech acts examined by Soroker *et al.* (2005). Production of requests showed a significant negative correlation with the extent of lesions in the right middle frontal gyrus. Nevertheless, the finding that basic speech acts are largely mediated by the left hemisphere is contrary to the widespread clinical view of the dominant role of the right hemisphere in natural language pragmatics.[19] To the extent that basic speech acts are fundamental to other more complex speech acts,[20] one might reasonably expect (prediction 1) to find some relationship between basic speech acts and the type of competence that enables a speaker to conversationally implicate a request (to have a window opened, for example) by means of uttering a statement ('It's warm in here'). Just such a relationship was established in a study of conversational implicatures in LHD and RHD patients by Kasher *et al.* (1999). According to Kasher's theoretical framework, conversational implicatures cannot be arrived at by means of a module. Rather, the recovery of implicatures depends on central cognitive processes:

> It is not assumed that implicatures are processed by a module. In particular, we do not posit that implicatures are processed by the Chomskian-Fodorian language module. On the contrary, according to Kasher's rationality framework for explaining Grice's maxims, implicatures are not created by a module but rather by the central cognitive system. (Kasher *et al.* 1999: 569)

To the extent that the central system is a general cognitive mechanism, one might reasonably expect (prediction 2) the ability to draw implicatures in these patients to vary with cognitive functions such as memory. Moreover, one might expect (prediction 3) to find no relationship between implicatures and more general language skills – if implicature processing occurs in a domain non-specific central system, then it should be dissociated from the linguistic processes of a domain specific language module. Also, the central system's lack of domain specificity might lead one to expect (prediction 4) no difference in how these subjects process verbal and nonverbal implicatures. These four predictions were largely borne out by the results of Kasher *et al.*'s study. In relation to the first prediction, most subtests of an implicatures battery[21] correlated positively and significantly with most subtests of a battery of basic speech acts in LHD patients. Also, both factors of the implicatures battery (verbal, nonverbal) correlated highly with all three factors of the basic speech act battery (verbal, nonverbal, execution-normative). While these findings suggest a relationship in the left hemisphere between the pragmatic competences that mediate basic speech acts and conversational implicatures (what Kasher terms a 'pragmatic processor'), the picture is more complicated in the right hemisphere. Only the nonverbal factors of both batteries correlated significantly in the RHD patients. This suggested 'the existence of several independent, material-specific means-ends pragmatic processors in the right hemisphere' (1999: 587).

The second prediction introduced above was also supported by Kasher *et al.*'s results. These investigators correlated patients' scores on the implicatures battery with scores on standardised neuropsychological tests.[22] These tests examined a number of the general cognitive functions (e.g. memory) that could be expected to reside in the central cognitive system, at least part of which Kasher believes to be responsible for the processing of implicatures.

The number of significant correlations reported by Kasher *et al.* was 20/40 and 16/40 in RHD and LHD patients, respectively. The presence of more significant correlations in RHD subjects, Kasher *et al.* argue, suggests that means-ends pragmatic processors in the right hemisphere are cognitive-specific. This finding thus serves to confirm the claim that 'implicatures are not governed by a modular system but rather by a "central" rationality process' (1999: 588). The third prediction was also upheld by Kasher *et al.*'s findings. To the extent that implicature processing takes place in a central cognitive system, one would not expect to find a correlation between subtests on the implicatures battery and more general language skills (the latter are mediated by a domain-specific language module). Indeed, no such correlation was found. In LHD subjects, only some implicatures correlated significantly with some language functions, as measured by the Hebrew version of the Western Aphasia Battery. These functions were naming, reading and writing. Correlations in RHD subjects were even weaker and involved different subtests. These results, Kasher *et al.* argue, suggest that the pragmatic processor in the left hemisphere does not extend 'to basic communicative abilities comprising standard aphasia batteries' (1999: 587). The fourth prediction – that a domain nonspecific central system would be equally adept at processing verbal and nonverbal implicatures – was also supported, at least in LHD subjects, by the findings of this study: 'Do implicatures share a set of basic cognitive mechanisms for performing unconventionalized means-ends analysis that are domain nonspecific and that apply to both the Verbal and Nonverbal Implicatures tests? There is good evidence for this in the LHD but not in the RHD patients' (1999: 587). Kasher *et al.* report that verbal and nonverbal implicatures intercorrelated highly in LHD subjects. However, this was not the case in RHD subjects, where there were strong correlations between verbal implicatures and between nonverbal implicatures but not between verbal and nonverbal implicatures. Kasher *et al.* conclude that the left hemisphere includes a general 'implicatures processor'.

Kasher *et al.*'s study can also help us address the third hypothesis that was introduced above. That hypothesis consisted in the claim that there is functional dependence between a central pragmatic capacity and a modular pragmatic capacity, in that the central system relies on a pragmatic module for its input. A corollary of this claim is that if the central system is receiving degraded input from an impaired pragmatic module, as may occur in subjects with brain damage, then impairments of central pragmatic phenomena such as conversational implicatures may be expected to vary with impairments of modular pragmatic phenomena such as speech acts. There is clear evidence of a functional relation between modular and central pragmatic capacities in at least some of the subjects in Kasher *et al.*'s study. For the LHD subjects in this study, most subtests of the implicatures battery correlated positively and significantly with most subtests of a battery of basic speech acts. Moreover, there was no relationship between the implicatures battery and general language skills, indicating that it was not a general language module that was providing input to the implicatures processor. Although Kasher *et al.*'s study did not examine the relationship between basic speech acts and general language skills in these LHD patients, we can reasonably predict on the basis of Soroker *et al.*'s findings that no such relationship would exist (Soroker *et al.* (2005) found no significant correlations between the four basic speech acts and a grammatical comprehension test in LHD subjects). In the absence of a language module providing input to the implicatures processor in the left hemisphere, the finding that there is no relationship between this module and the pragmatic competence that mediates basic speech acts, and the finding that implicatures are related to basic speech acts in LHD subjects, one might reasonably conclude that a discrete pragmatic module is functionally related to a central pragmatic capacity that is involved in the processing of implicatures in the left hemisphere. The third hypothesis generated by Kasher's framework is thus validated.

We have seen how Kasher's framework generates a number of interesting hypotheses about the neurocognitive basis of pragmatics, a significant number of which appear to be validated by the findings of recent empirical investigations. The type of systematic testing that this framework makes possible represents our best hope of making significant progress in addressing questions about the cognitive substrates of acquired pragmatic disorders. However, Kasher's framework is not without its difficulties. It will not have escaped the reader, for example, that different conceptions of the pragmatic input module are needed to support the second and third hypotheses considered above. In discussing the second hypothesis, there was a greater identification of the pragmatic module with a general language module than was the case when we examined the third hypothesis – in the latter, the pragmatic module was set apart from a language module. This reflects a deeper tension within Kasher's theory regarding the status of a pragmatic module. It cannot simply *be* the language module, as this is not supported by Soroker *et al.*'s finding that there is no significant correlation between basic speech acts (a function of the pragmatic module) and grammatical comprehension (a function of the language module) in LHD and RHD subjects. Also, such an identification would have the unfortunate consequence of making all pragmatic impairment (even central pragmatic impairments involving implicature, to the extent that the central system takes its input from a pragmatic module) secondary to language disorder. Yet, this does not conform with the clinical reality of pragmatic disorders – patients with poor structural language skills can have good pragmatic skills – or with results reported by Kasher *et al.* who found that patients' performance on an implicatures battery correlated most highly with aphasia tests other than Spontaneous Speech or Auditory Verbal Comprehension: this confirms, Kasher *et al.* argue, that 'the pragmatic deficit is not due to simple loss of basic language functions' (1999: 587). By the same token, the pragmatic module cannot be *entirely unrelated* to the language module. Such a pragmatic module could not explain Soroker *et al.*'s finding that there were significant correlations between all four basic speech acts in LHD subjects and almost all the components on the Western Aphasia Battery (Hebrew version). Also, it is clear that Kasher and his colleagues see the type of language functions that are tested by aphasia batteries as actually presupposing basic speech acts.[23] It would be difficult to envisage how this could be possible if the pragmatic input processes that mediate basic speech acts were not somehow related to other general language processes. Whatever is the solution to this tension and other difficulties in Kasher's framework, it is clear that in the attempt to address them, much will be revealed about the cognitive mechanisms that are involved in pragmatic disorders.

5.3   Cognitive theory

We have seen that pragmatic theories are still some way off providing an account of the cognitive basis of pragmatic disorders in adult subjects. Although these theories are increasingly generating hypotheses that are being tested in a range of clinical subjects, the focus of this research is still on the development of theoretical frameworks to explain pragmatics in normal subjects.[24] Clinical subjects have yet to move to the centre of theory construction, where they are not merely facilitating the development of accounts of normal pragmatics but they are the focus of theoretical explanation. Like pragmatic theories, cognitive theories have an important contribution to make to the development of an account of the cognitive substrates of pragmatic disorders. In section 5.1, we described how cognitive theories have largely been developed in a pragmatic vacuum. Not only do cognitive theorists display little appreciation of the types of phenomena that properly constitute pragmatics, but they also appear largely unaware of the significant contribution that cognitive theories can make to an explanation of pragmatic phenomena (see Chapter 4 for a similar point about cognitive theories in a developmental context). There is a very real sense in which cognitive theories may be said to lack pragmatic plausibility. It is only by fully engaging with cognitive theories, I believe, that pragmatists can hope to overcome this lack of pragmatic plausibility. We will see that discussions of cognitive theories in the context of adult clinical subjects have some interesting implications for the study of acquired pragmatic disorders. We will also see that pragmatics can play an important role in shaping those discussions. By encouraging a more dynamic, two-way exchange between pragmatics on the one hand and cognitive theory on the other hand, it is hoped that cognitive theories will begin to emerge over time as less pragmatically implausible after all.

5.3.1   Theory of mind theories

We saw in Chapter 3 how investigators are increasingly examining theory of mind (ToM) deficits in adults with acquired pragmatic disorders. However, in only very few of these cases has any attempt been made to relate pragmatic disorders to ToM deficits – in section 5.2.2, only five such studies were identified. This is all the more unusual when one considers that an ability to attribute mental states to others and to reason about those states is integral to pragmatic interpretation. It is clear that whatever lessons ToM theories hold for the study of pragmatic disorders, those lessons are still too abstract at the present time to be part of the routine explanations of pragmatic disorders by clinical investigators. Some consideration of ToM theories from a pragmatic perspective may well serve to establish greater relevance of these theories to those whose concerns are clinical in nature. We begin by examining the view that ToM skills are mediated by a cognitive module. Although this modular view is not the only contender to an explanation of theory of mind,[25] it is a position that has been growing in popularity in recent years. It is also consistent with the dominant cognitive scientific view of our mental architecture.[26] In this section, we examine what is involved in a modular account of ToM. We also discuss whether such an account is able to explain the type of mentalising abilities that must be exhibited by a speaker engaged in pragmatic interpretation. We then turn to consider the proposals of another theoretical perspective on theory of mind, those of simulation theory. In section 5.3.2, we consider the relationship of theory of mind to executive function skills in adults. We discuss whether the metarepresentational capacity that is ToM might not somehow be explained in terms of general executive function skills.

5.3.1.1   Modular ToM

In his discussion of the modularity of theory of mind, Segal (1996) draws a distinction between synchronic and diachronic modularity that is of relevance to our examination of ToM abilities in pragmatically disordered adults. In order to examine those abilities, we must first know something about ToM skills in the normal adult whose development is essentially complete. This is a different, though related, enterprise to examining how ToM develops in children over time. To the extent that fully acquired and developmental ToM capacities are both modular (this is, in effect, Segal's claim), Segal uses the terms 'synchronic' and 'diachronic' modularity of them, respectively. Segal goes on to examine four different notions of synchronic modularity which he uses to ground his discussion of the psychology faculty (what Segal calls the 'seat' of the psychological abilities that allow us to explain and predict our own and other people's actions on the basis of concepts such as belief and desire). While I do not wish to examine these four notions – intentional, computational, Fodor and neural modularity – in any detail, some consideration of their character is revealing of certain features of modular explanations of theory of mind. Moreover, if a ToM module is to play any role in an explanation of pragmatic interpretation, then we will need to ask if these same features reflect the essential characteristics of such interpretation. Segal begins his discussion of synchronic modularity by considering a feature of any psychological competence (he has in mind language and vision) that is to be given a modular explanation:

A precondition of any kind of modular explanation of the competence is that we have a reasonably clear idea of its domain of application ... These two domains of application [language and vision] are reasonably well demarcated and distinguishable from each other and from further cognitive domains. (1996: 142)

Clearly, for modular ToM theorists the psychology faculty is one such 'domain of application'. To the extent that modular status is being claimed for this faculty, it is relevant to ask how its demarcation from other cognitive domains is achieved. Demarcation is a function of certain restrictions on the flow of information between the psychology faculty (or psychology module) and other cognitive domains:

In particular, there may be a one- or two-way filter to information. In Jerry Fodor's (1983) terminology, intentional modules may be 'informationally encapsulated': some of the information in the subject's mind outside a given module may be unavailable to it ... And, going the other way, intentional modules may exhibit 'limited accessibility': some of the information within a module may be unavailable to consciousness ... I suggest that if a set of appropriately related psychological states exhibits either informational encapsulation or limited accessibility, then they constitute an intentional module. (Segal 1996: 143)

The features of informational encapsulation and limited accessibility, along with domain specificity, form the essence of a modular approach to ToM.[27] It is clear that Segal believes that the psychology faculty not only displays domain specificity and informational encapsulation but a number of other modular features besides.[28] He remarks that:

The psychology faculty certainly appears to be an intentional module. The faculty has a definite and self-contained body of knowledge that is framed in terms of a specific network of interrelated (and indeed, highly sophisticated and logically intriguing) concepts. Further, it appears to exhibit a degree of informational encapsulation. (1996: 147)

However, for our present purposes, a modular approach to ToM is only interesting to the extent that it can explain certain features of pragmatic interpretation. For example, a ToM module must be able to capture the relative ease with which a listener is able to draw upon beliefs about others' mental states in order to recover the implicature of an utterance. We will see that these beliefs are not domain specific or established in advance of interpretation, as they would have to be if they were mediated by the processes of a cognitive module. In fact, many of the beliefs that are integral to utterance interpretation are not even beliefs about our interlocutor's mental states (although, of course, many others are). We will also see that beliefs are revised, rejected and reinforced by a whole range of contingencies in the listener's environment and by other beliefs that are stored in memory or that are the product of more general inferential processes (not the specialised reasoning processes that are presumed to operate in a ToM module). It is difficult to see how these various contingencies and other beliefs can even get access to a ToM module, given its informational encapsulation. In the absence of such access, one cannot begin to imagine how a ToM module can capture the cancellability of implicatures and the defeasibility of presuppositions, for example. Yet these interpretive activities are effortlessly executed by most language users – we can readily identify when an implicature should undergo cancellation and the conditions under which a presupposition is defeasible. We examine each of these issues further below.

Consider the following exchange between Sam and Tom, in which Tom is bemoaning the state of the local park:

SAM: Do you come here often for a walk?
TOM: I hold down two jobs, so what do you think? It's not as nice as it used to be. Owners are letting their dogs foul the pavements and there's litter everywhere. It was local teenagers who vandalised the benches.
SAM: Actually, the benches are part of a modern art exhibition.

This exchange contains a number of features of pragmatic interest, all of which pose difficulties for a modular view of ToM. Clearly, Tom is implicating by way of his response 'I hold down two jobs' that he does not go to the park often for a walk. Sam is no doubt able to recover this implicature on the basis of several items of information, all of which must be salient to him and all of which must be brought together in a single processing environment. In this way, Sam must know that it is very time-consuming to do two jobs (item 1), that people who have two jobs have little spare time for leisure and other activities (item 2) and that walking in the park is a common leisure activity (item 3). Sam must also believe that Tom believes that doing two jobs is very time-consuming (item 4), that Sam will appreciate this fact (item 5) and that Sam will go on to conclude that Tom does not go for a walk in the park often (item 6). The first thing to notice about the items that have been listed here is that they are different types of knowledge. Items 1 to 3 are based on real-world knowledge. Item 4 is knowledge of Tom's belief states and is an example of first-order belief attribution. Items 5 and 6 are more complex still in that they involve second-order belief attribution – Sam believes that Tom believes that Sam believes that doing two jobs is very time-consuming. These different types of knowledge create a dilemma for a modular view of ToM which can be stated as follows. If

ToM truly is a domain-specific modular cognitive process that deals with certain types of knowledge (knowledge of mental states) to the exclusion of other types of knowledge (knowledge of the real world), then it will not have access to information that is vital in establishing the implicature of Tom's response (i.e. items 1 to 3). If, on the other hand, ToM does have access to knowledge other than that about mental states (i.e. items 1 to 3), then it does not exhibit the type of domain-specificity that is a feature of cognitive modules. In the absence of domain-specific knowledge, ToM cannot be a cognitive module.

A modular view of ToM has difficulty explaining another possible implicature of Tom's response to Sam in the above exchange. Tom may be taken to implicate that of course he goes to the park often for a walk – holding down two jobs is very stressful and he needs to go for regular walks in order to unwind. What makes this implicature less likely than the implicature we considered above is the rest of Tom's turn, in which he bemoans the poor state of the park. However, for this additional information to have any bearing on Sam's calculation of the implicature of Tom's utterance, it must be available to a ToM module. Yet, it is difficult to see how this can be the case, because only some of this information is even about Tom's mental states (i.e. Sam believes that Tom believes that the park is in a poor state). Other information based on visual perception (e.g. Sam can see litter everywhere) and retrieved from memory (e.g. Sam recalls a story in the local paper about residents' anger at the poor state of the park) is at least as likely to play a role in the recovery of Tom's implicature as any information based on Tom's mental states. Yet, this other information is unavailable to a ToM module, given its encapsulation from the cognitive processes of a visual perception module on the one hand and more general cognitive processes such as memory on the other hand. A similar difficulty surrounds the establishment of a referent for the spatially deictic expression 'here' in Sam's question. In this case, Tom will reason that Sam intends 'here' to refer to the place in which they are both physically situated (i.e. the park). So, clearly, some capacity on Tom's part to reason about Sam's mental states is required in order for Tom to establish the referent of 'here'. But in order to identify that referent as the park as opposed to, let's say, the children's play area in the park or a walled garden in the park, Tom must be able to process information gleaned from visual perception alongside information about Sam's mental states. Once again, it is difficult to see how this perceptual information can even get access to a ToM module, given the latter's encapsulation both from other cognitive modules and from more central cognitive processes.

Even if Sam had initially taken Tom to implicate that he went for walks in the park often, it is almost certain that Tom's further remarks about the poor state of the park would have brought about the cancellation of this particular implicature. Cancellability is not just an interesting feature of certain implicatures, but is a characteristic of utterance interpretation in general. Language users have little difficulty in assessing how new information relates to previously generated implicatures and in cancelling those implicatures when they are not consistent with that information. For example, Sam will readily determine that if Tom is unhappy about the state of the park, he is unlikely to want to spend much time in it. Sam will use this latter information to cancel his initial implicature that Tom often goes for walks in the park. In the same way, a presupposition of Tom's utterance 'It was local teenagers who vandalised the benches' is that Tom believes someone vandalised the benches. However, Tom will readily suspend his commitment to this presupposition when he learns from Sam that the 'vandalised' benches are actually part of a modern art exhibition. Language users have little difficulty in identifying the conditions under which presuppositions are defeated and implicatures are cancelled – the abilities that permit language users to make these identifications are simply part of our normal pragmatic competence. Yet, it is difficult to see how a ToM module, constrained as it is to process information relating to mental states, could even begin to simulate this competence. If it is discovered that what one had thought were vandalised benches are actually part of an art exhibition, this is not a discovery about a person's mental states, but a discovery about a state of affairs in the external world. It is exactly this world knowledge that Tom uses in order to reject his false belief that the benches have been vandalised. It is simply not conceivable that an informationally encapsulated ToM module has access to the world knowledge that Tom has so effortlessly drawn upon to defeat a presupposition of one of his utterances. It is equally inconceivable that this module could somehow recognise the real-world conditions that would have to exist to make Tom's belief about the benches false. Yet, without access to these conditions and this world knowledge, it is difficult to envisage how a ToM module can even begin to capture the interpretive processes at work in the defeasibility of presuppositions (equally, the cancellability of implicatures).

The reason that a ToM module is so vulnerable to objections of the type outlined above is that the modular view assumes that we can somehow demarcate in advance the knowledge that will be relevant to our deliberations concerning the mental states of others. But we have seen how information from a range of sources, including visual perception and memory, may not only be relevant to mental state reasoning, but may actually determine the outcome of that reasoning (such as occurred, for example, when Sam's perception that litter was lying everywhere in the park caused him to reconsider if Tom was in fact implicating that he often went for walks in the park). In short, mental state reasoning must be fully permeable to a whole range of cognitive processes and types of knowledge if it is to have any chance of capturing the competence that language users are drawing upon when they interpret speakers' utterances. Frye (2000) makes this same point when he describes Fodor's reasons for believing that the mind's central system must be informationally unencapsulated:

The reason that information cannot be restricted to domains is that we do not know in advance what is going to be related to what. The possibility that what is known in one domain can affect what is known in another is needed for scientific theorising, and it is similarly needed for the individual's understanding of the world. (2000: 150)

In the same way that Fodor does not believe it is possible to demarcate the knowledge that may be relevant to scientific theorising, I am arguing that we cannot circumscribe in advance of our interpretation of an utterance the knowledge that may be relevant to the interpretation of that utterance. However, unlike Fodor, who continues to support the existence of domain-specific cognitive modules (even if not as a model of how scientists develop theories), I believe that the lesson that we need to draw from the above considerations is that there is something inherently problematic about using cognitive modules to capture any aspect of our mental lives. This seems all the more true when that aspect involves something as fundamental as the ability to reason about the mental states of others, where notions such as belief and desire operate as part of a wider 'web' of knowledge (to use an expression of W.V.O. Quine). For further discussion of this point, the reader is referred to Chapter 5 in Cummings (2005).

5.3.1.2   Simulation theory   The view that ToM is a module is part of a 'theory-theory' explanation of theory of mind. Proponents of a 'theory-theory' explanation of ToM argue that our ability to establish the mental states of others and use those states to predict behaviour can be accounted for in terms of a folk psychological *theory* of minds.[29] Whether that theory is something comparable to a scientific theory (Gopnik[30]) or a cognitive module (Segal) is something that theory-theorists essentially disagree on. For simulation theorists, our mentalising abilities are not explained in terms of a theory, either developing as in children or fully acquired as in adults. Rather, when we simulate we are imaginatively projecting from our own mental activity (what we would think/believe/desire in a situation) to what someone else is likely to think etc. in a similar situation:

According to this view, what lies at the root of our mature mind-reading abilities is not any sort of theory, but rather an ability to project ourselves imaginatively into another person's perspective, *simulating* their mental activity with our own. (Carruthers and Smith 1996: 3; italics in original)

As with theory-theory, proponents of simulationism differ with respect to the details of how simulation comes about. According to Goldman, simulation requires first-person awareness of one's own mental states, with the inference from these states to the mind of another taking the form of an argument from analogy. Alternatively, simulationists like Gordon argue that recognition of one's own mental states is not a requirement of simulation and that the type of imaginative identification that occurs in simulation can take place without introspective self-awareness.[31] Of concern in the present context is whether simulation, achieved either through inference from one's own mental states of which one is aware or through imaginative identification in the absence of recognition of one's own mental states, can go any way towards explaining the type of mentalising abilities that are integral to pragmatic interpretation. Initial considerations suggest probably not. If all a listener has to base an interpretation of an utterance on is an analogical inference to the speaker's mental states (particularly, the speaker's communicative intention in producing the utterance) from the mental states that the listener would entertain if he had produced that utterance in a certain context, then it is clear that we have not explained interpretation, so much as we have simply given the problem of explaining interpretation a new form. We have transformed the problem of explaining how a listener can establish a speaker's communicative intention in producing an utterance into the problem of explaining how a listener can establish that intention using analogical inference from the type of communicative intention he might entertain if he produced the same utterance in the same situation. Nothing has really been explained here as we still don't have an account of how a listener arrives at the intention from which an analogical inference proceeds. To demonstrate this point further, consider the following utterance that is produced by a lecturer. The lecturer has just entered a room where he has arranged to meet a student in order to discuss the student's dissertation:

LECTURER: It's very warm in here.

According to simulation theory, the student identifies the lecturer's intention in producing this utterance, first by establishing the mental states that he would entertain if he had produced the same utterance in the same situation, and then by projecting (through analogical inference) those mental states onto the lecturer. For the sake of argument, let's imagine that as part of his simulation the student believes that if he were in the same situation as the lecturer and had produced the same utterance as the lecturer, then he would be intending to request that the heater in the room be switched off. So, similarly, the lecturer's intention in producing this utterance must be to indirectly request that the heater be switched off. But in order to identify this particular intention, the student's simulation would have had to use a number of contextual assumptions which it is the task of any theory of pragmatic interpretation to explain. For example, the student may have included in his simulation that the lecturer dislikes a very warm room and that the lecturer cannot concentrate in a warm room to the degree that is necessary to competently discuss a dissertation (all of which will be based on the student's own beliefs about how he would respond in the same situation). A simulationist account of the mentalising abilities that are involved in our interpretation of utterances thus has to assume the very thing that it should be attempting to explain. This is demonstrated by the fact that a simulation which makes use of different contextual assumptions could attribute to the lecturer a very different intention in producing the utterance (e.g. that he wants the meeting to be brief, that he wants to find another room to hold the meeting in, that he wants the student to get a glass of water). Sperber and Wilson (2002) make the same point against simulation theory as follows:

> Since the same sentence can be used to convey quite different meanings in different situations, a hearer who is simulating the speaker's linguistic action in order to retrieve her meaning must provide a considerable amount of contextualisation, based on particular hypotheses about the speaker's beliefs, preferences, and so on. Again, this would only work in cases where the hearer already has a fairly good idea of what the speaker is likely to mean. On this approach, the routine communication of genuinely unanticipated contents would be difficult or impossible to explain. (11)

Another difficulty with simulation theory as an account of the mentalising abilities that are integral to pragmatic interpretation is that such interpretation inevitably presupposes mental states such as belief. Consider Joan's response to Paul's question in the following exchange:

PAUL: Would you like more coffee?
JOAN: Coffee would keep me awake.

In order for Paul to recover the implicature of Joan's response, he must have a range of beliefs both about Joan's mental states and about the world. For example, in his calculation of the implicature that Joan does not want more coffee, Paul must subscribe to some combination of the following beliefs – that it is late at night, that people normally want to sleep at night, that Joan wants to go to sleep early, that coffee contains caffeine, that caffeine prevents some people from sleeping, that Joan is sensitive to caffeine, that Joan does not want to drink anything that will keep her awake, etc. Now, in performing a Joan simulation, Paul must take his own decision-making processes 'off-line' and feed Joan's mental states as 'pretend beliefs' into these processes.[32] But in order to decide which of Joan's mental states are relevant input beliefs to these processes, Paul must have prior beliefs about these states. For example, he must believe that Joan's belief that she is caffeine sensitive is a more relevant input belief to a Joan simulation than is her belief that the bus trip to work in the morning takes twenty minutes. Yet, these prior beliefs of Paul are deeply troubling to the simulation theorist, who is at pains to deny them a significant role within simulation. For example, one prominent simulation theorist, Robert Gordon, remarks that:

> Simulation as I understand it doesn't demand that one already possess intentional concepts and be capable of applying them in one's own case. I have also advanced the far

stronger suggestion ... that to ascribe to another individual x a belief that p is to assert that p within the context of a simulation of x. (Gordon 1995: 175)

So belief attribution for Gordon is tantamount to making an assertion, to stating something as a fact, within the context of a simulation. Nor do I agree with Fuller (1995) who charges the simulation theorist with circularity for his reliance on a prior concept of belief in the last stage of simulation, the stage at which Paul in our example above ascribes to Joan the belief that she does not want more coffee:

The circularity which I want to stress ... involves the last stage of simulation. It is not enough that I correctly simulate Mr Tees and go into the final stage of imagining, or pretending, that I am upset. I must also *ascribe* that state to Mr Tees. And this seems to require that I already have the, or at least *a*, concept of the mental state of being upset. In cases where the final state is one of pretend belief, I must likewise ascribe a similar state to the other, and that ability presupposes that I have the, or *a*, concept of belief. In ascribing my final state to the other, I am saying: the other is in a state similar to *this state* that I am in. Here again, 'this state' cannot mean any old state; it must mean 'this *belief* state'. (Fuller 1995: 25; italics in original)

Although Fuller fully acknowledges the priority of the concept of belief in simulation – something that is denied by Gordon – I contend that he is at least as mistaken as Gordon in believing that a prior concept of belief is something that is problematic ('circular') for simulation theory and hence should be avoided. This challenge to cognitive theorists such as Gordon and Fuller has its origins in the work of the philosopher Hilary Putnam (Putnam 1990, 1992, 1994a, b). I want to argue that both theorists are labouring under the misconception (Hilary Putnam would call it an 'illusion') that it is possible to step outside of our rational concepts of belief and knowledge in describing our core cognitive competence in attributing beliefs both to ourselves and to others. In doing so, all we are attaining is not a complete theory of our mentalising abilities but an *unintelligible* theory of those abilities – what sense can we even make of someone having mental states if we lack prior rational concepts of belief and knowledge with which to conceive of those states? In the same way, Joan's intention to implicate that she does not want more coffee will be unintelligible to Paul if he does not have prior concepts of belief etc. with which to interpret that particular intention. Putnam has mounted an extensive criticism of both philosophical and cognitive scientific theories that assume a 'metaphysical standpoint' in theorising on rationality (of which mindreading is a central element). Although this is not the context in which to outline Putnam's arguments in any detail,[33] it is clear that they have equal relevance to the cognitive ambitions of the simulation theorist. Whatever else the simulation theorist is explaining – and Putnam would say that at best it is a 'we know not what' – it is not an account of mindreading abilities that has any place in a theory of pragmatic interpretation.

5.3.2   *Executive function deficits*

Executive function deficits of various types were also reported in the clinical populations examined in Chapter 3. It is interesting to ask if these deficits might not somehow be able to account for the pragmatic disorders that were shown in that chapter to occur in adults. On first sight, there appear to be plausible grounds for the claim that at least some pragmatic disorders in adults are related to deficits in executive function. For example, the finding that schizophrenic adults exhibit problems with the inhibition of prepotent but irrelevant responses[34] may go some way towards explaining several pragmatic impairments in these adults. The schizophrenic adult may struggle to inhibit or suppress an intrusive thought with the result that he makes irrelevant contributions to a conversational exchange. Alternatively, he may fail to suppress the literal meaning of an utterance with the result that he is unable to recover a speaker's intended implicature. Problems with cognitive flexibility in TBI adults[35] may account for typical pragmatic deficits in the TBI population such as topic repetitiveness (Body and Parker 2005). The issues raised by these initially plausible connections between executive function deficits on the one hand and pragmatic disorders on the other hand are ultimately empirical in nature – it is only through extensive investigation of the relations between executive functioning and pragmatics in both normal and clinical subjects that we will be able to establish if there is any stronger warrant for these connections. Given the paucity of research in this area to date, it is clear that we will not be in possession of the type of knowledge that is needed to address these issues for some time to come.

A question of some interest to cognitive theorists is whether theory-theory and simulation accounts of theory of mind might not presuppose executive functions on some deeper explanatory level. By the same token, one may ask if executive dysfunction is ultimately responsible for the simulative and theory failures that occur in clinical subjects. These questions have been more extensively investigated in the developmental disorder of autism than in any acquired disorder.[36] Nevertheless, there are a growing number of studies that have attempted to address the relation of executive function to ToM in adult subjects. Bach *et al.* (2000) administered ToM stories and cartoons to a fifty-nine-year-old male (called G.O.) with closed head injury. These investigators report that this subject's ToM abilities were found to be intact and to be independent of executive functioning. This finding, they argue, provides support for the modular hypothesis of ToM: 'It has been suggested that ToM ability is dependent on general inferential ability. Nevertheless, G.O. demonstrates poor verbal abstract reasoning and this result therefore lends support to the domain specificity of theory of mind' (188). Fine *et al.* (2001) studied B.M., a thirty-two-year-old male with congenital left amygdala damage who had received psychiatric diagnoses of schizophrenia and Asperger's syndrome by adulthood. B.M. displayed a significant ToM impairment while his performance on all aspects of executive functioning was normal. Fine *et al.* conclude that 'the findings clearly suggest that theory of mind is neither mediated by nor necessary for executive functioning. Rather, the present findings suggest that theory of mind is mediated by a domain-specific, dedicated neural system' (2001: 295). On a different note, Henry *et al.* (2006) found that theory of mind was substantially correlated with performance on phonemic fluency (a measure of executive functioning) in sixteen adults who had sustained a TBI. These investigators conclude that executive impairments have a secondary impact on ToM performance.

Studies by Bach *et al.* (2000) and Fine *et al.* (2001) lend support to the view that general inferential processes of the type that belong to a Fodorian central system may not ultimately explain our mentalising abilities – there is dissociation of these competences in the subjects examined in these studies with ToM skills intact in the presence of poor verbal abstract reasoning (Bach *et al.*) and ToM skills impaired in the presence of normal executive functioning (Fine *et al.*). Recently, Wilson (2005) has argued that ToM is an essentially modular cognitive system using evidence of a developmental dissociation between mindreading skills and general-purpose reasoning abilities:

People with Williams Syndrome have good abilities for mind-reading and communication but poor general reasoning abilities ... This suggests that mind-reading cannot be a conscious, reflective process of the type illustrated in Grice's working out schema for implicatures, but depends on dedicated inferential mechanisms which may remain intact while general-purpose reasoning abilities are impaired. Dissociations are also possible in the opposite direction. For example, people with Asperger's syndrome may have good general reasoning abilities combined with serious impairments in mindreading abilities. (2005: 1135)

However, Wilson goes a step further than simply saying that mindreading is not a central cognitive competence which is subserved by general reasoning processes. She argues that pragmatics is a sub-module[37] of the mindreading module using evidence of dissociations between the ability for inferential communication and general mindreading ability (e.g. in children without autism who have pragmatic language impairment). Although I can see no reason for supposing that such a sub-module will fare any better against the criticisms of ToM modularity that were examined in section 5.3.1.1, it is clear that we cannot expect to make much progress on the question of the cognitive substrates of acquired pragmatic disorders without first addressing the status of our mindreading skills. As the discussion of this chapter has indicated, that status can only be established through an ongoing interaction between theoretical reflection and empirical investigation – reflection to establish the nature of mindreading as it pertains to pragmatic interpretation and empirical studies to finely tune those reflections to better capture human psychology, both normal and disordered. The pragmatic and cognitive theories examined in this chapter will undoubtedly continue to play a significant role in any future enquiry.

NOTES

1 Of course, as a relevance theorist Carston would argue that Sperber and Wilson's relevance theory is just such a 'cognitively plausible pragmatic theory'. In Cummings (2005), I argue that this is unlikely to be the case (see Chapter 4 in this volume for my argument that relevance-theoretic explanations of cognition and pragmatics are a form of scientific reductionism). We will examine the proposals of relevance theory later in this chapter.

2 Body *et al.* (1999) are concerned by the same lack of integration of cognitive theory and pragmatic theory, which they propose to resolve by 'grounding pragmatic theory in cognition'. They state that 'what we have ... are two distinct sets of theoretical constructs, provided by pragmatic theory and cognitive theory respectively, but so far virtually no mutual influence and certainly no superordinate framework to integrate the two' (89–90). They relate this lack of integration to the traditionally dominant role of parent disciplines such as philosophy in the field of pragmatics. For example, they remark of pragmatic theories that 'their rationale and area of focus have been by the concerns of their parent disciplines – principally philosophy, sociology, and linguistics – with the result that the relationship between pragmatics and areas such as cognition and neurology, both crucial in understanding communication pathologies, have been relatively little explored' (89). The views of Body *et al.* will be examined again in Chapter 7.

3 This is explained in large part by the fact that while delusions and hallucinations are considered 'core features' of schizophrenia, communication deficits are one of a number of 'related features' of the disorder. Frith (1992) states that 'in most diagnostic schemes, all schizophrenic patients have to show positive symptoms (hallucination and delusions) at some stage of their illness. We might refer to these as the core features of schizophrenia. Having defined schizophrenia in such a way, it is clear that there are a number of features that are often seen in association with this diagnosis ... incoherence [incoherent speech] is another related feature that is not found in all schizophrenic patients' (34, 36).

4 Carston (2002) makes this same point as follows: 'The two systems are closely related (if not one and the same, as some have claimed): the theory of mind system interprets the behaviour of others by attributing to them such intentional (that is, world-representing) mental states as beliefs, desires and intentions, and the pragmatic comprehension system interprets communicative behaviour in terms of an intention on the part of the speaker to bring about a certain belief state in the addressee' (132).

5 This is evident in the following views expressed by Kasher, and Sperber and Wilson. Kasher states that 'our main concern ... is how well does pragmatics fare with a certain general, psychological conception of the nature of human mind, viz. that of the modular approach, as put forward and discussed by Chomsky ... and Fodor' (1991a: 568). Sperber and Wilson remark that: 'we will argue that pragmatic interpretation is not simply a matter of applying Fodorian central systems or general mind-reading abilities to a particular (communicative) domain. Verbal comprehension presents special challenges, and exhibits certain regularities, not found in other domains. It therefore lends itself to the development of a dedicated comprehension module with its own particular principles and mechanisms' (2002: 5).

6 Fodor (1983) frames his modularity thesis in terms of a number of properties of the mind's input systems, which he characterises as modules. He enumerates these properties as follows: (1) input systems are domain specific; (2) the operation of input systems is mandatory; (3) there is only limited central access to the mental representations that input systems compute; (4) input systems are fast; (5) input systems are informationally encapsulated; (6) input analysers have 'shallow' outputs; (7) input systems are associated with fixed neural architecture; (8) input systems exhibit characteristic and specific breakdown patterns; and (9) the ontogeny of input systems exhibits a characteristic pace and sequencing.

7 Of course, Sperber and Wilson would deny such a claim for their own relevance theory (Sperber and Wilson 1986, 1995). In support of their relevance-theoretic account of utterance interpretation, they write: 'What the available psycholinguistic evidence shows is that, other things being equal, from a range of contextually-available interpretations, hearers tend to choose the most salient or accessible one, the one that costs the least processing effort to construct (Gernsbacher, 1995). This is also what many theoretical accounts of pragmatic interpretation (e.g. Lewis, 1979; Sperber and Wilson, 1986/1995) predict that hearers should do' (Sperber and Wilson 2002: 6–7). However, as Sperber and Wilson themselves state, the 'available psycholinguistic evidence' is consistent with several views of pragmatic interpretation, not all of which, as we will see, are consistent. So there is an important sense in which the available evidence does not provide any unique confirmation of the relevance-theoretic account of pragmatic interpretation.

8 According to Sperber and Wilson, utterances come with a presumption of optimal relevance: 'every utterance (or other type of ostensive stimulus ...) conveys a presumption of its own relevance' (2002: 17–18).

9 Sperber and Wilson very directly link their principle of relevance to features of human evolutionary development: 'We claim that relevance has been involved in two evolutionary transformations in human cognition: one continuous, and the other discrete. The continuous transformation has been an increasing tendency of the human cognitive system to maximise the relevance of the information it processes. The discrete transformation has been the emergence of a relevance-based comprehension module' (2002: 13).

10 'We will show how such a metacommunicative module might have evolved as a specialisation of a more general mind-reading module, and what principles and mechanisms it might contain' (Sperber and Wilson 2002: 5).

11 The dominant (literal) meaning serves as a prepotent response that schizophrenic patients have difficulty inhibiting. In a study of the understanding of non-literal speech in schizophrenic adults, Langdon et al. (2002) found that these patients had difficulty suppressing prepotent inappropriate information in a test of sequencing capture stories. Moreover, this difficulty was shown to predict both metaphor and irony hit rates in these patients: 'the better the patients were at suppressing prepotent inappropriate information when sequencing the *capture* stories, the more likely they were to recognise appropriate uses of metaphorical speech and ironical speech. The implication here is that some patients with schizophrenia may fail to understand non-literal uses of language because of a more pervasive problem with suppressing prepotent inappropriate information' (2002: 95).

12 The same is true of individuals with paranoid personality disorder (a disorder that can be distinguished from the paranoid subtype of schizophrenia by the presence of psychotic symptoms – e.g. delusions and hallucinations – in the latter). The

following account of paranoid personality disorder in DSM-IV-TR highlights the type of interpretive problems that occur in this disorder: 'They read hidden meanings that are demeaning and threatening into benign remarks or events. For example, an individual with this disorder … may view a casual humorous remark by a co-worker as a serious character attack. Compliments are often misinterpreted (e.g., a compliment on a new acquisition is misinterpreted as a criticism for selfishness; a compliment on an accomplishment is misinterpreted as an attempt to coerce more and better performance). They may view an offer of help as a criticism that they are not doing well enough on their own' (2000: 690–1).

13 Loukusa *et al.* (2007b) describe a similar failure to stop processing in two groups of children with Asperger's syndrome or high-functioning autism (seven- to nine-year-olds and ten- to twelve-year-olds). These investigators found that both groups of AS/HFA children were more likely to commit type 3 errors than control children when producing responses to questions. Type 3 errors occurred when a child produced a relevant response but then continued by drifting away from his or her original answer. Loukusa *et al.* conclude that 'some children with AS/HFA have difficulties in being optimally relevant and in stopping processing after they have given a correct answer' (2007b: 372).

14 Langdon *et al.* (2002) are explicit about the ultimate aim of their study, which is not to test the utility of relevance theory in explaining utterance interpretation problems in clinical subjects. Rather, they wish their study to contribute to investigations of the nature of the relationship between normal mindreading and normal pragmatics. They state that 'the proposal that everyday communication depends fundamentally on the on-line use of an ability to read minds would be strengthened considerably by evidence that there are forms of acquired cognitive dysfunction that can occur later in life and which are such that, if they impair the functional capacity of a mind to read other minds, then they also impair the functional capacity of a mind to use and understand language pragmatically' (2002: 75–6).

15 'The findings of this schizophrenia study suggest that not just a basic ability to attribute mental states but the more sophisticated mind-reading abilities of the kind needed to pass typical theory-of-mind tasks are critical for understanding ironical speech. In contrast, understanding of metaphorical speech may require only a very basic ability to represent mental states; this we know is intact in patients with schizophrenia' (Langdon *et al.* 2002: 97).

16 In 'Pragmatics and the modularity of mind', Kasher appears to be saying that a literal force is computed in all cases. However, in another publication in the same year, Kasher clearly states that a literal force may not always be computed: 'Notice also that exceeding the literal meaning does not necessarily mean first of all computing the literal meaning and then, as a result of some evaluation, making an attempt to identify the 'intended' meaning. It may well be the case that the need to go beyond the literal meaning is detected without a complete representation of the literal meaning being computed' (1991b: 395). Gibbs (2002: 457) remarks that 'most … psycholinguistic research shows … that given sufficient context people understand nonliteral meanings without first analyzing the complete literal meaning of an expression (i.e. the direct access view)'.

17 David (1993) describes 'the identification of a pair of cases where one has lost function X but has a normal function Y and the other has the opposite pattern of abilities/disabilities' as the 'magical double dissociation' (1). In the present case, the finding

that one subject was impaired in both the use and understanding of conversational implicatures, but observed politeness principles, while another subject displayed the reverse pattern of impairment, would constitute just such a dissociation.

18 It is interesting to note that Kasher and Langdon *et al.* have different theoretical conceptions of irony (sarcasm). Kasher clearly sees a significant role for a pragmatic module in sarcasm – sarcasm, Kasher argues, is 'conventionalized': 'Notice that sarcasm as well as certain forms of "indirect" speech act (e.g., 'Could you …'), are, in a sense, conventionalized, and we would, therefore, not be surprised if we find them to be dissociated from metaphorical expressions and "live", "indirect" speech acts' (1991b: 395). However, Langdon *et al.* argue that irony requires 'a high degree of mentalising ability'. Mentalising is the type of ability that Kasher would locate within a pragmatic central system. These different conceptions of irony reflect deeper theoretical differences between Kasher and Langdon *et al.* that stem from Langdon's use of relevance theory. Specifically, where Kasher has attempted to circumscribe mentalising abilities within a pragmatic central system, Sperber and Wilson assume that these abilities also play a role in what Kasher would describe as modular aspects of pragmatic interpretation: 'There are those who argue that most, if not all, aspects of the process of constructing a hypothesis about the speaker's meaning are closely related to linguistic decoding. These code-like aspects of interpretation might be carried out within an extension of the language module, by non-metapsychological processes whose output might then be inferentially evaluated and attributed as a speaker's meaning. On the other hand, there are those who see pragmatic interpretation as metapsychological through and through. On this approach, both hypothesis construction and hypothesis evaluation are seen as rational processes geared to the recognition of speakers' intentions, carried out by Fodorian central processes … or by a "theory of mind" module dedicated to the attribution of mental states on the basis of behaviour … We want to defend a view of pragmatic interpretation as metapsychological through and through' (Sperber and Wilson 2002: 4–5).

19 Kasher *et al.* (1999) state that 'it is often claimed that right-brain-damaged patients show selective deficits in natural language pragmatics, i.e., language use in context. Alleged right hemisphere involvement in pragmatics includes prosody; emotions and nonverbal communication; certain speech acts, especially indirect requests; and figurative language, including idioms and metaphors as well as humor, inferences and discourse' (567).

20 'Basic types of speech acts are interesting not just because they involve the use of marked sentences, but mainly because many other types of speech acts depend on them. Assertion has been argued to be the most basic speech act because every other speech act which is governed by rules that refer to the speaker's beliefs, depend on the availability of assertion' (Soroker *et al.* 2005: 215).

21 It is worth remarking on why Kasher *et al.* (1999) developed this implicatures battery. Zaidel *et al.* (2002) used a Hebrew version of the Right Hemisphere Communication Battery (RHCB, Gardner and Brownell 1986) in a study of natural language pragmatics in LHD and RHD patients. These investigators found that the functions of language use that were assessed by this battery were too 'heterogeneous, theoretically ill-understood, and pragmatically complex' to be of value in exploring the modularity of parts of natural language pragmatics. A new pragmatics battery, which 'systematically taps basic speech acts and implicatures both verbally

and nonverbally', was developed to overcome these shortcomings of the RHCB (Zaidel *et al.* 2002: 531).

22 The tests used in this study included the Picture Completion, Picture Arrangement and Block Design subtests of the Wechsler Adult Intelligence Scale (Wechsler 1981); some of the verbal subtests (Digit Span, Logical Memory I (Story A) and Verbal Paired Associates I) and nonverbal subtests (Figural Memory, Visual Paired Associates Part I, Visual Reproduction and Visual Memory Span) of the Wechsler Memory Scale (Wechsler 1987); the Coloured form of Raven Progressive Matrices (Raven 1965); the standard version of Benton's Line Orientation Test (Benton *et al.* 1983); the Star Cancellation subtest of the Behavioral Inattention Test (Wilson *et al.* 1987); and the Stroop (1935) test. A number of these tests had been adapted for Hebrew.

23 'We propose the radical interpretation that aphasia batteries commonly assess language functions, such as auditory language comprehension, naming, reading or speech, using formal tests that presuppose (but do not directly test) control over basic speech acts' (Soroker *et al.* 2005: 216).

24 That Kasher *et al.*'s (1999) study is a contribution to an account of pragmatics in normal subjects is clear from the following statement: 'Given the different modes in which right- and left-hemisphere damage affect the processing of conversational implicatures, it remains to be discovered how the two hemispheres interact to process natural language pragmatics in the normal brain in real time' (1999: 566). See also Langdon *et al.*'s comments in note 14.

25 An alternative to this modular view is that young children acquire a theory of mind by developing theories. Alison Gopnik is a proponent of this alternative position, which she calls 'theory-formation theory': 'My claim is that there are quite distinctive and special cognitive processes that are responsible both for scientific progress and for particular kinds of development in children ... It is my further claim that theories and theory changes, in particular, are responsible for the changes in children's understanding of the mind' (1996: 169). Gopnik and others challenge modularity on the grounds that cognitive modules are not deemed able to accommodate the developmental changes that take place in a child's theory of mind (modularity theories, Gopnik and Meltzoff (1997: 54) argue, are 'antidevelopmental'). See Scholl and Leslie (1999) for a refutation of this view of cognitive modules and for discussion of how developmental changes can occur in a module via parameterisation.

26 It is worth remarking that the original proponent of modularity – Fodor (1983) – would disavow the attempt to locate ToM skills within a domain-specific cognitive module. For Fodor, such skills are located within a non-modularised central system in the mind. Frye (2000) makes this same point as follows: 'An odd aspect of the view that theory of mind is domain specific is that it is one Fodor's (1983) own approach to modularity would explicitly disclaim' (149).

27 To the extent that computational modules realise intentional modules, they must display the same domain specificity, informational encapsulation and limited accessibility of intentional modules. Segal (1996) remarks that 'it is likely that every computational module realises an intentional module. That is because there exists a self-contained and definite description of what it does in purely intentional terms. The only further requirement is that it exhibit either informational encapsulation or limited accessibility. The former is almost inevitable, since any computer will have a characteristic set of inputs. And it is unlikely that any computer in someone's head has a range of inputs that allows it access to all the information in that head' (144).

28 Additional modular features that are satisfied by the psychology faculty are revealed when Segal asks if the psychology module is also a Fodor module: 'At present it seems to fit the criteria reasonably well, but not entirely. It does appear to be domain specific, informationally encapsulated, to fire obligatorily, to be reasonably fast and to have a characteristic ontogeny' (1996: 149). See note 6 for a full list of features of Fodor's input modules.

29 'So-called "theory-theorists" maintain that the ability to explain and predict behaviour is underpinned by a folk-psychological *theory* of the structure and functioning of the mind – where the theory in question may be innate and modularised, learned individually, or acquired through a process of enculturation' (Carruthers and Smith 1996: 1; italics in original).

30 Consistent with the view of the child as scientist, Gopnik argues that children undergo conceptual developments that are akin to scientific conceptual revolutions: 'We have argued that children, like scientists, may preserve a theory for some time by introducing ad hoc auxiliary hypotheses and that conceptual changes often have a "revolutionary" character, with one whole theory replacing another' (Gopnik and Meltzoff 1997: 213). Fodor (1992) challenges this view, arguing that no 'conceptual revolution' is required for the child to acquire an adult folk psychology. Instead, Fodor argues that developmental changes in a child's theory of mind can be explained in terms of performance factors: 'I will construct an account according to which the experimental findings are explained by assuming that the child's access to the computational resources required for problem solving increases with age. According to this account, the child's theory of mind, as such, undergoes no alteration; what changes is only his ability to exploit what he knows to make behavioral predictions. So what I have on offer is a "performance" theory of metacognitive development rather than a "competence" theory' (1992: 284).

31 Gordon (1996) captures these two positions as follows: 'There are basically two kinds of hot methodology theory that go under the name, "the simulation theory". According to one of these, one first recognises one's own mental states under actual or imagined conditions and then infers, on the basis of an assumed similarity or analogy, that the person simulated is in similar states. The recognition of one's own mental states is thought to be grounded in introspective access to these states, or at least in comparison of their qualitative features with a standard held in memory; and this is thought to require possession of the relevant mental state concepts ... I argue against this version of the simulation theory. Against the thesis that we make inferences from what we ourselves would do in the imagined circumstances to what the other will do, I emphasise imaginative transformation into the other ... what I oppose is the claim that simulation requires recognition of our own mental states *as such*, along with the corollary that it requires *possession of the concepts* of the various mental states simulated in others' (14–16; italics in original).

32 Gordon (1986) explains how simulation proceeds as follows: 'Our decision-making or practical reasoning system gets partially disengaged from its "natural" inputs and fed instead with suppositions and images (or their "subpersonal" or "sub-doxastic" counterparts). Given these artificial pretend inputs the system then "makes up its mind" what to do. Since the system is being run off-line, as it were, disengaged also from its natural output systems, its "decision" isn't actually executed but rather ends up as an anticipation ... of the other's behavior' (170). It should be emphasised that this off-line account is only one version of simulation theory for Gordon and that the

thing which is essential for him to all versions of simulation theory is imaginative identification (see note 31).

33 I have used Putnam's arguments to mount challenges to theories in pragmatics (relevance theory), argumentation and fallacy theory, Habermas's critical social theory and philosophy. The most recent versions of these challenges can be found in Cummings (2005).

34 Bellgrove *et al.* (2006) used a stop-signal task to assess response inhibition in twenty-one adolescent patients with early-onset schizophrenia. Patients were categorised into paranoid and undifferentiated subtypes. Undifferentiated patients had significantly longer stop-signal reaction times than either paranoid patients or controls. This finding was indicative of poor response inhibition in undifferentiated patients. Enticott *et al.* (2008) found that schizophrenic patients presented with significantly increased stop-signal reaction times, suggesting slower inhibitory responses.

35 De Guise *et al.* (2005) used the Neurobehavioral Rating Scale to assess cognitive function in 348 TBI patients at the time of their acute care stay. These investigators found that mental flexibility was one of the cognitive deficits most frequently observed on this scale. Johnstone *et al.* (1995) examined the extent of decline in several cognitive abilities following TBI in ninety-seven outpatients. The abilities examined were intelligence, memory, attention, speed of processing and cognitive flexibility. Cognitive flexibility was the cognitive ability that had declined most in these patients following TBI.

36 See Currie (1996) for discussion of how theory-theorists and simulation-theorists account for executive function deficits in autism.

37 It is worth remarking that Wilson is using a notion of module that is broader than that proposed by Fodor (see note 6). Specifically, Wilson's notion of module, which is influenced by evolutionary approaches to cognition, makes use of special-purpose inferential mechanisms that exploit certain regularities within the domain of intentional behaviour: 'More recently, a growing interest in evolutionary approaches to cognition has led to a reconsideration of the nature of modules and a questioning of Fodor's sharp distinction between modular input processes and relatively undifferentiated central processes. From an evolutionary perspective, what characterises a module is not so much the cluster of properties that Fodor (1983: 47–101) ascribed to input systems (being fast, mandatory, local, encapsulated, etc.), but the presence of dedicated mechanisms (typically biological adaptations to regularities in some domain) which cannot be seen as special cases of more general mechanisms operating in broader domains' (2005: 1131).

6 The assessment and treatment of pragmatic disorders

6.1 Introduction

At its most general level, the clinical management of clients with pragmatic disorders involves two main types of activity. In order to establish which pragmatic skills are impaired, clinicians must first engage in a process of assessment. Assessment is usually conducted over several sessions and can involve an extensive range of techniques. The results of assessment provide a basis for the planning of intervention as well as a baseline measurement of the client's pragmatic skills. We will see subsequently that this baseline measurement is vital in establishing a client's progress in therapy and in determining the efficacy of a particular programme of intervention. An equally eclectic group of techniques is used in the intervention or treatment of pragmatic disorders. These techniques often reflect the particular experience of a clinician and the availability of resources. Certainly, few of these techniques have been the subject of efficacy studies. There is a very important sense, therefore, in which most interventions of pragmatics lack the type of clinical validation that we have come to expect of interventions in areas such as phonology and syntax. In this section, we examine the full range of methods that are available to the clinician who is charged with the assessment and treatment of pragmatic disorders in children and adults. In doing so, we will make a distinction between formal and informal assessment methods. We will consider the types of clients that may be assessed and treated using these methods. We will also discuss the question of efficacy studies in the area of disordered pragmatics. Before engaging with these issues, however, a few more introductory comments are in order about the nature of assessment and treatment in pragmatically disordered clients.

Although most assessment is undertaken at the outset of the management of a client, it is not unusual for assessment to be conducted concurrently with intervention. In fact, assessment and intervention are very rarely conducted in two discrete phases of activity. Rather, assessment is often integrated into many intervention activities. For example, in an intervention activity designed to elicit the use of verbal requests by a child, the therapist may place a toy out of the child's reach in order that he or she will have to ask for it. One can easily imagine how this activity can be extended to increase the pragmatic complexity of the request. If the toy is a doll, the therapist can place two dolls beside each other and out of the child's reach (the proximity of the dolls will preclude the use of pointing as a means of requesting the doll). In order to receive a doll, the child must then specify an exact referent of the word 'doll' – for example, the doll with the blonde hair, the doll with the red dress, etc. So an intervention activity that is designed to elicit verbal requests can have an assessment component integrated within it – the assessment of referential communication skills. The close integration of pragmatic assessment and treatment has a number of clinical benefits. It permits pragmatic skills to be assessed in as naturalistic a manner as possible. The child who fails to comply with more formal assessment activities will be completely unaware of the clinician's assessment agenda in the above example. Also, assessment that is undertaken in the first couple of contact sessions with a child is unlikely to reflect this child's typical use of language – the presence of an unfamiliar clinician may inhibit the use of many pragmatic skills. By delaying some aspects of assessment until the child is relaxed in the clinician's presence, a more complete account of that child's skills can be obtained. Finally, by continually assessing pragmatic skills, clinicians can rapidly adjust treatment activities in ways that can usefully extend a client's skills.

In treating a pragmatic disorder, the clinician must have in mind a number of considerations. Some of these considerations also apply to the treatment of any language disorder. For example, the clinician must be continually aware of the interaction between pragmatics and other levels of language. The production of verbal requests is only a viable treatment objective for the client who has the phonological, syntactic and semantic skills that are necessary to issue requests. If these skills are lacking, the clinician may have to prioritise the treatment of certain language structures before any direct targeting of pragmatic skills can be attempted. By the same token, specific cognitive deficits may adversely affect a client's pragmatic language skills. A neuropsychological intervention that targets cognitive deficits (e.g. in the adult with a traumatic brain injury) may have to take place before or alongside an intervention that targets pragmatic impairment. Socialisation deficits, such as occur in individuals with autistic spectrum disorder, may play a significant role in a pragmatic language disorder. For example, the autistic child who is unable to develop peer relationships appropriate to his or her developmental level will lack the experience of social interaction that is so important for the development of pragmatic language skills. Mental retardation will place limits upon the rate and extent of learning of new skills in therapy, while sensory impairments (e.g. hearing loss) and concomitant communication disorders (e.g. dysarthria) will also have implications for the types of activities undertaken as part of treatment. In short, when planning any pragmatic intervention, clinicians must consider a whole range of factors that are likely to impact more or less directly on a client's use of pragmatic language skills.

When treating language pragmatics, clinicians must be aware of areas of strength in clients and of how these areas can best be exploited to assist intervention for pragmatic deficits. It is frequently observed, for example, that visual processing skills are an area of relative strength in Down's syndrome subjects.[1] A visual processing route can be incorporated into most pragmatic language assessments and interventions. Depending on the age of the subject, a wordless picture book or a cartoon strip may be used to elicit narrative production in the Down's syndrome child. Similarly, the relatively intact social knowledge and understanding of Down's syndrome subjects[2] can be exploited in activities designed to increase comprehension and use of a range of non-literal and implied meanings (e.g. indirect requests, sarcasm). Even so-called deficits (e.g. restricted interests in autism) may be gainfully employed to develop pragmatic language skills. The verbal autistic child with an interest in trains may be encouraged to engage in conversational interaction with others on this particular topic. During this interaction, skills that are more or less directly related to pragmatics (e.g. turn-taking, perspective taking, use of a range of speech acts) may be rehearsed in a naturalistic context. Of course, as well as non-pragmatic areas contributing to the treatment of pragmatic language skills, these same skills may also be used to compensate areas of linguistic deficit. Paradis (1998b) remarks, for example, that 'therapy may try to capitalize on the dysphasic patient's preserved right hemisphere-based pragmatic aspects of verbal communication by using paralinguistic features such as intonation, gestures, and facial expressions and a greater reliance on inference to aid the comprehension and production of verbal messages and thus circumvent the loss of linguistic structure' (7).[3]

Finally, one of the most significant changes ushered in by the 'pragmatic turn' in the study of language disorders has been an emphasis on the notion of context in all aspects of clinical assessment and treatment.[4] Clinicians and researchers have become increasingly aware of the substantial variations that can occur in an individual's communicative performance across different contexts of language use. More specifically, an individual's communicative performance in the setting of a clinic is now no longer assumed to be representative of how that same person communicates at home with family members or in a social setting with friends. An emphasis on context has led practitioners and researchers to develop naturalistic techniques of assessment and treatment and to make a number of other substantial adjustments to the clinical management of clients. For example, therapeutic techniques that involve the participation of a client's key communicative partners and that try to simulate the communicative demands of everyday situations are now commonplace in the treatment of clients. The rapid ascendancy of assessment techniques such as conversation analysis and discourse analysis is a direct consequence of the need to understand language disorders within the wider social, physical, linguistic and epistemic contexts in which they are found. We will see in subsequent sections that some assessment and treatment approaches have been more successful than other approaches in designing and implementing techniques with considerations of context in mind. In Chapter 7, we critically evaluate a number of clinical studies that have attempted to study the role of context in language processing.

6.2   Pragmatic language assessment

Assessments of pragmatics are now more numerous and diverse than at any time in the past. Yet, the increasing number and range of pragmatic assessments available to the clinician belie the fact that certain pragmatic language skills are still poorly assessed and many pragmatic assessments lack clinical validity and reliability. In this section, I consider the different types of instruments that are used to assess pragmatic language disorders in children and adults. These instruments include pragmatics profiles and communication checklists. They also include assessments of narrative and other forms of discourse, techniques based on conversation analysis and formal tests of pragmatic skills.[5] Many of these assessments have been published and are commercially available to clinicians. Other assessments are devised by individual clinicians and may draw more or less extensively on published sources. Some procedures have undergone extensive investigation to establish their utility as methods of clinical assessment. Where validation studies of particular assessment techniques exist, we review their findings. Many more assessments, however, are used extensively in clinical settings, despite the fact that there is little or no evidence on hand to support their continued clinical use. For each assessment, we describe the types of clients who may be assessed through the use of a particular procedure.[6] We also discuss how these assessments are administered to clients and the various factors that must be considered by clinicians when deciding which assessment procedure to adopt (e.g. ease of administration, time constraints, training required). Finally, I describe the merits and drawbacks of different forms of assessment for the planning of treatment or intervention.

6.2.1   Pragmatics profiles and checklists

Within this category of pragmatic assessment I include any instrument that contains a descriptive taxonomy of pragmatic behaviours. Based on observation of a client's communication skills and/or interview with a client's relative or carer, an examiner (usually a speech-language pathologist) determines if these behaviours are a feature of an individual's communicative repertoire. Three of the most prominent assessments in this category are Dewart and Summers's (1995) Pragmatics Profile; Prutting and Kirchner's (1987) Pragmatic Protocol; and Bishop's (2003b) Children's Communication Checklist. Similar descriptive profiles can also be found in formal language tests and in assessments of functional communication.[7] As its name suggests, the Pragmatics Profile is a direct attempt to place pragmatics at the centre of an investigation of children's language and communication skills. Through a structured interview, which is conducted informally with a parent, teacher or other carer, investigators can glean information on the following broad communicative areas: communicative functions, response to communication, interaction and conversation and contextual variation. The profile is intended for use with school-age children between five and ten years of age, although other versions are available for use with preschool children up to approximately four years of age and for use with adults. The Pragmatics Profile is not a standardised measure of language and communication skills, but a descriptive, qualitative approach to the study of children's everyday communicative behaviours.[8] Dewart and Summers (1995) state that 'we believe that a descriptive approach that relies on information from people who know the child well can have considerable value, at least as a first step in the investigation of pragmatics' (14).

This particular assessment tool has been used to assess communication and plan intervention in a range of child clients, including children with delayed language development, specific language impairment, hearing impairment, visual impairment, physical difficulties, learning disabilities and autism. It is also relevant to nonverbal children and bilingual children (Dewart and Summers 1995). Chandler et al. (2002) used the Pragmatics Profile, along with a range of other assessment and diagnostic techniques, in a study designed to evaluate a home-based intervention in autistic children. Ten autistic children, who were aged 1:10 to 2:9 at assessment, underwent an intervention consisting of home visits, modelling, workshops and written information and in which parents performed the role of therapists. Information from the Pragmatics Profile and other techniques (e.g. play-based assessment) was used not only in making the diagnosis, but also in establishing a baseline and individual objectives for intervention. The Pragmatics Profile was used by Parkinson (2006) in a study of pragmatic functions in thirty-five children, aged six to eleven years, who had a history of epilepsy and demonstrated autistic features, ASD or autistic regression. Semi-structured interviews with key workers were used to examine conversational engagement, paralinguistic features and the children's ability to recognise and convey communicative intentions. Johnston and Stansfield (1997) used the Pragmatics Profile to establish parental perceptions of the pragmatic skills of six preschool children with Down's syndrome. Stojanovik and James (2006) used the Pragmatics Profile in an investigation of the development of early social communication skills in a child with Williams syndrome.

Prutting and Kirchner's Pragmatic Protocol has been in use since the early 1980s. It contains thirty pragmatic parameters that are organised according to three categories: (1) verbal aspects (e.g. variety of speech acts), (2) para-linguistic aspects (e.g. vocal quality) and (3) nonverbal aspects (e.g. physical proximity). Assessors judge each parameter as being either appropriate or inappropriate. A parameter is appropriate if it facilitates the communicative interaction or is neutral. An inappropriate parameter detracts from the commu-nicative interaction and penalises the individual. A third category of response is used when there is no opportunity to observe a particular parameter. Prutting and Kirchner (1987) applied the protocol in a comparative study of pragmatic impairment in four clinical populations – forty-two children with articulation disorders, forty-two children with language disorders, eleven aphasic adults and ten adults with right-hemisphere lesions. Forty-two children with normal language development and ten adults with normal language were also included in the study. At least six subjects were drawn from each of these groups to obtain interobserver reliability data. To obtain these data, two investigators independently completed the protocol after observing conversational inter-action. Reliability for all groups in the study exceeded 90%. Reliability ranged between 93% and 100% in children with articulation and language disorders (mean of 94.4% for judgements of appropriate parameters and 92.3% for judge-ments of inappropriate parameters). For adults with left- and right-hemisphere damage, reliability ranged between 90.9% to 100% (mean of 95.6% for judge-ments of appropriate parameters and 93.1% for judgements of inappropriate parameters). For both judgements of appropriate and inappropriate parameters, reliability was 100% for normal children and adults.

Since Prutting and Kirchner's early work, the Pragmatic Protocol has been used to assess pragmatic skills in a wide range of clinical groups. McCabe *et al.* (2007) used the protocol to assess the pragmatic skills of five men living with AIDS. Representative portions of a semi-structured interview were rated for pragmatic appropriateness by ten experienced assessors. Fyrberg *et al.* (2007) used the protocol to assess eight severely brain-injured children and youths during an intensive six-week rehabilitation period. A speech-language path-ologist and a rehabilitation assistant independently rated the pragmatic behav-iours of these subjects. Aubert *et al.* (2004) assessed nonverbal communication in four men with TBI using the protocol. All four men were assessed more than seven years after having sustained a severe TBI. The protocol was used by Meilijson *et al.* (2004) to obtain a general profile of pragmatic abilities in forty-three subjects with chronic schizophrenia. Mentis and Lundgren (1995) used the protocol to assess discourse-pragmatic components of language in five children who were prenatally exposed to cocaine. McNamara and Durso (2003) examined the pragmatic communication skills of twenty patients with Parkinson's disease using the protocol. Avent *et al.* (1998) used the protocol in a study that examined the relationship between language impairment and pragmatic performance in twenty aphasic adults. It is perhaps a sign of the widespread appeal of this particular pragmatic assessment that it has also been used to assess pragmatic skills in other domains. Scherz *et al.* (1995), for example, used the protocol to assess the communicative effectiveness of doctor–patient interactions. Some fourteen family practice residents and seventy patients were rated using the protocol.

The Children's Communication Checklist (CCC) was first used in 1998 to examine pragmatic language impairments in children (Bishop 1998). Since this original study, a second edition of the checklist has been published (Bishop 2003b). Such is the popularity of the CCC that it has 'rapidly become the instrument of choice for the identification of pragmatic language impairment' (Adams 2002: 976). The seventy-item questionnaire is intended for use with children aged four to sixteen years. It may be completed by a caregiver, speech and language therapist or teacher. Raters respond to a series of statements with one of the following: (a) does not apply, (b) applies somewhat, (c) definitely applies or (d) unable to judge. The checklist contains the following ten scales: (A) speech, (B) syntax, (C) semantics, (D) coherence, (E) inappropriate initiation, (F) stereotyped language, (G) use of context, (H) nonverbal communication, (I) social relations and (J) interests. Standard scores and percentiles are provided for these scales. The checklist contains two composites which are based on these scales. The General Communication Composite (scales A to H above) is used to identify children who are likely to have clinically significant communication problems. The Social Interaction Deviance Composite (scales A to E and H to J) is used to identify children who may merit further assessment for an autistic spectrum disorder. In a study of the first edition of the checklist, Bishop and Baird (2001) found that reliability, as measured by internal consistency, was 0.7 or higher for most scales, when checklists were completed by parents and professionals. Correlations between ratings for parents and professionals on the individual pragmatic scales of the checklist ranged from 0.30 to 0.58, with a correlation of 0.46 for the pragmatic composite.[9] When the checklist is completed by teachers and speech and language therapists, Bishop (1998) reports interrater reliability and internal consistency of around 0.80 on the five pragmatic subscales. In a validation study of the second edition of the checklist, Norbury *et al.* (2004) report good interrater agreement (r = 0.79) on the Social Interaction Deviance Composite.[10]

The Children's Communication Checklist has been used extensively in the study of different clinical populations. One of these populations is children with autistic spectrum disorder. Bishop *et al.* (2006b) used the checklist to examine the broader phenotype of autism in the siblings of children with autistic disorder and pervasive developmental disorder, not otherwise specified (PDD,NOS). Verté *et al.* (2006) examined if the checklist could be used to differentiate children with high-functioning autism, Asperger's syndrome and PDD,NOS. Farmer and Oliver (2005) used the checklist to differentiate between groups of children diagnosed as having autism, autistic spectrum disorder/Asperger's syndrome, pragmatic difficulties and other types of specific language impairment. Towbin *et al.* (2005) screened children for symptoms of ASD in the setting of a mood disorders research clinic using the checklist. The checklist was one of several follow-up assessments used by Michelotti *et al.* (2002) to examine eighteen children who were first assessed at a mean age of 4;4 years and then four years later at 8;7 years. At the initial assessment, all the children had severe developmental language delay/disorder and some autistic features (although not sufficient to meet diagnostic criteria for childhood autism). In a study aimed at determining if pragmatic language impairment is just another term for autistic disorder or PDD,NOS, Bishop and Norbury (2002) used the checklist to subdivide twenty-one children aged six to nine years into thirteen cases of PLI and eight cases of typical SLI. The checklist was used by Norbury and Bishop (2003) in a study of narrative skills to establish the diagnostic status of children (specific language impairment or autistic spectrum disorder).

Several non-autistic populations have also been assessed using the Children's Communication Checklist. James and Stojanovik (2007) examined the communication skills of eight children with congenital blindness using the checklist. Helland and Heimann (2007) used the checklist to determine the prevalence of pragmatic language impairments among children who were referred to child psychiatric services. Gilmour *et al.* (2004) used the checklist to examine pragmatic language impairments in a group of children with a predominant diagnosis of conduct disorder (children with a diagnosis of an autistic spectrum condition were also included in the study). In a study of mental state verbs, Spanoudis *et al.* (2007) used the pragmatic composite score on the checklist to identify children with pragmatic difficulties. Glennen and Bright (2005) used the checklist to examine language and pragmatic skills in a group of six- to nine-year-old children who had been adopted from Eastern Europe. The checklist was used by Geurts *et al.* (2004) to investigate if children with attention deficit hyperactivity disorder (ADHD) experience pragmatic language problems and to establish if the checklist can be used to differentiate ADHD children from children with high-functioning autism. Botting (2004) examined if different subgroups of communication disordered children scored differently on the checklist. The subgroups examined in this study were children with an autistic spectrum disorder, those with typical specific language impairment,[11] the generally impaired and those with a clinical history of primary pragmatic language impairment. The checklist has also been used to examine pragmatic language impairments in children and adults with Williams syndrome (Laws and Bishop 2004).

6.2.2   Pragmatics tests

While most areas of pragmatic assessment have experienced considerable growth in recent years, tests of pragmatic language skills are still relatively few in number. Little test development has occurred because of the wide-spread view that few aspects of pragmatics permit of formal testing. However, not all clinicians and researchers subscribe to this view in its entirety. Adams (2002), for example, believes that some aspects of pragmatics can be formally assessed: 'Formal testing of pragmatics has limited potential to reveal the typ-ical pragmatic abnormalities in interaction but has a significant role to play in the assessment of comprehension of pragmatic intent' (973). Nevertheless, it remains the case that few formal tests of pragmatics exist and such tests as do exist must be supplemented by a range of informal techniques in order to obtain a reliable picture of an individual's pragmatic functioning. Adams (2002) remarks that 'in practice there are … no really satisfactory single tests of language pragmatics which cover all the aspects one would wish to assess with an individual child. Tests will always need to be supplemented by obser-vations and elicitation procedures' (976). In this section, we examine several assessment procedures that purport to test one or more aspects of pragmatics. I use the term 'test' loosely to apply to procedures that are fully standardised, as well to procedures that are not standardised but which have the format of a test (a subject is required to perform a task on which there is only one cor-rect outcome). We review the Test of Pragmatic Language (Phelps-Terasaki and Phelps-Gunn 1992), the only currently available test that is exclusively dedicated to the assessment of pragmatics. We also examine tests that are not dedicated to the assessment of pragmatics, but which nevertheless examine specific aspects of pragmatics (e.g. figurative language) or which examine lan-guage skills in subjects with known pragmatic deficits (e.g. subjects with right-hemisphere damage).

The Test of Pragmatic Language (TOPL) is an individually administered instrument that examines six core subcomponents of pragmatic language: physical setting, audience, topic, purpose (speech acts), visual-gestural cues and abstraction. These various components are motivated by the operational framework of the Model of Pragmatic Language. This test is designed for use by a range of professionals, including speech-language pathologists, teachers, psychologists and mental health professionals. It may be used to examine prag-matic language skills in a wide range of client groups, including adults with aphasia, children and adolescents with language delays or disorders and chil-dren, adolescents and adults with learning disabilities. Norms are provided for students from five to twelve years of age. Although the performance of older individuals can be compared to the highest age norms, the test's authors sug-gest that it might be equally effective to use the results to highlight individual areas of strength and weakness. Test items, many of which have corresponding pictures, are read by the examiner and answered by the student. This test is a reliable, valid assessment of language pragmatics. Phelps-Terasaki and Phelps-Gunn report several reliability statistics for the TOPL. All but one internal consistency coefficients are in the acceptable range (approximates or exceeds 0.80). An interscorer reliability coefficient of 0.99 was obtained. Systematic and controlled item selection and analysis were used in the development of TOPL to ensure the content validity of this assessment. For example, items that produced unsatisfactory item discrimination and difficulty statistics were deleted from the first experimental version of the test. A coefficient of 0.82 is reported by the test's authors for the concurrent validity of the TOPL test score. The TOPL score is also reported to have good construct validity.

Recently, Young *et al.* (2005) investigated if the TOPL could be used to differentiate pragmatic language disorders in children with autism spectrum disorders (ASDs) from controls matched on verbal IQ and language fundamentals. The TOPL was administered to thirty-four matched ASD subjects. Results showed that ASD subjects obtained significantly poorer scores than controls on the TOPL. Young *et al.* concluded that the TOPL was effective in differentiating pragmatic language disorders in children with autism spectrum disorders when performance was compared to matched controls.

One area of pragmatics that has been extensively tested is figurative language. Tests of idiom and metaphor are quite commonly employed in clinical studies, although few if any of these tests appear in a published format. Qualls *et al.* (2004) used an Idiom Comprehension Test (Qualls and Harris 1999) in a study of adolescents with language-based learning disabilities. Subjects were presented with idioms in two test conditions. In a story condition, subjects were presented with an idiom in a short story following which they were asked a question about the idiom's meaning. They were presented with a choice of four responses, only one of which was correct. In a verification condition, subjects were asked a question about an idiom's meaning (e.g. Does 'skate on thin ice' mean to be in a dangerous situation?). Subjects were required to demonstrate their agreement or disagreement with the meaning of the idiom by circling either a 'yes' or a 'no' response. Papagno (2001) used an idiom and a metaphor test (Papagno *et al.* 1995) in a study of patients with probable early Alzheimer's disease. Subjects were required to give verbal explanations of a number of nominal metaphors (e.g. 'Marco è un leone' Mark is a lion) and opaque idioms (e.g. 'essere al verde' to be completely out of money – literally, to be at the green). In a later study, Papagno *et al.* (2003) tested idiom comprehension in fifteen patients with mild probable Alzheimer's disease using a sentence-to-picture matching task. Subjects were read sentences containing idioms. They had to choose from two pictures the one that corresponded to a sentence's idiomatic meaning (the other picture represented the sentence's literal meaning). Similar tests have been used to examine idiom comprehension in aphasic patients (Papagno and Caporali 2007), schizophrenic and depressive patients (Iakimova *et al.* 2006), children with spina bifida meningomyelocele (Huber-Okrainec *et al.* 2005), children with learning disabilities (Abrahamsen and Burke-Williams 2004) and children with communication disorders (Norbury 2004).

Aspects of language pragmatics are frequently disrupted in right-hemisphere language disorder. One prominent assessment of the language disorder in right-hemisphere damage (RHD) – The Right Hemisphere Language Battery (RHLB; Bryan 1995) – examines several language functions that draw on pragmatic language skills.[12] The seven tests in the battery include tests of spoken and written metaphor appreciation, verbal humour appreciation, comprehension of inference, production of emphatic stress and lexical semantic comprehension. There is also a comprehensive discourse analysis (see section 6.2.4). The administration of the two metaphor tests follows the same procedures as those outlined above – subjects have to select one picture (spoken metaphor) or sentence (written metaphor) that corresponds to the correct meaning of eleven common metaphors incorporated into short contextual sentences. A similar test procedure is used to examine the appreciation of humour – subjects are required to select from a choice of four punchlines an ending that would make jokes funny (jokes and punchlines are presented on cards). To assess comprehension of inferred meaning, subjects are asked to listen to and read short paragraphs printed on cards. Following each passage, responses to four questions are recorded. All questions require subjects to draw inferences. The psychometric properties of the RHLB have been extensively investigated. Bryan (1995) reports that RHD subjects made significantly more errors than controls and more errors than subjects with left-hemisphere damage (LHD) on all the language tests (the one exception was the lexical-semantic test in LHD subjects). Pearson correlation coefficients were calculated to examine reliability of the discourse analysis. High interrater reliability was obtained ($r = 0.89$). Test–retest reliability coefficients, as measured by the Pearson Product Moment Correlation Coefficient, were highly significant for RHD subjects on all tests.

6.2.3   Conversation analysis

Pragmatics tests have an advantage over other forms of pragmatic assessment in being relatively quick and easy to administer. The same, however, cannot be said of approaches that make use of conversation analysis (CA). The recording, transcription and analysis of even small amounts of conversation can be a challenge to the busy clinician.[13] Notwithstanding these practical difficulties, conversation is a rich arena in which to assess the pragmatic language skills of clients. For the clinician who can surmount the time constraints of this approach, the rewards in terms of understanding a client's pragmatic skills can be considerable. It is possible to discover, for example, the particular triggers of communicative breakdown in the conversation of the aphasic client. More often than not, these triggers may reside in the conversational style of a communicative partner (Beeke *et al.* 2007). The impression that a client's conversational contributions are tangential or somewhat bizarre can be grounded by examining the 'goodness of fit' with other utterances in a conversational exchange. This is the basis of the concept of meshing in the Analysis of Language Impaired Children's Conversation, a conversation analytic approach proposed by Bishop and coworkers and examined in Chapter 7. The skills that are needed to monitor a listener's state of understanding in conversation and reformulate a message when a lack of comprehension occurs can only be adequately examined in the interactional to and fro of dyadic conversation. Conversational exchanges are really the only naturalistic context in which a speaker's ability to represent shared background knowledge within the presuppositions of an utterance can be examined. In short, the clinician who pursues a conversation analytic approach to the assessment of pragmatic language skills will find his or her commitment of time and effort well rewarded.

The clinician who opts for an assessment approach based on conversation analysis is faced with a staggering array of techniques.[14] Some techniques are aimed at specific clinical groups. For example, the Conversation Analysis Profile for People with Aphasia (CAPPA; Whitworth *et al.* 1997) is specifically designed for use with aphasic adults and their conversational partners.[15] This assessment tool aims to establish the perceptions of both these parties of the aphasic client's current conversational abilities and to relate these perceptions to what actually occurs during conversation, to determine the strategies used by aphasic speakers and their partners as well as establish their success, and to assess changes in pre-morbid communication styles in persons with aphasia. To this end, the CAPPA includes a structured interview that is conducted with the aphasic client and his or her key conversational partner, an analysis of a ten-minute sample of conversation between the person with aphasia and his or her partner and a summary profile that brings together information obtained from the interview and conversation analysis. In the conversation analysis component of CAPPA, the three key areas of conversational management that are assessed are (1) initiation and turn-taking, (2) repair and (3) topic management. Many of the concepts that inform this analysis – notions such as transition relevance place, self-initiation versus other-initiation of repair and self-repair versus other-repair – are taken directly from the work of Harvey Sacks and Emanuel Schegloff, two founding figures in conversation analysis. The information gleaned from these various investigations is used to guide intervention either through the reinforcement of existing conversational strategies and the development of new strategies or through the identification of those behaviours that are most disruptive to interaction and which may become targets for deficit-focused therapy.

Beeke *et al.* (2007) used the structured interview from CAPPA during a conversation analysis of the interaction of two aphasic clients with their respective spouses. A second CA-based analysis – Supporting Partners of People with Aphasia in Relationships and Conversation Analysis (SPPARC; Lock *et al.* 2001a) – was used as a framework for collecting and analysing data and planning intervention. In one exchange, a woman called Connie, who had a non-fluent Broca's aphasia, produced phonemic errors that became the focus of other-repair introduced by her husband Sam. These other-repairs initiated a correct production sequence which Sam continued, even to the point where Connie became distressed. Part of this extract is reproduced below:

```
 8   SAM: what hand?
 9   CONNIE: lef hands.
10   SAM: lef:T
11   CONNIE: lef  ⌐⌐ hands
12   SAM: ⌊/t/⌋
 •

 •

33   SAM: lef:t,
34   CONNIE: lef,
35   (0.3)
36   SAM: hand.
37   CONNIE: hand.
38   ⌐(5.5)
39   ⌊((CONNIE LOOKS UPSET))
```

Both Connie and Sam felt that these other-repair sequences were disruptive to the flow of conversation and that they would like to change them. Intervention took the form of four two-hour sessions during which Connie and Sam were first made aware of these correct production sequences and were then introduced to alternative conversational strategies. In a second exchange, the wife of a seventy-three-year-old aphasic man called Jim frequently asked him 'test questions' and used cueing during their conversations. Two of these questions are evident in lines twenty-two and twenty-six of the extract below:

```
22   SANDRA: where- where- where was it being set (.) wuh- what's the
         name of the book
23   ⌐(1.9)
24   JIM: ⌊((puts his hand to his face))
25   WELL I (1.2) I DUNNO.=
26   SANDRA: =can- can you remember who wrote it
27   JIM: (1.2) uh yes I- I- I've got to think but yes I-
28   SANDRA: and (.) well the name of the book (0.6) is A Passage to India
29   JIM: oh. (.) yeah.
```

This problematic questioning strategy was addressed during intervention along with other strategies that were intended to facilitate Jim in making contributions to conversation and in influencing the topic of conversation. Post-intervention videos of Jim and Sandra's conversations revealed no examples of Sandra's earlier use of test questions and cueing. Instead of cueing Jim, Sandra provided him with the word. Moreover, Sandra now regularly left silences during which Jim could self-select and contribute to the conversation. We will examine further the role of CAPPA and SPPARC in intervention with aphasia clients in section 6.3.1.

Aside from aphasia, conversation analysis has been used to assess pragmatic language skills in a number of other clinical populations. Dobbinson *et al.* (2003) used conversation analysis to examine the interactional significance of formulaic utterances in individuals with autism. Using conversation analysis, Damico and Nelson (2005) analysed several examples of problematic behaviours in autism as a type of compensatory adaptation. In a study of an adolescent girl with an autistic spectrum disorder, Stribling *et al.* (2007) used conversation analysis to explore the sequential contexts in which two different forms of repetition occurred. The two forms of repetition that occurred very frequently in the verbal output of this girl were prior-turn repeats (repetition of turn-final lexical items from another speaker's immediately prior talk) and within-turn repeats (repetition of the first item within a turn such that the turn consists solely of repeated items). Dobbinson *et al.* (1998) used the methodology of conversation analysis to examine the conversation of an adult diagnosed as autistic. Features such as topic movement, topic maintenance, repairs, overlaps, latching, pauses and interference from earlier structures and common collocations were used to highlight differences in conversational style between this adult and a researcher. Tarling *et al.* (2006) used conversation analysis in a study of a twelve-year-old boy with Williams syndrome. This boy displayed conversational strengths that were not predicted by his results on standardised language tests. Friedland and Miller (1998) used conversation analysis to examine pragmatic deficits in a speaker with a closed head injury. These investigators found that CA was a sensitive tool for the identification of these deficits. Conversation analysis helped investigators establish if language impairments identified on formal tests were evident in functional communication. Furthermore, CA could be used to reveal how different interlocutors responded to language difficulties in conversation and helped explain why some interlocutors were more successful than others in adapting to these difficulties.

Although conversation analysis is by nature a qualitative approach to the assessment of conversation, some investigators have integrated quantitative analysis within this approach.[16] For example, during the structured interviews in CAPPA, interviewees are asked to rate the frequency with which particular conversational behaviours occur. These ratings of frequency allow quantification 'which can be used to examine change over time as well as for comparison with problem severity ratings' (Whitworth *et al.* 1997: 48). It is worth remarking that data on the reliability and validity of various conversational measures are often lacking or highly variable. For example, when Oelschlaeger and Thorne (1999) applied correct information unit (CIU) analysis to the naturally occurring conversation of a speaker with moderate aphasia, they found that reliable CIU measures could not be obtained. Low intrarater reliability for CIU and percentage CIU was obtained (72 per cent). Interrater reliability was never higher than 63 per cent. 72 per cent of rater disagreements in the application of the CIU analysis resulted from insufficiencies in the scoring rules. The remaining 28 per cent of disagreements were caused by human error in the application of the rules. Adams and Bishop (1989) obtained conversational samples from fifty-seven SLI children aged eight to twelve years, fourteen of whom fitted the clinical description of semantic-pragmatic disorder. These investigators found that exchange structure, conversational repair, turn-taking and use of cohesive devices could be assessed with adequate interrater and test–retest reliability. Hux *et al.* (1997) used four methods to compute the reliability of Clinical Discourse Analysis (Damico 1985).[17] The results of this study suggest 'some apparently contradictory conclusions' with some methods (generalisability coefficients) indicating good reliability and other methods (interobserver agreement percentages for target behaviour occurrences and Cohen's kappa) indicating that agreement between raters was due to chance and high frequency non-occurrence of target behaviour.

6.2.4   Discourse analysis

Many pragmatic language disorders that are too subtle to be detected on standardised language batteries are often revealed through the study of extended language use in discourse analysis. This is particularly true in the case of traumatic brain injury (TBI), where performance on standardised batteries may give little cause for concern, yet communication skills are still noticeably disorganised and tangential.[18] In section 6.2.3, we examined how one form of discourse, conversation, draws upon a range of pragmatic language skills and is now the focus of assessment efforts by clinicians and researchers. In this section, we will discuss how noninteractive or monologic forms of discourse, of the type encountered in telling a story or describing a pictured scenario, may also be used to examine pragmatic language skills in children and adults. An assessment of narrative, for example, can be used to examine an individual's ability to distinguish between given and new information (and represent given information as presuppositions), monitor a listener's understanding of the events in a story, use cohesive devices and observe maxims of relevance, quantity and manner. These same pragmatic skills can also be observed during procedural discourse of the type needed to explain the rules of a game or describe steps in an activity (e.g. making a meal). Of course, satisfactory narratives and other forms of discourse can only be produced if a range of non-pragmatic skills and competences are also intact – structural language skills and cognitive abilities, most notably. Many discourse activities also draw extensively on an individual's world knowledge. The study of discourse thus provides assessors with a valuable context in which to assess the interaction of world knowledge and language and cognitive skills with pragmatics.

The elicitation of monologic discourse can be quite easily achieved in the setting of a clinic. A number of different discourse genres should be sampled including procedural, descriptive and narrative discourse. A child client can be asked to explain how a familiar game should be played (procedural discourse) or to describe the people and events in a pictured scenario (descriptive discourse). Wordless picture books, cartoon strips and sequences of pictures may be used to elicit narratives in children. Older clients may relate a funny story to which they were party. The clinician must select pictures and choose activities with a child's language level and knowledge in mind – the child who has no experience of playing the card game Happy Families or who lacks the vocabulary to describe a scene at the post office is unlikely to produce much in the way of procedural and descriptive discourse, respectively. Picture-based narratives have the advantage that the clinician is aware of the target vocabulary that the client is attempting to produce and the client does not have to recall a story from memory. This is particularly helpful if the client has problems with intelligibility (e.g. the aphasic client with dysarthria) or has a number of cognitive deficits (e.g. memory problems in the TBI client). All elicited discourse should be audio- or video-recorded. This will ensure accurate transcription and help the clinician assess the client's reliance on gesture (e.g. pointing to pictures) and use of suprasegmental features such as intonation and stress. The length of a recorded discourse can vary depending on a number of considerations (expressiveness of child, cooperation of client, etc.). Notwithstanding this variation, Coelho (2007) states that a spoken narrative should ideally be five sentences in length.

The analysis of discourse can proceed on a number of levels. Coelho (2007) characterises these levels as microlinguistic, microstructural, macrostructural and superstructural. At the microlinguistic level, investigators are concerned to perform within-sentence analysis. Measures at the microlinguistic level include productivity (e.g. words per T-unit[19]), grammatical complexity (e.g. subordinate clauses per T-unit) or tallies of propositions and content units (Coelho 2007). These measures have been used extensively in studies of discourse in a range of clinical subjects. Ward-Lonergan *et al.* (1999) examined the verbal retelling abilities of twenty adolescent boys with language-learning disabilities. The performance of these boys was compared with that of boys with normal language abilities on a number of measures, including number of T-units, subordinate clauses per T-unit and T-units per second. Scott and Windsor (2000) found that total T-units (productivity) and words per T-unit (grammatical complexity) were both significantly lower in the narratives and expository discourse of school-age children with language-learning disabilities than in the discourse of chronological- and language-age peers. Coelho (2002) elicited narratives from fifty-five adults with closed head injury in two story tasks (retelling and generation). Words per T-unit was one of two discourse measures that distinguished the performance of these CHI subjects from that of non-brain-injured adults. Coelho et al. (2005) used a measure of semantic complexity – the propositional complexity index – in a study of story narratives in TBI subjects. To obtain this index, these investigators tallied the number of propositions in each language sample which was then divided by the number of T-units. In a study of thirty-two aphasic subjects, Williams et al. (1994) used number of T-units and number of words and clauses per T-unit to measure amount of verbal output and grammatical complexity, respectively, during story retell and procedural discourse tasks.[20]

Microstructural or across-sentence analysis examines how well sentences are linked to each other within an extract of discourse. Sentences may be conjoined in a number of different ways, with the type of cohesive ties used varying, depending on the nature of the text and the ability and style of the speaker (Coelho 2007). Some cohesive ties may be judged to be more adequate than others. For example, a speaker who produces the utterance 'She lives alone' as part of a narrative when there is no obvious referent of 'she' in prior discourse (e.g. Jane, the young woman, etc.) has failed to adequately link this sentence to those that precede it. Halliday and Hasan (1976) proposed a system of five cohesive categories – reference, lexical, conjunctive, ellipsis and substitution – that has been widely adopted in clinical studies of discourse. Van Leer and Turkstra (1999) examined three cohesive markers (reference, conjunction and lexical) in the narratives of six adolescents with traumatic brain injury. Crosson and Geers (2001) found that narratives produced by children who had at least four years of cochlear implant experience achieved cohesion from the correct use of conjunctions and referents. Cohesion during narrative production has also been examined in adults with right-hemisphere damage (Marini et al. 2005), left-hemisphere stroke (Ellis et al. 2005) and traumatic brain injury (Coelho et al. 1995) and in children with early-onset hydrocephalus (Dennis et al. 1994). Investigators have also examined the use of cohesive devices in conversational discourse. Ripich et al. (2000) found that subjects with early to midstage Alzheimer's disease (AD) produced more referent errors during conversation than non-demented elderly, but otherwise made similar use of cohesion devices. A subset of AD subjects who were followed up at eighteen months post-entry to the study showed a significant decline in the number of ellipses and conjunctions.

Measures of local and global coherence are integral to a macrostructural analysis of discourse. Local coherence and global coherence describe the relationship of the meaning or content of an utterance to the preceding utterance and the general topic of discourse, respectively (Coelho 2007). A range of informational or content measures are also included in a macrostructural analysis of discourse. Such measures include content units, correct information units and propositions, as well as ratios that relate information units to time such as correct information units per minute (Coelho 2007). Coherence and informational measures have also featured extensively in clinical studies of discourse. Nicholas and Brookshire (1993) assessed the informativeness and efficiency of the connected speech of twenty aphasic adults using correct information analysis. Jensen *et al.* (2006) examined the number and type of information units produced during a picture description task by subjects with chronic nonthalamic subcortical lesions following stroke and subjects with Huntington's disease. Davis and Coelho (2004) examined logical coherence and accuracy of narration of six stories produced by adults with closed head injury. The logical coherence of these stories was based on the identification of causal relations between propositions. Accuracy was assessed relative to a story's theme and point. Logical coherence and accuracy of narration were also assessed by Davis *et al.* (1997) in a study of narrative production in eight adults with right-hemisphere dysfunction. Local and global coherence were among eight measurements recorded by Wilson and Proctor (2002) in a study of written discourse in adolescents with closed head injury (see also Wilson and Proctor 2000). Glosser and Deser (1991) examined global and local coherence of spoken narratives produced by patients with closed head injury, patients with probable Alzheimer's disease and patients with fluent aphasia following a left-hemisphere CVA.

Story narratives may undergo an analysis of story grammar at the superstructural level. Story grammar describes 'the purported regularities in the internal structure of stories that guide an individual's comprehension and production of the logical relationships between characters and events (temporal and causal)' (Coelho 2007: 125). Episodes are integral to an analysis of story grammar. According to Stein and Glenn (1979), an episode must consist of (a) an initiating event that causes a character to formulate a goal-directed behavioural sequence, (b) an action, and (c) a direct consequence marking attainment or nonattainment of the goal. These three components must be logically related. An episode is judged to be complete only if it contains all three of these components. As well as obtaining counts of the number of complete episodes in a story narrative, clinicians and researchers can derive efficiency scores for story narratives such as the number of T-units within episodic structure. Studies have undertaken story grammar analysis of narratives in a range of clinical subjects, including children with specific language impairment (Pearce *et al.* 2003; Newman and McGregor 2006), children with attention deficit hyperactivity disorder (Lorch *et al.* 1999), young deaf children following cochlear implantation (Nikolopoulos *et al.* 2003),[21] children and adults with closed head injury (Coelho *et al.* 1991; Jordan *et al.* 1991) and students with learning disabilities (Montague *et al.* 1990). Coelho (2002) found that adults with closed head injury produced significantly fewer T-units within episode structure than non-brain-injured adults. Merritt and Liles (1989) assessed narratives produced by language disordered children aged 9;0 to 11;4 years. These investigators found that more story grammar components and complete episode structures were produced by these children in a story retelling task than in a story generation task.

Notwithstanding the various benefits of discourse analysis in a clinical setting, the reader should also be made aware of a number of drawbacks of this assessment approach. The recording, transcription and analysis of narrative and other forms of discourse is a costly process in terms of time and effort. At the present time, there are no computer-based programs that can perform transcription or the type of analyses described previously (Coelho 2007).[22] Although some investigators are attempting to address these issues,[23] it remains the case that the commitment of time required to perform discourse analyses may reduce their feasibility as an assessment method for many clinicians. Another drawback of discourse analysis is that assessment findings fail to translate readily into a particular treatment approach. Coelho (2007) remarks that the 'primary deterrent' to the widespread use of discourse analysis in adults with neurogenic disorders, more than even time constraints, is the failure of researchers to demonstrate how findings of discourse deficits can be used for the planning of treatment. The reliability of some discourse analytic procedures has also been found to be highly variable. In a study of narrative discourse production in older language-impaired learning-disabled children, Henshilwood and Ogilvy (1999) reported that cohesive ties (anaphoric reference, ellipsis) and cohesive adequacy (anaphoric reference, lexical tie) were not stable across testing sessions and were therefore not considered reliable (high interrater reliability (95% to 98%) and intrarater reliability (98%) were obtained). John *et al.* (2003) reported interrater reliability of 87% for the story grammar components and 81% for the coding of C-units in the Strong Narrative Assessment Procedure (Strong 1998). However, these investigators were not able to substantiate Strong's claim that the stimulus stories were equivalent and could be used for test–retest purposes.[24]

6.3   Pragmatic language intervention

Having conducted a detailed assessment of a client's pragmatic language skills, the speech and language therapist is then in a position to institute a programme

of intervention. Assessment may lead the therapist to conclude that direct intervention is unnecessary. More often than not, however, some form of intervention will be recommended. This may simply take the form of one or more
advice-giving sessions, during which, for example, the therapist may instruct
the parent of the language disordered child on how to create the communication situations that will encourage greater use of a range of speech acts. In cases
where pragmatic deficits are severe, are unlikely to resolve spontaneously or
are having an adverse impact on an individual's social and occupational functioning, a more direct form of pragmatic intervention may be required. The first
thing one notices when surveying the literature on pragmatic language intervention is that there is a complete lack of consensus amongst clinicians and
researchers on the question of how pragmatic disorders should be treated. This
lack of consensus has led to the development of quite distinct approaches to
pragmatic intervention. Adams (2001) remarks that 'approaches to pragmatic
therapy currently in use tend to be eclectic and a "method" of intervention
would currently be difficult to identify' (301). The second thing one notices
is that there is little and, in some cases, no research evidence to support the
use of these approaches.[25] Indeed, the choice of approach is motivated more
by the availability of resources[26] and by therapists' experience of particular
techniques than by the application of well-validated principles. Adams *et al.*
(2005) state that:

There is ... some consensus that therapy is resource- rather than principle-driven, due to
the research vacuum. Practitioners rely on judgement and experience to select an intervention programme. There is little or no existing guidance to support these decisions.
There is certainly no significant evidence for them. (2005: 229)

Notwithstanding the eclectic nature of treatment approaches in pragmatics and
the lack of clinical rationale for many treatment techniques, we will attempt in
this section to examine the main approaches to the intervention of pragmatic
disorders. The remediation of conversation skills in both children and adults is
a frequent target of clinicians. We saw in section 6.2.3 how the methodology of
conversation analysis is being used by clinicians to assess a range of conversation skills in adults with aphasia. This same methodology is increasingly being
used by clinicians to address areas of conversational breakdown in interactions
involving aphasic clients and their key conversational partners. We resume discussion of this particular intervention approach from section 6.2.3. A major
impetus of conversation analytic approaches to the treatment of aphasia is
the recognition that impaired use of language in aphasia has some of its most
adverse consequences on a client's sense of himself as a social being.[27] The
adverse social consequences of pragmatic disorder are also well recognised
in other clinical groups[28] and are the principal motivation for the inclusion of
pragmatics in social communication interventions. We examine several of these

interventions in this section. As the discussion of earlier chapters makes clear, investigators are increasingly interested in the link between theory of mind deficits and pragmatic disorders in children and adults. Although it is too soon to say definitively that ToM deficits are the cause of pragmatic impairments, investigators have nonetheless operated on the assumption that by 'teaching' ToM skills to individuals who have mind-reading deficits, some improvement in pragmatic skills can reasonably be expected. We examine treatments that attempt to teach ToM skills as well as consider if any evidence exists to support the role of these treatments in pragmatic language interventions.

6.3.1   Conversation skills

Remediation of conversation skills is typically part of most pragmatic language interventions. This includes techniques that attempt to train subjects in how to use particular conversation skills without appeal to a wider methodological framework. It also includes techniques that draw upon the methodology of conversation analysis. These latter techniques implement the findings of CA-based assessments such as CAPPA, which were examined in section 6.2.3. We will examine both types of conversational approach in this section.

Several published studies have now reported on the use of CA-based approaches such as CAPPA and SPPARC to guide conversational intervention in aphasic adults. Whitworth et al. (1997) describe the case of J.B., who sustained an intracerebral bleed at the age of fifty-nine which had resulted in a fluent aphasia. At the time of his bleed, J.B. had been living in Australia. Subsequently, he returned to Scotland to live with his brother R.B. The CAPPA interview was conducted with R.B. A conversational sample between J.B. and his brother was recorded at home. By combining information from the interview and conversation analysis, investigators were able to determine that R.B. displayed a high level of acceptance of J.B.'s problems and had considerable insight into them (agreement between J.B.'s report and evidence from the conversation analysis was relatively high at 70 per cent). For example, R.B. reported that J.B. had a wide range of linguistic impairments, which was reflected in a score of 68 per cent for this area. This was supported by the conversation analysis which confirmed R.B.'s report of problems in nine out of eleven areas. Notwithstanding the frequency of these behaviours, R.B. only rated them as 9 per cent on the problem severity rating scale. A similar pattern – a CA-confirmed high frequency rating for a behaviour combined with a low score on the problem severity scale – was observed for repair, initiation and turn-taking and topic management (only certain aspects). It was clear that in a relatively short space of time – J.B. had only been living with R.B. for six months at the time of CAPPA administration – R.B. had attained considerable insight into J.B.'s communication problems and had developed strategies for coping with them. Whitworth *et al.* remark that 'an important part of management would be to acknowledge and value the high level of skill that J.B. and his brother already have in coping with the consequences of aphasia' (1997: 57).

It emerged from the interview with J.B.'s brother, and was confirmed by conversation analysis, that R.B. often encouraged J.B. to correct his aphasic errors. Booth and Perkins (1999), who also examined J.B., report that 78 per cent of major conversational turns during pre-intervention conversation were involved in repair sequences. R.B. admitted that this repair strategy only had a positive outcome on some occasions (only 39 per cent, according to Booth and Perkins, were reported by R.B. as having the desired outcome). Moreover, only some of this repair work was even necessary to allow the exchange to continue. More often than not, R.B. knew J.B.'s intended target and it was possible to continue the conversation without the disruption caused by lengthy repair sequences. It was decided that a reduction in this particular conversational strategy may result in less frustrating and more socially rewarding conversations for J.B. It was also expected that by reducing the impact of this strategy on conversation, J.B. might be willing to assume a more active role in conversation. Intervention therefore focused on providing R.B. with information on the effective use of collaborative repair and on the potential negative effects on J.B.'s self-image of withholding this collaboration. Other areas addressed during intervention were the psychosocial consequences of aphasia and J.B.'s linguistic processing abilities (Booth and Perkins 1999). Repair was addressed by encouraging R.B. to consider the face-threatening nature of other-corrections in conversation and to adhere to the principle of least collaborative effort[29] when carrying out repair work. Short samples of conversation were examined with R.B. having to suggest the repair initiator that most accurately reflected his state of understanding at particular points in the conversation. This was intended to achieve more rapid resolution of repair. The disruption of lengthy repair sequences to topic development was also discussed. Conversation analysis revealed that only 29 per cent of major turns were involved in repair work following intervention. There were no instances in the post-intervention analysis of R.B. initiating repair to correct J.B.'s aphasic errors. Instead, repair was used only to resolve trouble sources and permit J.B. turns to contribute to the conversation. There was also some evidence of J.B. initiating repair on R.B.'s conversational turns following intervention.

CAPPA-based intervention has also been implemented in a group setting. Booth and Swabey (1999) recruited four aphasic adults and their key conversational partners (their carers) into an intervention that involved six weekly communication skills groups, each of two hours' duration. CAPPA interviews and conversation analyses were conducted. An analysis of collaborative repair management was also undertaken. Group activities consisted of lectures, discussions and workshops. Participants also analysed short written and video-recorded conversation samples and discussed impairments, turn-taking and repair. Individualised advice was delivered to partners through the use of written advice sheets. A repeat CAPPA and repair analysis were undertaken upon completion of intervention. These analyses revealed a significant increase in agreement scores post-intervention (i.e. reports of problems by carers were confirmed by the conversation analyses). This suggested a greater awareness of the aphasic speakers' difficulties on the part of carers following intervention. Although severity scores decreased for each aphasic client, decreases were not statistically significant. Notwithstanding the fact that three of the four partners reported an increase in the frequency scores for the conversational management procedure of repair, all partners reported a reduction in the problem severity rating for this area. In two of the aphasic–carer dyads, there was a significant decrease in the number of turns spent on collaborative repair. In one dyad, the average length of the repair trajectory decreased from thirty-five to eight turns. Qualitative analysis of repair produced some variable results. For example, while the carer in one dyad used more efficient strategies post-intervention which reduced the amount of metalinguistic work that was devoted to repair, the carer in another dyad often refused to offer assistance, preferring instead that the aphasic person self-repair. Booth and Swabey (1999) conclude that although more research is needed in this area, the results of this study appear to confirm the usefulness of CAPPA and a quantitative/qualitative analysis of repair management in motivating individualised advice to carers and targeting conversation management in a group setting. These techniques also had demonstrated value in measuring the effectiveness of intervention.

Another intervention that is based on conversation analysis is Supporting Partners of People with Aphasia in Relationships and Conversation (SPPARC; Lock *et al*. 2001a). Conversations between aphasic speakers and their partners are video- or audio-taped in the speakers' own homes. At least ten minutes of talk are recorded and transcribed. This can include several short conversations, depending on the participants' conversational style. Assessment focuses on areas of conversation that are most often problematic in aphasia, such as the use of repair, the construction of turns and sharing of the conversational floor and topic management (Lock *et al*. 2001b). For example, the aphasic speaker may be subject to numerous requests for repair which serve to highlight his or her lack of linguistic competence. He or she may frequently use minimal turns such as 'mm hm' or lose the conversational floor owing to silences related to word-finding difficulties. It may be difficult for the aphasic speaker to initiate topics and guide the direction of conversation. The clinician will be concerned to examine patterns of behaviour as well as assess the frequency and location of particular behaviours. Behaviours that will benefit from training include those that indicate that the couple is relying excessively on a particular pattern of interaction (e.g. the use of test questions), the assumption of certain roles (e.g. the aphasic speaker's partner assuming the role of teacher or therapist) and behaviours that cause distress to the aphasic speaker, as evidenced by emotional reactions. For each area that is addressed during training, participants are led through three progressive stages. These stages are designed to help participants gain insight into conversational patterns, to reflect upon these patterns and to identify and actively experiment with options for change.

The first stage of raising awareness of and insight into a particular conversational pattern can be achieved by a number of activities. If the behaviour that is problematic to interaction is overlap of the aphasic speaker by the partner, the clinician should first introduce and explain the concept of overlap during turn-taking in conversation. Teaching videos can be used to demonstrate examples of the behaviour to be targeted, as can the use of handouts and written exercises and role-playing activities (these resources are available in SPPARC). Once the behaviour is reliably identified using these various resources, the aphasic speaker and conversational partner should be encouraged to reflect upon their own use of overlap during conversation. The effects of overlap on the interaction should be considered and will be the basis upon which the couple makes decisions about the retention or modification of this particular behaviour. The Conversation Training Programme of SPPARC includes methods that are aimed at achieving these ends, including examining examples of the target behaviour in the couple's own video-taped conversation, discussing transcripts of this conversation and monitoring conversations at home with the help of written guides and activities. In order to avoid a prescriptive stance on the part of the clinician, behaviours that are to be targeted for change must emerge from discussion with the couple.[30] Strategies for change may be identified and practised between the aphasic speaker and partner, with the clinician or with members of a group. The use of new strategies during conversations at home should also be encouraged by the clinician. The knowledge and insight gained through the Conversation Training Programme should enable the aphasic speaker and partner to reflect on the success of these strategies (Lock *et al*. 2001b). Recent studies that have used SPPARC to guide intervention with aphasic clients include Lock *et al*. (2001a) and Burch *et al*. (2002), both of which are reported in Beeke *et al*. (2007). Turner and Whitworth (2006) have also used SPPARC in a study that has examined clinicians' perceptions of candidacy for conversation partner training.

Other conversational interventions with aphasic adults are currently available, including the use of Supported Conversation for Adults with Aphasia (SCA).[31] This approach is motivated by a model that emphasises goals of social participation for the aphasic adult. SCA makes use of volunteers who receive training in techniques that will help them reveal the competence of speakers with aphasia. In a recent efficacy study, Kagan *et al*. (2001) administered SCA training to twenty volunteers. A further twenty control volunteers were simply exposed to people with aphasia. On ratings of acknowledging competence and revealing competence in their aphasic partners, the trained volunteers scored significantly higher than the untrained volunteers. Moreover, a positive change in ratings of social and message exchange skills in aphasic speakers was observed, despite the fact that these speakers did not participate in training. Rayner, H. and Marshall, J. (2003) also examined the efficacy of SCA in the treatment of conversation skills in aphasic adults. Six adults with moderate to severe aphasia participated in this study. Aphasic subjects were aged between fifty-six and seventy-nine years and were between one and thirteen years post-onset of aphasia. Six volunteers in an aphasia group in Milton Keynes, England were recruited into a training course. This course drew on a number of Kagan's techniques, including viewing of videos and role play, presentation of information using different media and group discussions. Although the main aims of the study were to establish the impact of training on the volunteers in the study, a further aim of the study was to increase the participation of aphasic subjects in conversation. Questionnaires were completed by volunteers before and after training. Videos of the volunteers in conversation with aphasic speakers were also rated by speech and language therapists who used nine-point rating scales. Questionnaire scores and therapists' ratings of the volunteers' videos revealed significant improvements after training. Comparable gains in aphasic subjects' participation in conversation also occurred after training.

Beyond aphasia, conversation skills have been the focus of intervention in a number of other clinical groups. Chief amongst these groups are clients with autism and schizophrenia, where conversation is most often targeted as part of a social skills training programme. Barry *et al.* (2003) included conversation in an outpatient clinic-based social skills group intervention with four high-functioning elementary-aged children with autism. Chin and Bernard-Opitz (2000) attempted to train conversational skills in three high-functioning children with autism. The children in this study were taught how to initiate a conversation, maintain and change conversational topics appropriately, take turns during conversation and listen attentively. Charlop and Milstein (1989) examined the effects of video modelling on the acquisition and generalisation of conversational skills in three autistic boys. Videotaped conversations between two people who discussed specific toys were observed by these boys. To assess generalisation of conversational skills, untrained topics, new stimuli (toys), unfamiliar persons, siblings and autistic peers and other settings were used. Chien *et al.* (2003) included conversation skills in social skills training of thirty-five schizophrenic subjects. Conversation was also part of social skills training of outpatients with persistent and unremitting forms of schizophrenia in a study conducted by Liberman *et al.* (1998). These studies have resulted in highly variable conversation outcomes. For example, while Chien *et al.*

observed that conversation skills improved significantly in their schizophrenic subjects with treatment and were superior to a control group at intratreatment, post-treatment and follow-up, Barry *et al.* noted 'less clear improvements' in the conversation skills of their high-functioning children with autism in an outpatient clinic setting and little or no generalisation of skills outside of this setting.

6.3.2   Social communication

Clinical and academic interest in social communication has never been greater. Much of this interest has been generated by a significant increase in the number of diagnosed cases of autistic spectrum disorders.[32] There are marked social communication impairments in ASD children and adults. Certainly, the study of these disorders has generated most of our knowledge of the different processes and skills that constitute social communication (see Chapter 3 in Cummings 2008). It is becoming increasingly clear that at least some of these processes and skills are pragmatic in nature. However, while clinicians and researchers are in general agreement that pragmatics has a role to play within social communication, there is much less agreement on what the extent of that role should be. For some practitioners, pragmatics is the major component of social communication, so much so in fact that these terms have often come to be used interchangeably. A somewhat different view of the relationship of pragmatics to social communication is taken by Adams (2005). Pragmatics, Adams argues, 'has for too long been used synonymously with social communication when it is in fact only one of four aspects of development that contribute to social communication that practitioners need to consider in speech-language intervention' (2005: 182). According to Adams, 'social communication development is founded on the synergistic emergence of social interaction, social cognition, pragmatics (verbal and nonverbal aspects), and language processing (receptive and expressive)' (182). In this section, we leave aside the question of the relationship of pragmatics to social communication – this question will be addressed again in Chapter 7. Instead, we examine social communication interventions that have targeted pragmatic language skills to a greater or lesser extent.

Within social communication intervention, Adams (2005) employs a meta-pragmatic approach to the remediation of pragmatic deficits. As Adams describes this approach, 'intervention focuse[s] on direct work on the formal aspects of pragmatics at a reflective level, explicitly talking about rules and conventions and putting these into practice' (2005: 184). The 'aspects' of pragmatics that Adams addresses in this approach are conversational conventions, topic management, speech acts, turn-taking, linguistic cohesion and matching style to context (e.g. politeness). Adams *et al.* (2005) describe the use of metapragmatic therapy techniques in the treatment of two children with social communication impairment. These children were 9;9 and 8;01 years of age at the start of intervention. One of the priorities for intervention with the older child was 'to use his above average language skills to reflect upon his own conversational and nonverbal interactional style' (2005: 235). During individual structured sessions with the younger child, conversation rules were demonstrated as metapragmatic constructs and practised in role play. The child was encouraged, for example, to identify conversational breakdown during a sabotage role play in which puppets were scripted to interrupt, switch topic and talk too much. Andersen-Wood and Smith (1997) describe a similar approach to the remediation of pragmatics within metapragmatic awareness training.[33] The emphasis of metapragmatic awareness teaching is on thinking about the process of communication: 'Metapragmatic awareness is *conscious* knowledge of what is required in communicative interactions: for example, being consciously aware that it is necessary to take turns in a conversation, rather than simply being able to do so in a conversation' (107; italics in original). The requirement for reflection in this approach means that it may not be suitable for all clients. Adams (2005) states that it is rare for children who are functioning below seven years of age in terms of their language processing skills to participate successfully in a metapragmatic approach.

The versatility of social communication intervention is demonstrated by its application to quite diverse clinical groups. Clegg *et al.* (2007) conducted two phases of speech and language therapy in a fifty-three-year-old adult male schizophrenic patient who presented with severe poverty of speech. Desensitisation of this patient to verbal communication was the focus of the first phase of therapy. The aims of the second phase of therapy were to increase the patient's awareness of his social communication skills, and to develop language productivity. Three social communicative behaviours were chosen as targets: (1) the establishment and maintenance of eye contact with the relevant partner in communicative settings, (2) the initiation and return of greetings, and (3) the increase of facial expression by smiling. Timler *et al.* (2005) undertook social communication intervention in a school-age child with a complex cognitive and behavioural profile secondary to a diagnosis of a foetal alcohol spectrum disorder. Social cognitive skills and mental state verb production were targeted during intervention. Intervention proceeded by means of group role play of social scripts and used a checklist to elicit statements from the child about others' perspectives and strategies for completing the social script. These two studies are typical of social communication interventions in general, in that each is targeting a very different set of skills – Clegg *et al.* are focusing on conversational and nonverbal behaviours, while Timler *et al.* are emphasising theory of mind skills (theory of mind false belief tasks were used by Timler *et al.* to examine mental state verb use during probe sessions). Perhaps these studies serve to exemplify the type of approach advocated by Adams, in which four aspects of development contribute to social communication and intervention can target one or two of these aspects over others.[34] Whatever their ultimate rationale, the rather eclectic nature of social communication interventions and the still largely uncertain role of pragmatics within these interventions precludes any definitive conclusions about their contribution to the remediation of pragmatics at this time.

6.3.3   Pragmatic skills training

While many interventions attempt to teach pragmatic skills from within a social communication framework, the focus of other interventions is on the development of pragmatic skills within a social skills training group approach. The techniques employed in this latter approach have been extensively outlined elsewhere (Andersen-Wood and Smith 1997). In this section, we describe the basic features of pragmatic skills training as well as examine several studies that have adopted this approach to pragmatic remediation. Training typically occurs within a group setting and involves extensive use of role-playing activities.[35] Such activities, Andersen-Wood and Smith contend, require a level of skill that is not commonly seen in children under 3;6 years. However, some children of four years of age and many five-year-olds are able to participate in these types of activities. The presence of several participants in a group setting confers numerous benefits on the training of pragmatic skills. The opportunity to practise pragmatic skills in the presence of other clients is more akin to everyday speaking situations and thus has ecological validity that is largely lacking in client–therapist interactions. Other clients can provide constructive feedback on an individual's use of particular skills in a non-threatening environment. Clients who have strengths in particular areas of pragmatic functioning (e.g. turn-taking) can provide good models to individuals with impairments in those areas. As well as benefits, group training has a number of disadvantages. Clients who present with disruptive behaviours (e.g. the child with attention deficit hyperactivity disorder) can be difficult to manage in a group and can pose a distraction to other participants. Shy clients may respond poorly to role-playing activities which demand performance in front of other group participants. Also, some clients may require more intensive intervention than can be provided in a group setting. In short, group intervention presents a range of unique challenges that only a highly experienced clinician can address.

With these various considerations in mind, two studies that have used pragmatic skills training will be outlined. Hyter *et al.* (2001) describe a classroom-based pragmatic language intervention in children diagnosed with emotional and behavioural disorders. Six boys participated in the intervention. These boys were aged between 8;6 and 12;11 years and attended a specialised educational facility for children with emotional and behavioural disorders. Intervention took the form of thirty-minute sessions that were conducted twice weekly over a period of eight weeks (a total of sixteen sessions were undertaken). Four pragmatic skills were targeted during intervention: describing objects, giving directions, stating personal opinions about inappropriate behaviour and negotiating for desired outcomes. The describing objects activity was a type of referential communication task in which children had to describe objects to naïve listeners who could not see the objects in question. In the giving directions activity, children had to tell a novel listener the various steps, correctly sequenced, in a familiar activity (e.g. getting ready to go to school). In stating opinions about inappropriate behaviour, children were required to say if a particular behaviour was inappropriate (e.g. violated a school rule) and how they would respond to someone who committed such a behaviour. In negotiating for some desired outcome, children were required to give reasons why they wanted a certain object, activity or outcome (e.g. state why the child should be allowed to play a little longer with a friend's toy). In a lesson, children were first introduced to an activity, received oral and written step-by-step instructions of the activity and were given a role-played model of the desired communication. During role play, a speech-language pathologist and special education teacher modelled appropriate and inappropriate responses for the children. In the first lesson of each week, children worked in small groups of two or three students. During the second lesson each week, smaller groups were brought together as the whole classroom.

Wiseman-Hakes *et al.* (1998) performed peer-group training of pragmatic skills in six adolescents, aged fourteen to seventeen years, with acquired brain injury. All six adolescents achieved a rating of three or less on each subdomain of the Rehabilitation Institute of Chicago Rating Scale of Pragmatic Communication Scale (RICE-RSPCS; Burns *et al.* 1985) prior to intervention. Wiseman-Hakes *et al.* taught four modules of the training programme Improving Pragmatic Skills in Persons with Head Injury (Sohlberg *et al.* 1992) during an intervention that ran for six weeks, four days a week, for an hour each day. These modules included Initiation, Topic Maintenance, Turn Taking and Active Listening. This training programme, which is designed for individual therapy, was modified for use in a group setting. These modifications included the training of adolescent subjects in how to give feedback to peers on their communication performances. No negative feedback was permitted. To increase awareness of communication and to improve self-monitoring, adolescents rated their own and others' communication performance. A range of exercises was used to practise conversational exchanges with each other. Subjects were first given the opportunity to view appropriate and inappropriate pragmatic behaviours on videotapes that had been previously prepared by the investigators. Later, role-playing exercises, initially between the therapist and research assistant and then between adolescents, were carried out. These exercises targeted specific communication goals and were videotaped and reviewed by the group. Each of the four modules that were taught during intervention consisted of an awareness phase, a practice phase and a generalisation phase. In order to facilitate generalisation, the adolescents in this study were encouraged to practise pragmatic skills outside of therapy with peers, staff and parents. Age-appropriate activities and realistic contexts were selected for this purpose.

The techniques used in both these pragmatic interventions were evidently successful. Before intervention, all of Hyter *et al.*'s child subjects scored in the below-average range (80–89) on the Test of Pragmatic Language. Following intervention, three of the six subjects in this study had increased their scores on this test to the average range (90–110) and three had improved to the above-average range (111–120). Error scores decreased in the four areas of TOPL that directly related to the pragmatic skills targeted during classroom intervention (i.e. describing information, expressing judgement, considering the listener and understanding the listener). Interactive communication sample data revealed that five of the six subjects improved their scores on the describing objects activity and four of the six improved their scores on the activity that involved giving step-by-step directions. On both these pragmatic behaviours, differences in pre- and post-test scores were statistically significant. Moreover, the children in this study significantly increased their number of speaking turns following intervention. Similarly positive outcomes in terms of pragmatics were reported for the brain-injured adolescents in Wiseman-Hakes *et al.*'s study. From pre-treatment to post-treatment, the mean score for the RICE-RSPCS subscales increased by an average of 44 per cent. Statistically significant changes occurred in four RICE-RSPCS subscales following intervention. These subscales were Nonverbal Communication, Use of Linguistic Context, Organisation of a Narrative and Conversational Skills. No significant differences were found on the RICE-RSPCS subscales between post-treatment and at follow-up six months after the programme. The mean scores on the Communication Performance Scale (CPS; Ehrlich and Sipes 1985)[36] increased by 32 per cent during the pre-treatment to post-treatment interval but did not change between post-treatment and follow-up. This represented a statistically significant change during the course of the study. For one fifteen-year-old, known as M, who participated in the study, considerable functional gains were reported. M's mother described how he had poor turn-taking skills, and produced egocentric comments that were inappropriate to the context of conversation prior to intervention. Following intervention, he was able to make comments that were relevant to the topic under discussion, initiate interaction with family members, join in conversations and make appropriate comments to other unfamiliar teenagers.

6.3.4   Teaching theory of mind

A number of interventions have attempted to remediate pragmatic impairments by treating cognitive deficits that are believed to be related to those impairments. One such group of deficits, at least in individuals with autistic spectrum disorders, involves the ability to attribute beliefs and other mental states both to one's own mind and to the minds of others (so-called 'theory of mind' deficits). The guiding rationale of these pragmatic interventions is that if gains can be made in a client's theory of mind skills, then these gains might reasonably be expected to generalise to the type of belief attribution (specifically, attribution of communicative intentions) that is the basis of all pragmatic interpretation. Training programmes that directly target ToM skills are now used extensively to treat social and communication impairments in autistic clients and in clients with schizophrenia. In this way, Parsons and Mitchell (2002) state that 'recent, cognitive approaches to teaching social skills to people with ASDs have included older children, and adults. These approaches tend to be based on the "theory of mind" (TOM) hypothesis of autism and provide an alternative to behaviour-based techniques' (431). However, empirical studies are increasingly revealing that although autistic clients can be taught to pass tests of false belief, gains in the ToM skills that are assessed by these tests tend not to lead to improvements in non-trained areas of social and communicative functioning: 'it appears that people with autism can be taught to pass false belief tasks, but the benefits of this understanding are restricted to tasks on which instruction has been given' (Parsons and Mitchell 2002: 435). In this section, we review the findings of some of these studies. We will also be interested in the techniques that are used by investigators to teach ToM skills to autistic individuals and other clients.

Several techniques have been successfully used to teach ToM skills to individuals with autism. A pictorial augmentation methodology, in which mental states are made concrete by associating them with a tangible counterpart in reality (e.g. a photograph), is one of the main paradigms for teaching ToM skills to autistic clients (Parsons and Mitchell 2002). Hadwin *et al.* (1997) taught mental state understanding in three areas to thirty children with autism. The three areas in question were the understanding of emotions, understanding belief and pretend play. Children in the emotion teaching group were first taught the external indicators of others' emotions (e.g. facial expression) and then that emotions can have internal, cognitive causes such as beliefs and desires. Perspective-taking and belief tasks were used to train children in the belief teaching group. Teaching in the emotion and belief groups consisted of a question–answer structure with corrective feedback. The teacher also explicitly stated a general principle that governed the understanding of the target mental state. To teach pretend play to children, a combination of modelling and verbal guidance was used. This required the teacher to take on a pretend role during play and make comments and suggestions to encourage children to play. All three teaching groups made gains in their respective areas of mental state understanding, with significant gains observed in the emotion and belief groups.

In a social skills training programme, Ozonoff and Miller (1995) borrowed an approach from Baron-Cohen and Howlin (1993) to teach ToM skills to five adolescent males with autism. This approach emphasises that perception influences knowledge (in other words, that a person only knows what he or she hears or sees). To illustrate principles of this type, autistic subjects participated in role plays that mirrored standard first-order and second-order false belief tasks. For example, in a role play targeting first-order belief attribution, two children hide a toy together. One of the children changes the location of the toy outside of the other child's view. Group members are then asked to predict where the latter child will look for the toy. The performance of autistic children who received ToM training on a theory of mind composite improved at post-treatment assessment, while that of an autistic control group did not. The effect sizes of the group difference on the theory of mind composite and change scores (i.e. pre-treatment minus post-treatment composite) was medium to large and very large, respectively. This suggested that the intervention was effective in improving performance on false belief tasks. Roncone et al. (2004) performed cognitive exercises in ten schizophrenic adults with ToM deficits using Feuerstein's (1980) Instrumental Enrichment Programme. One of the sub-objectives of this programme 'consisted of the realisation, in role-play sessions, of social situations in which first and second order ToM issues were present' (2004: 427). Schizophrenic subjects were required to recognise and describe the hidden beliefs of people in these social situations, particularly their beliefs about other people. Intervention lasted for up to one hour each week for twenty-two weeks, following which subjects were re-evaluated. After six months of metacognitive rehabilitation, these schizophrenic subjects displayed statistically significant improvements in first- and second-level ToM abilities.

These studies clearly demonstrate that autistic and schizophrenic subjects who receive ToM training can make significant gains in performance on false belief tests and other ToM tasks. However, the difficulty for intervention approaches based on ToM training is that these gains seldom generalise to areas such as social and communicative functioning. So while the autistic children in Hadwin et al.'s (1997) study made significant gains in the understanding of emotion and belief, these children failed to develop improved conversational skills as a result of intervention or to use more mental and internal state words in speech.[37] Hadwin et al. state that 'the results show that children, through teaching, did learn to pass tasks concerning emotional and belief understanding. However, there was no corresponding advance in social communication skills' (1997: 533). Similarly, the adolescent males with autism in Ozonoff and Miller's (1995) study displayed improvements on a theory of mind composite following ToM training. Yet, these subjects did not display significant change in parent and teacher scores on the Social Skills Rating System (SSRS; Gresham and Elliott 1990) following intervention. Also, their SSRS scores did not differ from untreated autistic subjects at post-treatment follow-up. In fact, negative correlations were found between performance on the theory of mind composite at post-treatment follow-up and SSRS scores following intervention. This indicated that subjects with high scores on ToM measures were given low ratings by parents and teachers on general social skills. Ozonoff and Miller state that 'the change seen in theory of mind performance after treatment ... did not extend to more general ratings of social competence made by important figures in the subjects' lives' (1995: 430).[38] In the absence of greater generalisation of gains in theory of mind skills to areas such as social and communicative functioning, treatments that adopt ToM training still have limited clinical value as pragmatic interventions.[39]

NOTES

1 In relation to children with Down's syndrome, Buckley and Le Prèvost (2002) remark that 'visual short-term memory is not impaired relative to non-verbal mental abilities and is described as a relative strength' (71).
2 Loveland and Tunali (1991) examined the ability of high-functioning verbal individuals with autism or Down's syndrome to respond appropriately to social scripts that involved a distressed individual. During a tea party situation, an examiner told subjects about an unhappy personal experience that he or she had experienced (e.g. a stolen wallet). If the subject did not contribute an acceptable response after several probes (e.g. 'My money has gone; now I can't buy groceries'), the examiner modelled a sympathetic response and then produced more probes. While autistic subjects gave a significantly greater percentage of responses relating to the tea party, subjects with Down's syndrome produced a significantly greater percentage of relevant suggestions and sympathetic comments. Significantly more autistic subjects than Down's syndrome subjects needed models.
3 Although in Chapter 7 I challenge accounts in which gestures and facial expressions are characterised as pragmatic in nature, Paradis's point is nonetheless well made.
4 Penn (1999) states that 'as sensitivity to task and context is the essence of pragmatic competence, multitask and context evaluation should be the hallmark of pragmatic assessment' (543).
5 In keeping with standard use, the terms 'formal' and 'informal' are applied to assessment tools that are standardised and non-standardised, respectively. Some clinicians and researchers use the term 'formal' of any *published* assessment tool, regardless of whether the tool is standardised. Such usage is evident in the Young *et al.* (2005) study discussed in section 6.2.4 – the Strong Narrative Assessment Procedure is a non-standardised tool, yet is described by these investigators as a formal assessment.

6 Some pragmatic assessments have been designed for use with specific clinical subjects. The Profile of Communicative Appropriateness (Penn 1988), for example,
was specifically designed for use with people with aphasia. A total of forty-five
parameters are grouped into six main categories: response to interlocutor, control of
semantic content, cohesion, fluency, sociolinguistic sensitivity and nonverbal communication. Each parameter is assessed according to a five-point scale: inappropriate, mostly inappropriate, some appropriate, mostly appropriate and appropriate. A
response of 'could not evaluate' is also possible.

7 A Pragmatics Profile has been included in the latest (fourth) edition of the Clinical
Evaluation of Language Fundamentals (CELF-4; Semel *et al.* 2003). The profile
contains a checklist of descriptive items in three areas: rituals and conversational
skills; asking for, giving and responding to information; and nonverbal communication. Pragmatic skills are also assessed in the Functional Communication Profile –
Revised (Kleiman 2003), a descriptive tool that evaluates communication skills
in individuals with developmental and acquired delays across age ranges. Some
of the pragmatics items in this profile are communication intent, initiates communication, answers questions and topic initiation. The Functional Assessment of
Communication Skills for Adults (FACS; Frattali *et al.* 1995) also assesses pragmatic skills. For example, the section in this assessment on social communication
contains items on the understanding of intent (e.g. 'It's getting late' implies that
it's time to go), the understanding of non-literal meaning and inference (e.g. 'He
has a heavy heart' or other culturally appropriate idiom) and items that relate to
the use and understanding of speech acts (e.g. requests information of others). This
assessment is designed for use with adults who have speech, language and cognitive
communication disorders. In a web-based survey of speech-language pathologists,
Simmons-Mackie *et al.* (2005) found that FACS was the most frequently reported
functional assessment tool used to measure outcome in aphasia (this assessment
comprised some 25 per cent of reported functional tools).

8 The descriptive, qualitative nature of the profile means that 'reliability and validity must be approached differently from typical quantitative methods' (Dewart and
Summers 1995: 15). The consistency of an interviewee's responses, Dewart and
Summers contend, can be tested in informal ways (e.g. asking a similar question
again at a later time). The examiner can attempt to validate responses by obtaining
information from other sources (e.g. by interviewing someone else or by using other
approaches to assessment in the area of pragmatics). The process of triangulation is
thus essential to validating responses in the Pragmatics Profile.

9 The first edition of the checklist contained a pragmatic composite that was based on
the following five scales: coherence, inappropriate initiation, stereotyped conversation, use of context and rapport. In the second edition, the pragmatic composite was
replaced by the Social Interaction Deviance Composite.

10 Bishop *et al.* (2006a) assessed the internal consistency, interrater reliability and
validity of the CCC scales in a study that examined the effectives of the checklist in
identifying heritable language impairment. Internal consistency was 0.7 or greater
for most scales. Two exceptions were the use of context and interests scales in the
parent- and teacher-completed questionnaires and the social relationships scale
in the parent-completed questionnaire. The internal consistency of the pragmatic
composite was 0.89 and 0.91 in the parent- and teacher-completed questionnaires,
respectively. Interrater reliability between parent and teacher ratings was generally

weak with correlations exceeding 0.5 on only the speech, syntax and coherence scales and on the General Communication Composite. Validity was assessed in terms of how the CCC compared with psychometric tests in terms of their ability to distinguish children with a language impairment risk from children at low risk of language impairment. The speech, syntax and coherence scales and the General Communication Composite were at least as effective as psychometric tests at discriminating these two groups of children.

11 Conti-Ramsden and Botting (2004) found that pragmatic language difficulties, as measured on the Children's Communication Checklist, were most strongly related to poor social outcome in SLI children and to expressive language related to victimisation.

12 The following extract from Bryan (1995) highlights the central role of pragmatics in right-hemisphere language disorder: 'the results of work on RH language processing, particularly at the semantic, discourse and prosodic levels of language, provide support for clinical observations of the failure of certain RHD patients to appreciate humour, connotative aspects of meaning and paralinguistic cues. Their overall impairment in comprehending and using contextual information to derive meaning may partly explain their insensitivity to the pragmatic aspects of communication. They seem unable to fully appreciate the speaker's intentions, the purposes of the exchange or their listener's needs. In addition they are unable to extract and isolate key elements, see the relationships among them, integrate them into an overall structure, and draw inferences based on these relationships both in complex structured linguistic tasks and in discourse' (1995: 9–10).

13 Coelho (2007) states that 'to transcribe and analyze a 15-minute sample of conversation may require 3 hours' (126). Adams et al. (2006) remark that the transcription and coding time for ten minutes of conversation in Bishop's Assessment of Language Impaired Children's Conversation is approximately two hours for a skilled coder.

14 It should be emphasised that some conversation analytic techniques do not explicitly align themselves with the CA principles which are discussed by Damico et al. (1999) and which have their origins in the pioneering work of Harvey Sacks and his collaborators, Emanuel Schegloff and Gail Jefferson. For example, Dorothy Bishop has developed a quantitative approach to the analysis of conversation known as the Assessment of Language Impaired Children's Conversations. Adams (2002) states that this conversational coding system is based on the work of Coulthard (1985) and McTear (1985).

15 The CAPPA is based on the Conversation Analysis Profile for People with Cognitive Impairment (CAPPCI; Perkins et al. 1997). The CAPPCI was developed for two research projects that examined cognitive impairments in dementia (Whitworth et al. 1997).

16 Beeke et al. (2007) state that 'quantitative analysis is possible within CA, but it should always follow on from a qualitative analysis of particular examples in context and not stand alone as a mere count of language forms, for example' (138).

17 Damico states that although his Clinical Discourse Analysis (CDA; Damico 1985) applies many of the principles from ethnography of speaking and conversation analysis, it is only a 'superficial hybrid' of these more elaborate and interpretive research methodologies. The inclusion of CDA in this section is motivated more by the fact that this framework examines *conversational* discourse than by its adherence to the

principles of conversation analysis. In listing the procedures to follow when using CDA, Damico states that a spontaneous language sample 'should be collected during conversational interaction rather than in simple picture description activities. This is essential in order to analyze the individual's discourse abilities' (1985: 184). Although CDA was originally developed by Damico to assess language abilities in older school-age children, the technique has now come to be applied to other clinical groups. Snow *et al.* (1998) used a modified form of Damico's CDA to assess the conversational abilities of a group of severely injured TBI speakers.

18 Coelho (2007) remarks of TBI speakers that 'examining performance by means of such batteries may give the impression that communicative skills are intact. However, when individuals with disordered pragmatics are engaged in interactions, the listener has the impression that they are off target, disorganized, or tangential. Thus, the communicative behavior of interest lies beyond the level of single words or sentences, which such individuals have little difficulty with, but rather involves longer units of language such as discourse' (123).

19 T-units (terminable units), as described by Hunt (1965), are obtained prior to analysis of discourse. A T-unit is defined as 'one main clause with all the subordinate clauses attached to it. The number of subordinate clauses can, of course, be none' (1965: 20).

20 A published assessment of narrative discourse – the Strong Narrative Assessment Procedure (Strong 1998) – employs C-units (communication units) in a number of its analyses of length (number of C-units) and syntactic complexity (average number of words per C-unit; number of clauses per C-unit). C-units were introduced by Loban (1976) to analyse oral samples (Hunt's T-units were originally used only for written samples). However, it is clear from Loban's definition of the C-unit as 'each independent clause with its modifiers' (1976: 9) that C-units and T-units are functionally equivalent.

21 Nikolopoulos *et al.* (2003) used the Stories/Narratives Assessment Procedure (SNAP) to elicit narratives from the children in this study. SNAP-Dragons (Lloyd-Richmond and Starczewski 2008) is a narrative assessment that uses a story retell technique. Although this assessment was originally developed for use with deaf children from preschool to nine years of age, it has also been successfully used with children with communication difficulties and learning difficulties. The assessment makes use of two levels of analysis, story grammar and semantic combinations.

22 Coelho (2007) states that two programmes that have been applied to adult discourse – SALT (Miller and Chapman 2006) and CHILDES (MacWhinney 2000) – require extensive coding of transcripts before they can undergo computer analysis.

23 Recently, Armstrong *et al.* (2007) addressed the issue of the time-consuming nature of the transcription process by examining the validity and reliability of transcription-less discourse analysis. Ten aphasic subjects were audio- and video-recorded performing tasks in three different discourse genres (conversation, procedural discourse and picture description). An analysis of discourse produced by these subjects and transcribed in the usual way was compared with an analysis of discourse that was made directly from recordings (transcription-less discourse analysis). Comparison of the two types of analyses revealed that transcription-less discourse analysis was a valid and reliable procedure. There were no significant differences between scores from the two methods on any of the seven measures employed – gesture use, topic use, turn-taking, repair, conversational initiation, topic initiation

and concept use – thus demonstrating the validity of transcription-less discourse analysis. The transcription-less method also produced acceptable interrater reliability: it was strongest for the gesture totals (intraclass correlation coefficients (ICCs) were between 0.80 and 0.90) and varied among the attributes of turn-taking (ICCs were between -0.05 and 1.00) and repair (ICCs were between -0.07 and 0.82).

24 While John et al. (2003) were unable to demonstrate the equivalence of the SNAP stories, Peña et al. (2006) found that two wordless picture books elicited narratives that were equivalent with respect to total story scores and productivity. Peña et al. state that these results provide evidence of parallel-forms reliability.

25 Adams et al. (2005) state that 'relatively little research has focused on appropriate intervention strategies or on the efficacy of current management for children with pragmatic language impairment. Certainly no intervention research has been carried out which reflects the heterogeneous character of the group and the way in which this impinges on research methods in therapy studies' (228).

26 Published resources for pragmatic language intervention are now widely available. They include practical activities and supportive texts. Some examples are Andersen-Wood and Smith (1997), Bliss (1993), Johnston et al. (1991), Paul (1992), Naremore et al. (1995) and Rinaldi (2001).

27 In their discussion of the theoretical background of CAPPA, Whitworth et al. (1997) remark that 'in aphasia, the compromised ability to engage in social life results, from a psychosocial perspective, in a handicap that is acutely experienced in virtually every aspect of daily living' (3).

28 The link between pragmatic disorders and poor social skills is well attested to in the literature. Conti-Ramsden and Botting (2004) examined the social and behavioural status of 242 SLI children aged eleven years who were first examined at seven years of age. These investigators found that pragmatic language difficulties, as measured on the Children's Communication Checklist (Bishop 1998), were most strongly related to poor social outcome in these children. Bruce et al. (2006) administered questionnaires to the parents of seventy-six children (mean age eleven years) with ADHD. These investigators found that problems with language and pragmatics appeared to be associated with the typical problems in social skills seen in ADHD children. Laws and Bishop (2004) report significant levels of pragmatic language impairment and difficulties with social relationships in nineteen children and young adults with Williams syndrome.

29 The principle of least collaborative effort is taken from Clark and Schaefer's (1987, 1989) CA-motivated model of conversational contributions. As Booth and Perkins (1999) define this principle, it requires that 'participants strive to minimize the total effort spent on a contribution in both the presentation and acceptance phases' (286). The presentation phase describes the presentation of an utterance by a contributor; the acceptance phase is initiated by the listener and involves both participants in working to establish that the listener has an adequate understanding of the speaker's contribution for current purposes.

30 Lock et al. (2001b) state that 'the clinician should be wary of being prescriptive about what is "good/to be retained" or "bad/to be changed" about any conversation. Partnerships vary both in terms of what their conversational style as a couple was before the onset of aphasia and also how comfortable they feel about their conversations at the time of the programme. It is therefore important to be participant-driven in choosing targets for change, and to allow the partner/couple to comment

on which aspects of their conversations are problematic for them and would benefit from intervention' (29).

31 In 1998, the journal *Aphasiology* hosted a clinical forum on Supported Conversation for Adults with Aphasia. The reader is referred to volume 12, issue 9 of this journal.

32 Some indication of the extent of this increase is provided by the following studies. Powell *et al.* (2000) found that incidence rates for classical childhood autism increased by 18 per cent per year between 1991 and 1996. A much larger increase (55 per cent per year) was seen for other ASDs. Kaye *et al.* (2001) found that the incidence of newly diagnosed autism increased sevenfold, from 0.3 per 10,000 person years in 1988 to 21 per 10,000 person years in 1999. Powell *et al.* attribute their observed rise in incidence rates to clinicians 'becoming increasingly able and/or willing to diagnose ASDs in preschool children' (2000: 624).

33 Metapragmatic awareness training also includes pragmatic skills training and assertiveness training in addition to metapragmatic awareness teaching. Andersen-Wood and Smith state that although teaching metapragmatic awareness overlaps pragmatic skills training and assertiveness training, there are differences in these approaches. For example, although role-playing is used in pragmatic skills training, it is of secondary importance in teaching metapragmatic awareness. Andersen-Wood and Smith outline a number of activities that may be used to develop metapragmatic awareness. The therapist can be critical of communication errors that are committed by puppets without this criticism threatening the therapist's relationship to younger clients. The opportunity for young children to reflect on these errors and advise the puppets on how they should behave can help them acquire metapragmatic awareness. Andersen-Wood and Smith describe a range of other puppet activities that can be used to teach politeness, figurative and literal meanings and the use of socially appropriate styles through metapragmatic awareness.

34 Certainly, this is the type of approach that Adams appears to adopt. In this way, Adams *et al.* (2005) describe the case of a child aged 9;9 years who had significant social and pragmatic deficits in the presence of excellent formal language skills and above average comprehension of inference. In view of this child's intact language skills, it was decided that intervention should aim to improve social interaction and nonverbal aspects of social cognition by using metapragmatic therapy techniques.

35 Heyer (1995) describes the contribution of role-playing to the assessment and treatment of pragmatic skills in one clinical population, children with attention deficit hyperactivity disorder: 'if a decision is made to include a child on the caseload … role-playing can be an effective way to both assess and address difficulties with pragmatic skills … information gained from role-playing can provide concrete information on where to begin the intervention phase when addressing pragmatic skills' (286).

36 The CPS is a behavioural rating scale that contains thirteen pragmatic behaviours which are typically impaired following brain injury. These behaviours include intelligibility, prosody/rate, body posture, facial expression, lexical selection, syntax, cohesiveness, variety of language uses, topic, initiation of conversation, repair, interruption and listening.

37 Four categories were used to analyse the sample of conversation that was obtained by the children telling a story from a picture book: (1) an answer category (if the child produced a one-word or a one-sentence response to a prompt), (2) a development

category (if an utterance was produced that was two or more sentences), (3) a per-severative category (if a response was echolalic or repetitive) and (4) an unclear category (if a response was unclear or unrelated to the book). Mental state words included emotion words, perception words (e.g. watch), cognition words (e.g. thinking) and volition words (e.g. want). Hadwin *et al.* (1997) found that there was 'no discernible overall difference' for each conversational category before and after intervention for all teaching groups. Similarly, there was 'no appreciable difference' in the number of mental and internal state words used before and after training for all teaching groups.

38 Of course, a possible interpretation of these findings is that the ToM skills that are tested by false belief tasks are not the same as the ToM skills that are needed for social and communicative functioning. Some support for this interpretation comes from a study of three high-functioning children with autism conducted by Chin and Bernard-Opitz (2000). The children in this study received training in five types of conversational skills: making a conversation, turn-taking in conversation, listening, maintaining a conversation topic and changing a topic appropriately. Although the conversational skills of these children improved as a result of training, there was no corresponding increase in their performance on false belief tasks (a score of 0 on these tests remained constant throughout all sessions). Chin and Bernard-Opitz conclude that 'a child may acquire a ToM through specific training programmes and still not improve in performance in standard ToM tasks ... this implies that we should be careful in our inference of an individual's social communicative ability based on his or her performance on standard ToM tasks' (2000: 579).

39 I emphasise 'greater' generalisation, as some studies have demonstrated social gains following intervention that teaches theory of mind skills. In this way, the schizo-phrenic subjects studied by Roncone *et al.* (2004) displayed statistically significant improvement in first- and second-level ToM abilities following six months of treat-ment. However, these subjects also showed statistically significant improvement on a social function measure after treatment. Roncone *et al.* state that their results 'showed a statistically significant association between social cognition measures and increase in social functioning' (2004: 431).

7   A critical evaluation of pragmatic assessment and treatment techniques

7.1   Introduction

Since its inception as a branch of linguistic enquiry, pragmatics has been the focus of numerous debates about its scope of study. While such debates have brought about necessary refinement of core concepts, they have also resulted in uncertainty about exactly which linguistic phenomena are pragmatic in nature. This uncertainty has come to characterise the related discipline of clinical pragmatics, with many investigators labelling as 'pragmatic' behaviours that are not pragmatic on any reasonable interpretation of this term. In this chapter, I examine a number of clinical studies in which behaviours have been incorrectly characterised as pragmatic. These studies will be classified according to several categories of error. The implications of these erroneous characterisations for the assessment and treatment of pragmatic language disorders will be discussed. Finally, a number of criteria are advanced which, it is expected, will constrain the tendency of clinicians and theorists alike to incorrectly identify behaviours as pragmatic.

7.2   The domain of pragmatics

In addition to obvious differences in the content of their respective enquiries, pragmatics is unlike other branches of linguistics in one further fundamental respect. While theorists in fields such as syntax and semantics can at least agree on what it is that they should be studying – if not on how they should be studying it – theorists in pragmatics lack even this most basic consensus on what constitutes their domain of study. This lack of consensus is evident in the many widely differing definitions of pragmatics, no two of which appear to agree on the exact parameters of the field. In a recent definition by Cruse (2000), the non-conventional and contextual aspects of pragmatics are emphasised:

Pragmatics can be taken to be concerned with aspects of information (in the widest sense) conveyed through language which (a) are not encoded by generally accepted convention in the linguistic forms used, but which (b) none the less arise naturally out of and depend on the meanings conventionally encoded in the linguistic forms used, taken in conjunction with the context in which the forms are used. (2000: 16)

However, in Mey's definition of the same subject area, no mention is made of the contribution of conventional meaning to pragmatics (a prominent feature of Cruse's definition), while context is construed in social terms. Moreover, Mey (2001) introduces the notion of communication between speakers and hearers, an aspect that is noticeably lacking from Cruse's definition:

Pragmatics studies the use of language in human communication as determined by the conditions of society. (2001: 6)

In a definition of pragmatics advanced by Stalnaker (1998), the field is characterised so broadly that it is not clear what it is intended to exclude. Although pragmatics is defined as 'the study of linguistic acts and the contexts in which they are performed', when elaborated the notion of context includes cognitive, linguistic, temporal, semantic and communicative factors:[1]

The various properties of the context in which the act is performed [include] the intentions of the speaker, the knowledge, beliefs, expectations or interests of the speaker and his audience, other speech acts that have been performed in the same context, the time of utterance, the effects of the utterance, the truth value of the proposition expressed, the semantic relations between the proposition expressed and some others involved in some way. (1998: 58)

This lack of consensus on the scope of pragmatics need not unduly concern theorists in the field, who at least can be afforded the luxury of debating where the subject's boundaries should lie. Indeed, some of these theorists have even challenged the necessity of establishing such boundaries. In this way, Mey (2001) asks 'why do we need clear, sharply demarcated boundaries at all, when pragmatics is in constant development, so that boundary markers, once placed, will have to be moved all the time?' (7). However, while theorists can treat the question of boundaries as an interesting academic point that is worthy of discussion, clinicians who are working with clients with pragmatic language disorders must address an altogether more urgent set of demands. For such clinicians, the institution of clear boundaries on the field of pragmatics is essential if the impaired communicative performance of their clients is to be accurately assessed and successfully treated. In fact, the failure of theorists in pragmatics to establish these boundaries has led to a number of adverse consequences for the clinical management of clients with these disorders. We will discuss some of these consequences subsequently. In the meantime, we examine a number of clinical investigations in which behaviours have been incorrectly identified as pragmatic in nature. To assist this examination, these behaviours will be grouped according to several categories of error, each of which can be seen to reflect a more fundamental problem in the definition and delineation of pragmatics itself.

7.3   Clinical studies of pragmatics

Pragmatics has been an active area of clinical linguistic investigation for the past twenty-five years.[2] In that time, numerous studies have claimed to reveal significant pragmatic deficits in a range of child and adult clinical populations. However, upon closer scrutiny of these studies, it is clear that a sizeable number fail to accurately characterise the so-called pragmatic phenomena that are at the centre of these investigations. Errors in identification range from describing as pragmatic, behaviours that are not pragmatic on any reasonable interpretation of this term to a failure to capture the essential pragmatic character of behaviours that are genuinely pragmatic in nature. Several categories of these errors will be discussed in this section along with studies that exemplify the particular error in question. In each case, it will be shown how conclusions describing the pragmatic deficits in the child and adult subjects of these studies are not warranted on account of these errors.

Error 1: treating nonverbal behaviours as pragmatic   One of the most unfortunate consequences of the failure to institute boundaries around the field of pragmatics has been the tendency to apply the term 'pragmatics' in a rather undiscerning way to every aspect of communication. This tendency is pervasive in the clinical literature with everything from pragmatic language assessments to intervention studies exhibiting it to some degree. In a recent study of an intervention programme in autistic children, Chandler *et al.* (2002) include a diverse array of behaviours within pragmatics. However, their account of 'the pragmatics of language' mentions few, if any, linguistic behaviours and focuses almost exclusively on nonverbal phenomena:

They include: body language (facial expression and eye contact, gesture, posture or stance), listening skills (including maintaining attention to body language as well as speech, and knowing who is being addressed), using intonation to understand and express meaning, adapting volume and emphasis to the attentional state of the other person, understanding intention (tuning in to personal meaning, as in teasing), sharing understanding, attention, intention and interest and reciprocal turn-taking. (2002: 50–1)

The justification for such a wide-ranging list of behaviours can be nothing more than that they have something to do with communication. However, even given the lack of disciplinary boundaries in pragmatics, it is clear that most theorists have something altogether more specific than this in mind when they use the term 'pragmatics'. Definitions of pragmatics that emphasise communication, such as that advanced by Mey, may be responsible in part for the type of approach exemplified by Chandler and others. Yet, even these definitions emphasise the central role of language in pragmatics. Loveland *et al.* (1988) similarly subordinate language to nonverbal aspects of communication in their study of pragmatic deficits in autistic children. The first sign that this

subordination is occurring can be seen in the terminology used by these investigators. The distinctly linguistic phenomenon of 'speech acts' appears in the
title of Loveland *et al.*'s article, only to be replaced shortly thereafter by 'communicative acts'. Presumably, this shift in terminology is undertaken in order
to accommodate the largely nonverbal behaviours of the autistic children in
this study. Certainly, the significant findings of this investigation all relate to
nonlinguistic aspects of communication. Loveland *et al.* found that the autistic
children in this study were less likely to use gesture and affirming, turn-taking
vocalisation and had more incidents of no responses than mental-age-matched
children with developmental language delay and normally developing two-
year-olds. On the basis of these findings, these investigators conclude that
the autistic children in this study have 'pragmatic deficits'. However, none of
these so-called pragmatic deficits is even describing a linguistic behaviour. It
is only a very loose conception of the field of pragmatics, specifically one that
identifies pragmatics with wider communication (verbal and nonverbal communication included) that makes it seem that these nonverbal behaviours are
pragmatic in nature.

With the publication of Prutting and Kirchner's pragmatic protocol, the
tendency to identify pragmatics with communication assumed widespread
legitimacy. The protocol is a descriptive taxonomy that is intended to assist
clinicians and researchers in identifying pragmatic deficits in a range of clinical populations. In this way, Prutting and Kirchner (1987) applied the protocol
in a comparative study of pragmatic impairment in four clinical populations –
children with articulation disorders, children with language disorders, aphasic
adults and adults with right-hemisphere lesions. It was found that the aphasic
subjects in this study had a greater mean percentage (18 per cent) of inappropriate pragmatic parameters than subjects from the other three clinical groups.
However, when these supposed areas of pragmatic deficit are examined, it is
clear that they are not so pragmatic after all. Of the five pragmatic parameters
identified by Prutting and Kirchner as being impaired in the aphasic sample,
two parameters – fluency and pause time in turn-taking – are not pragmatic in
any sense of this word. Speech fluency is a function of many variables, only
some of which are linguistic.[3] Similarly, abnormal pause times in turn-taking[4]
may have a number of sources, ranging from cognitive delays in the planning
of utterances to an inability to programme the articulators to produce speech
movements. Neither dysfluency nor abnormal pause times in turn-taking are
indicative of an impairment in language, let alone an impairment in the pragmatic aspects of language. Prutting and Kirchner also identified a number of
impairments in the aphasics in this study in areas that are truly pragmatic in
nature. Speech acts, for example, have been included in accounts of pragmatics without contention since Austin and Searle first characterised them. The
subjects with aphasia in this study who exhibit problems with specificity and

accuracy of expression, and quantity and conciseness of messages are strug-gling to observe Gricean maxims of quantity, quality, relevance and manner. And no one, least of all myself, is wishing to challenge the centrality of Grice's thinking to the field of pragmatics. However, the fact that non-pragmatic fea-tures such as fluency and pause times are grouped alongside these clear areas of pragmatic deficit is evidence again of the tendency to equate pragmatics with communication in general, nonverbal communication specifically included.

Error 2: attributing communicative intentions where none exist   We saw in section 7.2 how Stalnaker's definition of pragmatics presupposed a notion of context that included, amongst other things, the 'intentions of the speaker'. Communicative intentions are an explicit or implied component of some definitions of the field.[5] This fact is not overlooked by clinicians, who have attempted to include an assessment of speakers' communicative intentions within their respective investigations of pragmatic skills in clients. Most com-monly, these investigations involve studies of the comprehension of indirect speech acts, implicatures and idioms, where a speaker's intentions must be established in order to obtain the intended (implied) meaning of an utterance.[6] While most of these studies succeed in testing the communicative intentions that are integral to notions like implicature, a significant number falsely attrib-ute these intentions to the participants in communicative exchanges. This can be seen in recent theory of mind research into the pragmatic deficits of autism. Baron-Cohen *et al.* (1999) set out to investigate the recognition of faux pas by children with Asperger's syndrome (AS) or high-functioning autism (HFA). Twelve children with AS or HFA, and sixteen normal controls were presented with ten short stories on audio cassette. In one of these stories, a woman called Jill has just put up curtains after moving into a new house. Her friend Lisa visits and, not realising the curtains are new and have been put up by Jill, says to her 'Oh, those curtains are horrible. I hope you're going to get some new ones'. Subjects were then asked a series of questions. One of these questions was designed to assess if subjects had detected the faux pas in the story ('In the story, did someone say something that they should not have said?'). A further question required subjects to identify the faux pas ('What did they say that they should not have said?'). A third question tested subjects' understanding of the language used in the story, while a fourth question aimed to assess if subjects were aware that the faux pas was a consequence of a false belief on the part of the speaker in the story.

There can be little doubt that this task is testing a range of language and cog-nitive skills in the autistic children in this study. It is far from clear, however, that the ability to recognise Lisa's mistake in the above scenario is a form of *pragmatic* interpretation. The only thing that can be said about this scenario is that Lisa has made a mistake – she has a false belief about the curtains, a belief which leads her to describe the curtains in somewhat unpleasant terms in front of Jill. In failing to detect this faux pas, autistic children are failing to detect Lisa's false belief. But this particular failing is something quite different from the recognition of communicative intentions that is integral to pragmatic interpretation. Indeed, as Baron-Cohen *et al.* (1999) define faux pas, it is clear that no *intentional* communication is involved in either its production or recognition: 'A working definition of faux pas might be when a speaker says something *without considering* if it is something that the listener might not want to hear or know, and which typically has negative consequences that the speaker *never intended*' (408; italics added). Moreover, it is unsurprising that the autistic subjects in this study failed to detect instances of faux pas.[7] For the detection of faux pas is none other than the detection of false belief, and this particular theory of mind skill is known to be impaired in autism.[8]

Nor is the tendency to falsely attribute communicative intentions to speakers confined to studies of pragmatic deficits in autism. In a study of pragmatic skills in a forty-seven-year-old woman who sustained a traumatic brain injury, Body *et al.* (1999) produce this somewhat bizarre analysis of her tendency to swear during conversation with a therapist:

> Her use of swear words might be interpreted as implicating 'Pat is being aggressive/overly familiar/impolite', though [the therapist's] awareness of Pat's case history will presumably lead him instead to infer the overriding implicature 'Pat is head-injured', and also that these potential and actual implicatures are not intended by Pat. (1999: 106)

As Body *et al.* characterise Pat's swearing behaviour, it is motivated by certain communicative intentions – Pat is taken to implicate either that she is aggressive (overly familiar or impolite) or that she is head-injured. However, it is certain that Pat intends to communicate no such thing. Her swearing behaviour is clearly the result of her post-traumatic cognitive deficits, particularly her poor impulse control and failure to monitor her verbal behaviour. The entire framework of implicature is totally unsuited to the analysis of this case. Pat is not implicating anything by means of her swearing behaviour. Nor does she have a set of communicative intentions when she swears, which her listener, the therapist, is expected to recover through reasoning. The question must be asked: why have the notions of implicature and intention been so seriously misapplied by Body *et al.*? It can only be because they are operating with a rather loose understanding of key pragmatic concepts such as implicature and intention, an understanding that allows these terms to be applied to non-intentional behaviours as well as to intentional communicative behaviours.[9] We must also ask: how has such a loose understanding of pragmatic concepts come about? Although it is difficult to give a definitive answer to this question, it is at least reasonable to suppose that an answer may be found in the lack of delineation in pragmatics itself.

Error 3: missing the pragmatic point of an exchange   The case of autism also exemplifies the third type of error that occurs in clinical studies of pragmatics. Theory of mind researchers have also been concerned to examine the ability of autistic children to recognise violations of Gricean maxims. In a study of high-functioning children with autism, Surian *et al.* (1996) remark that 'if children with autism have deficits in ascribing mental states, and particularly ascribing intentions, then they should fail to recognise when such Gricean maxims are being violated' (58). One of the examples used in Surian *et al.*'s study is the following violation of the quantity maxim:

A: What would you like for breakfast?
B: A hard boiled egg cooked in hot water in a sauce pan.

In this case, B has provided an excessively informative response to A's question. However, this exchange is only pragmatically interesting to the extent that B's excessively informative response can be used by A to recover an implicature. In this way, B is likely to be implicating by way of his detailed instructions that A is not particularly competent at even basic food preparation (of course, to obtain this particular implicature, we are assuming that A has had previous problems with cooking and that B is aware of this fact). The recognition that a response is excessively informative is an important step in the inferential process by means of which implicatures are recovered during pragmatic interpretation. However, it is only a first step in this process. Such interpretation is only fully achieved when a listener is able to use his recognition that a response is excessively informative to derive a speaker's intended or implied meaning. Surian *et al.* found that while most children with autism performed at chance on this maxim task, all children with specific language impairment and all normal controls performed above chance. Yet, this finding lacks any real implications for our knowledge of pragmatic functioning in autism, given the failure of this maxim task to assess the processes that are integral to pragmatic interpretation.

Surian *et al.*'s study has missed, in an important way, the pragmatic point of the above exchange. The pragmatic significance of this exchange rests, not in the detection or recognition of the violation[10] of a Gricean maxim, but in the use of that recognition to derive the speaker's intended or implied meaning. This same error accounts for a further bizarre analysis of Pat's pragmatic skills by Body *et al.* (1999). During one of Pat's assessment tasks, she is instructed by the therapist to enquire about her next appointment when an alarm sounds. The exchange unfolds as follows:

T: I'm going to set this alarm to go off in 20 minutes. When it rings
    I want you to ask me about your next appointment.
P: It's on Wednesday.

According to Body *et al.*'s analysis of this exchange, 'Pat could be said to be sometimes unable to identify the intended illocutionary force of T's utterances' (1999: 105). To the extent that Pat interprets the therapist's instructions as a question about the date of her next appointment, there is a sense in which she is missing the pragmatic point of this exchange. However, viewed in a different light, Pat's utterance in the above exchange is not so pragmatically inappropriate after all. Pat's depressed performance on the Test for Reception of Grammar (Bishop 1983) indicates that she has difficulty decoding syntactic and semantic constructions. In the presence of such difficulty, Pat is likely to fall back on a range of strategies to help her understand T's utterance (see section 1.7 in Chapter 1). For example, she will use her knowledge of conversational structure, and particularly her knowledge of the types of turns that occur in therapist–client exchanges, to help her decode T's set of instructions. Such interactions are characterised by question–answer exchanges, in which the therapist poses a question that the client is then expected to answer. This is especially true when a formal assessment is taking place, as is happening in the present case. Under these circumstances, it is hardly surprising that Pat treats the therapist's instructions as a question to which she duly responds.

So it emerges that Pat's utterance in the above exchange is not so pragmatically inappropriate as Body *et al.* are claiming. Indeed, if anything her response to the therapist reveals considerable pragmatic ingenuity on her part. The question that I am concerned to address in the present context, however, is less whether Pat has missed the pragmatic point of the exchange than if Body *et al.* have done so. This question can be answered affirmatively, I believe, on the basis of the following consideration. It is surely a precondition on the asking of any sincere question that (a) the person asking the question does not already know the answer and that (b) the person who can provide an answer must believe that the questioner does not know the answer but wants to be given this information. However, neither aspect of this precondition is satisfied in the above exchange between the therapist and Pat. In relation to (a), Pat is being compelled by the requirements of this particular assessment task to ask about the date of her next appointment when she already knows that this will take place on Wednesday. The exchange makes little more sense from the perspective of the therapist, because (s)he knows that Pat already knows the answer to the question about the date of her next appointment and that she is unlikely to want to be told something she already knows (feature b). Put quite simply, the requirements of the therapist's assessment task effectively distort every reasonable pragmatic constraint on the asking of questions. It is little wonder, therefore, that Pat ends up treating the therapist's instructions as a question to which she responds with an answer. It is also unsurprising that she resorts to asking later in the exchange 'Will it be Wednesday? Will I see you on Wednesday?'

For Pat has quite sensibly reasoned that if the therapist is asking about the date of her next appointment, then (s)he must not know the date. Thus, Pat's questions about the date of the appointment late in the exchange are not evidence that she has understood the therapist's instructions after all. Rather, they indicate an attempt by her to confirm a date about which she believed there was a mutual understanding.

It emerges that Pat has shown considerable pragmatic resourcefulness in this exchange with the therapist. When confronted with an assessment task in which expected constraints on the asking of questions have been violated, Pat responds with an altogether impressive level of pragmatic ingenuity. In failing to detect Pat's pragmatic skills in this situation, and preferring to read this exchange as evidence of pragmatic impairment on Pat's part, it is not Pat who has missed the pragmatic point of the interaction so much as Body *et al.* These researchers have completely overlooked the consequences of the violation of certain expectations on the exchange of questions for the development of a conversation. The question of why this has occurred, particularly when some of the other analyses undertaken by Body *et al.* do indicate that they understand how pragmatic concepts operate, cannot be answered with certainty. However, it seems likely that a general lack of clarity about the extent of the field of pragmatics, and a concomitant uncertainty about the concepts to include in this field (e.g. expectations around the exchange of speech acts) may provide at least part of the answer.

Error 4: distorting the notion of context in pragmatic interpretation   Although there is disagreement about the extent of the notion of context, there is a general consensus that some notion of context is integral to the definition of pragmatics.[11] Context's central role in pragmatics is not lost on clinical researchers, many of whom have attempted to test aspects of context, either directly or indirectly, in their studies of language-impaired subjects. Researchers who are concerned to validate the weak central coherence theory of autism are chief amongst those investigators who have performed direct experimental studies of context. This theory states that the underlying cognitive deficit in autism is related to a certain cognitive processing style, one in which subjects exhibit a preference for the processing of parts over wholes. In relation to language, an autistic subject who exhibits weak central coherence may neglect aspects of context and fail to understand the meaning of a sentence, yet be able to reproduce the sentence verbatim. In a study of normally intelligent adults with either autism or Asperger's syndrome, Jolliffe and Baron-Cohen (1999) found that clinical subjects were less likely than normal controls to use sentence context spontaneously in order to obtain the context-appropriate pronunciation of a homograph (e.g. *lead*; *read*). The following experimental task was used to establish this finding. Subjects were asked to read aloud sentences that contained homographs. Each homograph had a frequent and rare pronunciation. An accompanying sentence or part of a sentence favoured one pronunciation over the other and appeared either before or after the homograph. Two of the test items for the homograph *lead* are as follows:

Rare pronunciation; before context:
It was lead in the box that made it so heavy.

Frequent pronunciation; after context:
Mary wanted to take the dog for a walk, so she went to the cupboard and took the lead.

Jolliffe and Baron-Cohen (1999) also found that clinical subjects were less able than normal controls to use context to interpret ambiguous sentences that were presented auditorily. An Ambiguous Sentence test was used to establish this finding. Subjects were required to listen to pairs of sentences. The last sentence in each pair was either lexically or syntactically ambiguous. In each case, the ambiguity could be resolved by the preceding sentence that acted as a disambiguating context. Each ambiguous sentence was presented twice, with the preceding sentence biasing disambiguation towards either a rare or a common interpretation. Subjects were asked a question about the ambiguous sentence to which they had to choose one of three possible responses. These responses represent a context-appropriate interpretation, a context-inappropriate interpretation and an erroneous interpretation. One of the test items used in this study is given below:

Lexical ambiguity, rare interpretation: The boiler house was very noisy.
The roar of the fans disturbed the team.
Question: What happened?
Possible responses:
   (1) football fans disturbed the team
   (2) football fans helped the team
   (3) cooling fans disturbed the team

Norbury (2005) examined lexical ambiguity resolution in children aged nine to seventeen years who had autistic spectrum disorder (ASD) with normal language abilities, ASD plus language impairment or language impairment without ASD. Two experiments were conducted.[12] The first was designed to establish subjects' knowledge of the dominant and subordinate meanings of ambiguous words. The second experiment investigated subjects' ability to use preceding linguistic context to either facilitate word meaning identification or suppress irrelevant meanings. In the contextual facilitation condition, subjects' accuracy and response times to picture judgements that followed either a neutral sentence or a biased sentence were recorded. For the test item *bank*, the sentences used as the preceding linguistic context were as follows:

Neutral sentence: He *ran* from the bank – picture *money*
Biased sentence: He *stole* from the bank – picture *money*

Similar experimental techniques have been used to examine the ability of autistic subjects to use context to establish the meanings of homophones (see discussion of Hoy *et al.* (2004) in section 4.5 of Chapter 4).

The tasks described above are typical of the experimental methodology that
is employed to investigate the claims of the weak central coherence theory of
autism. In each task, subjects must draw upon linguistic context, usually an
accompanying sentence, to achieve the disambiguation of a word or sentence
or the correct pronunciation of a homograph. The assumption of studies that
use these tasks is that language interpretation proceeds on the basis of a tightly
circumscribed notion of context that is somehow determined in advance of
interpretation. However, this assumption is mistaken for at least two reasons.
First, context is a sprawling notion that evades all attempts to place limits on it.
The potentially infinite range of factors that may be employed in the recovery
of an implicature of an utterance is evidence enough of context's capacity to go
beyond boundaries.[13] It is in this respect that the inferential process involved in
pragmatic interpretation is a truly global process.[14] It is simply not possible to
throw a net over those aspects of one's linguistic and other knowledge that may
be deemed relevant to the interpretation of a word or sentence. Even less is it
possible to represent these diverse aspects within a single sentence or part of a
sentence, as the studies discussed above would appear to be claiming. Second,
pragmatic interpretation is a dynamic process in which language users must
create a context for the understanding of utterances. This context is not ready-
made or somehow determined in advance of interpretation, as experimental
tasks on the disambiguation of homophones would lead one to believe (recall
that in Hoy *et al.*'s homophone task a disambiguating context in the form of a
sentence is provided for subjects). Two prominent theorists of pragmatic interpretation, Dan Sperber and Deirdre Wilson, subscribe to the view of context
as an essentially dynamic construct in their relevance theory. Cruse (2000)
remarks of this theory that 'the proper context for the interpretation of an utterance is not given in advance; it is chosen by the hearer' (370). It emerges that
in an effort to establish how autistic subjects process aspects of context, central
coherence studies end up distorting the very notion of context that they are
aiming to examine.

Although the discussion of this fourth type of error has concentrated on
studies of autistic subjects, the distortion of context that occurs in these studies
is also to be found in investigations of other clinical populations. In this way,
Qualls *et al.* (2004) used an Idiom Comprehension Test to assess the effects of
context and familiarity on the comprehension of idioms in twenty-two adolescents with language-based learning disabilities (LBLD). Two context conditions were used, a story task and a verification task. It was hypothesised that
LBLD subjects would find an enriched context (the story task) a disadvantage
when comprehending idioms and that these subjects would comprehend idioms

best in the verification condition.[15] In the story task, subjects were required to read a series of short stories, each of which contained an idiom. A question at the end of each story probed the subjects' understanding of the idiom's meaning. To indicate the meaning of each idiom, subjects selected one response from a choice of four possible answers. This story task can be shown to involve the same problematic notion of context that undermined the central coherence studies of autism discussed above. Each of the short stories presented to the LBLD subjects was intended to circumscribe the context used by these subjects to arrive at an interpretation of the idioms in the passages. This experimental method makes two assumptions, first, that it is possible to circumscribe the informational context that subjects will use to obtain the meaning of these idioms and, second, that the context is somehow ready-made and determined in advance of interpretation (the hearer doesn't actually create a context of interpretation). However, neither assumption is correct. For example, to establish that 'to talk through one's hat' in the following story means 'to talk foolishly', a subject may well mark as salient the fact that John is a practical joker and that he produces ridiculous statements in class. However, this subject is equally likely to recall a mother's frustrated reprimand from the previous day ('Mary, will you stop talking through your hat?') or a teacher's earlier attempt to explain the idiom's meaning. Neither of these aspects are part of the context presented in the story. Nevertheless, they are part of the wider informational context that the subject will bring to bear upon an interpretation of the idiom in this story:

It seems that every class has a practical joker. Well, John was that person in Mrs Jones' fifth grade class. He would say things like the earth is nearer to the sun in the summer. Mrs Jones told him, 'You're *talking through your hat*'.

The second assumption stated above is also problematic. In challenging the first assumption of this experimental method, I portrayed the subject in this experiment as someone who was actively involved in creating the contexts against which the various idioms of these stories would be interpreted. In constructing a context for the interpretation of the idiom 'to talk through one's hat' in the above story, the subject draws upon not only the content of the story, but also upon a wider informational context consisting of knowledge and beliefs. This wider context contains information relating to the subject's prior linguistic practice and knowledge of people and events in the world. Aspects of this wider context reflect not only the subject's own interests and values, but also the specific purposes for which interpretation is undertaken (in this case, to obtain the meaning of a particular idiom).[16] As was demonstrated above, these features of context may play a more significant role in the interpretation of the idiom in the story than any content of the story itself. The important point here is not that the story plays no part in the interpretation of the idiom – it clearly does through its raising of the salience of certain aspects of the wider informational context. Rather, it is that the story is merely providing a starting point in a very active process of context construction on the part of the subject.

The question arises: if the dominant experimental method for examining context in these studies is serving only to distort this notion, then why is this method in such widespread use amongst experimental psychologists and clinical researchers? To respond that these investigators simply don't understand the notion of context is too easy a reply. A more enlightened analysis of the situation requires that we consider how context is defined and discussed by workers within pragmatics. Perhaps simplistic characterisations of context by these workers can explain the distorted notion of context that drives the experimental studies of psychologists and clinical researchers. Several points about the discussion of context in the pragmatics literature are worth commenting upon. First, the use of the definite article in relation to context ('the context') in definitions of pragmatics conveys the false impression that we are dealing with some type of bounded entity – recall Stalnaker's definition of pragmatics as 'the study of linguistic acts and *the contexts* in which they are performed'. This notion of a bounded context is in stark contrast to the view of context proposed here, one in which context is a dynamic, evolving entity that is constrained only by the interests and values of the language users whom it serves. With context presented as a bounded entity, either implicitly or explicitly, in most definitions of pragmatics, it is hardly surprising that clinical researchers have chosen to represent context in an equally bounded fashion in their respective investigations.

Second, when workers in pragmatics discuss what should constitute their respective notions of context, the assumption is that each part of context is essentially isolable from the other parts. In reality, however, cognitive, linguistic and social components, amongst others, are inextricably linked together, with no one component capable of being separated from the other components. This was seen in the example discussed above, where the subject's linguistic practice was as relevant as cognitive factors (e.g. world knowledge of practical jokers) to the interpretation of the idiom 'to talk through one's hat'. The standard practice of experimental and clinical researchers is to take one part of context and extract it from all other parts. This extracted component is then labelled 'the context' in studies that are designed to assess the ability of clinical subjects to use context to achieve the disambiguation of words, for example. Although this standard practice serves only to distort the notion of context, the error in this case is at least an understandable one that can be related ultimately to how workers in pragmatics compartmentalise the notion of context.

Third, to the extent that experimental and clinical researchers represent context most often in their investigations in the form of a single sentence, they are in good company. For when most workers in the field of pragmatics attempt to demonstrate pragmatic concepts, the examples they employ also simplify context by reducing it to a single preceding utterance in a conversational exchange. To appreciate this point, we need only consider how the concept of implicature is standardly explicated in introductory texts in pragmatics. These books are awash with examples such as the following:

A: Would you like more coffee?
B: Coffee would keep me awake.

The ensuing analysis usually involves statements to the effect that B is conversationally implicating that he does not want more coffee and that A recovers this implicature through reasoning using a context consisting of the utterance in the exchange, amongst other things. The effect is that linguistic context tends to assume significance while other factors, such as A's mental states, are altogether less prominent. Even in more advanced texts, the same privileging of linguistic information in accounts of context occurs. For example, Sperber and Wilson (1995) remark that 'the context used in interpreting a given utterance generally contains information derived from *immediately preceding utterances*' (16; italics added). Yet, it can be easily demonstrated that linguistic information in the form of preceding sentences or utterances is often less important in interpretation than other features of context. Consider again the above exchange between A and B. I characterised the implicature in this exchange as one in which B was implicating that he did not want more coffee. However, this same exchange is consistent with quite a different implicature, that B wants more coffee in an effort to stay awake. The factor that is decisive in determining these interpretations is not the linguistic context provided by A's question – after all, this remains the same in both interpretations. Rather, the decisive factor is the different interests, values and purposes that motivate these alternative interpretations – if A is aware that B wants to sleep some time later, then B will be taken to implicate that he does not want more coffee. Discussions of implicature in pragmatics tend to overstate the significance of linguistic context and to subordinate other, quite legitimate factors to this context. It is hardly surprising, therefore, that experimental and clinical researchers have decided to follow the lead of workers in pragmatics by privileging linguistic context (often in the form of a disambiguating sentence, for example) over other aspects of context.

7.4   Implications for the management of pragmatic disorders

It has been argued that many of the pragmatic impairments that have been identified and examined by clinical researchers are not pragmatic impairments after all. In some cases, behaviours that are not pragmatic in any sense of the word have been inaccurately identified as pragmatic in nature. In other cases, studies of pragmatic impairment in clinical subjects have rested on inaccurate conceptions of notions such as context, with the result that the findings of these studies must be treated with some scepticism. The conceptual and theoretical arguments that have been used to support these claims may seem far removed from the concerns of the clinical practitioner, whose job it is to assess and treat individuals with a range of pragmatic impairments. However, no practitioner can afford to overlook the significance of these arguments for their own clinical practice, because if they are correct, then it is clear that clinicians have been inappropriately treating some clients and failing to treat other clients. In this section, I outline some of the implications of the arguments of the previous section for the management of pragmatic disorders.

7.4.1   Pragmatic language assessment

Assessment is a necessary first step in the management of any communication disorder. Clinicians have long recognised that formal tools, such as those used to assess structural aspects of language (i.e. syntax, semantics), are particularly poorly suited to an assessment of pragmatic language skills. Although such tools exist for the assessment of pragmatics (see section 6.2.2 in Chapter 6), most clinical and research effort has been directed towards the development of informal methods of assessment. These methods include a diverse array of techniques, ranging from conversation analysis and narrative assessment to the use of communication checklists and pragmatics profiles. Each assessment tool, it is argued, can be used to identify pragmatic impairments.[17] However, examination of the content of these assessments reveals that many informal techniques perpetuate the same misunderstandings about pragmatic phenomena that weakened the various investigations examined in section 7.3. Consider in this regard the types of conversation analytic approaches that are used to examine pragmatic impairments in children and adults. These approaches range from simple orthographic transcriptions of conversation in which speech acts, implicatures and other noteworthy pragmatic phenomena are analysed to highly developed conversational systems in which each turn is coded and other behaviours are classified. As an example of the former type of approach, we return to Body et al.'s analysis of conversational and pragmatic skills in a female subject who sustained a traumatic brain injury. This subject, known as Pat, is engaged in a conversation with a therapist about her house key. The conversation develops as follows:

1. T: sets up video camera
2. P: waves to camera, smiles
3. P: Hi.
4. P: rummages in handbag

5. P: Do you mind if I use your telephone, please? I want to telephone my daughter at home
6. to tell her I haven't got a house key.
7. T: Do you need to do that straight away?
8. P: If you don't mind.
9. T: Will she not be … what's she going to do today?
10. P: She'll be ironing.
11. T: So isn't she likely …
12. P: stands up, starts to leave room
13. T: …to be at home anyway?
14. P: Yes, but not for much longer.
15. P: leaves room.

As Body *et al*. analyse this exchange, Pat has failed to establish the communicative intention underlying the therapist's question in line 9 – if Pat's daughter is at home, then presumably she can let Pat into the house in which case a key is not required. However, upon further examination of this exchange, it is clear that this particular interpretation is unwarranted. For Pat's utterance in line 14 indicates quite clearly that she is aware of the therapist's communicative intention. Yet that intention, Pat is indicating, is effectively cancelled by an additional item of knowledge that only she has had access to up until line 14 in the exchange – the knowledge that her daughter will not be at home for much longer. Viewed in this enlarged knowledge context, Pat's responses are both intelligible and pragmatically appropriate. In fact, it is to the notion of context that we must turn in order to understand the error in Body *et al*.'s analysis. Body *et al*. see only one context at work in the above exchange. This context consists of the therapist's knowledge and beliefs, for example, knowledge that to gain access to a house, one needs a house key. While some of the therapist's beliefs are undoubtedly shared by Pat, Pat's utterances appear not to contribute to the development or enlargement of the therapist's context. Pat's additional knowledge that her daughter will not be at home for much longer should be able to permeate and change the therapist's context (and in the actual interaction between Pat and the therapist, this 'new' information almost certainly altered the therapist's context). However, within Body *et al*.'s analysis of the exchange, Pat's contribution of new and relevant information in line 14 is quite simply overlooked. The notion of context that motivates Body *et al*.'s analysis of this exchange is static and non-collaborative and is in stark contrast to the dynamic, evolving context that is actually developing between Pat and the therapist. It emerges that in an attempt to qualitatively analyse the exchange between Pat and her therapist, Body *et al*. end up distorting the notion of context that is central to this exchange.[18]

In reality, Pat's pragmatic skills are considerably more sophisticated than Body *et al*.'s analysis of them would tend to suggest. Quite apart from being pragmatically impaired, Pat is able to ascertain her interlocutor's communicative intentions and demonstrate the relevance of new information to those intentions. These areas of pragmatic strength are not recognised by Body *et al.* because they have approached the analysis of this exchange with a distorted notion of context. Just such a distortion is the basis of the fourth category of error identified in section 7.3. Of course, the above qualitative procedure is only one approach to conversation analysis which, in turn, is only one method of analysing pragmatic language skills in communication-impaired subjects. It remains to be seen if other forms of pragmatic assessment can accurately identify pragmatic impairments without succumbing to the errors of the previous section.

While a qualitative approach to conversation analysis can tell us which pragmatic skills are impaired in a subject, this approach is of limited value in measuring a subject's progress in therapy or in determining the efficacy of a particular intervention. These latter concerns are quantitative in nature and can only be adequately addressed through the use of a quantitative conversation analytic procedure. Just such a procedure has been developed by Bishop and coworkers (Bishop and Adams 1989; Bishop *et al.* 2000). The Analysis of Language Impaired Children's Conversation (ALICC) provides a communicative profile of behaviours such as turn-taking skills, responsiveness and initiation of topics, which can then be used to plan intervention and evaluate therapy.[19] Additionally, it contains a method for examining the goodness of fit between first and second parts of interactions or exchanges. Known as meshing, it 'remains one of the best characterisations of the bizarre quality of interactions with children who have pragmatic language disorders' (Adams 2002: 980). With its quantitative orientation, ALICC has certainly been hailed as a welcome development in the field of pragmatic language assessment.[20] Yet, it is far from clear that this particular conversation analytic approach is even assessing pragmatic language skills. Consider in this regard the ALICC category of responsiveness. Bishop *et al.* (2000) recently used this category to examine conversational responsiveness in eighteen children with specific language impairment. Half of these children were judged to have pragmatic difficulties on the basis of ratings on a teacher checklist and were described as having pragmatic language impairment (PLI). The children's responses to adult soliciting utterances were coded according to (1) the type of responses produced and (2) the extent to which responses meshed with adult information-soliciting utterances. However, examination of the various codes used to perform these analyses reveals considerable misunderstandings about the scope of pragmatics on the part of these investigators. In relation to analysis (1), codes incorrectly identify nonverbal responses as pragmatic for no other reason than that they seem to involve the communication of some intent. But this is not enough for nonverbal behaviours such as nods and shrugs to be classified as pragmatic.

For a behaviour to be genuinely pragmatic in nature, it is not the mere fact that an individual's intent has been communicated that is important. Rather, it is that that intent is being revealed, often indirectly, *through the language used* (equally, from the viewpoint of the listener, that the speaker's intent is capable of being recovered through a process of reasoning that *originates in language*). Bishop *et al.*'s understanding of pragmatics in this context appears to obviate a role for language in this area of behaviour. In reality, however, it is through language that pragmatic phenomena derive their significance (the notion of a speech act, for example, would be entirely meaningless if we could not envisage linguistic utterances performing acts such as promising, warning, etc.). It is helpful at this point to remind ourselves of certain uncontested features of pragmatics. It is perhaps revealing of the conceptual confusion that currently pervades the field of clinical pragmatics that I should draw on the words of one of the authors of the present study to make this reminder: 'The term "language pragmatics" refers to a group of behaviours that are concerned with how *language* is used to convey meanings' (Adams 2002: 973; italics added).

Like other clinicians and researchers before them, Bishop *et al.* are overlooking the essential role of language in pragmatics in their analysis of conversational responsiveness. An alternative way of construing the same error is to say that these investigators are identifying pragmatics with communication in general, nonverbal communication specifically included. However, further examination of responsiveness in the ALICC system indicates that this is not the only misunderstanding about pragmatics on the part of Bishop *et al.* In the second analysis in the study, children's responses to adult information-soliciting utterances were coded in terms of how well they addressed the expectations of those utterances. Responses that addressed those expectations adequately – that 'meshed' with adult utterances – either provided the information that was requested or indicated through the use of expressions such as 'don't know' that a response could not be provided (the latter in a context where an adult may be unable to provide a response, e.g. in answer to 'Where are you going on holiday next year?'). Included in this category of adequate responses were those where the requested information was not explicitly stated by the child but could be readily inferred by the adult. The following exchange between an adult (A) and a child (C) provides an example of such a response (Bishop *et al.* 2000: 188):

1.1: A: has your dad got a 'car?
1.2: C: got a 'van.

Although C does not say that his dad doesn't have a car, this can be readily inferred by A on hearing the response 'got a van'. Bishop *et al.*'s category of 'adequate response' is problematic in the following respect: responses that indicate a high level of pragmatic ability on the part of a child are grouped alongside responses that place relatively few demands on a child's pragmatic competence. This category thus fails to distinguish pragmatic behaviours in conversation from behaviours that draw upon other competences and skills (knowledge of syntax, for example). This can be demonstrated using the above examples. The child who responds 'don't know' to the question 'Where are you going on holiday next year?' is certainly drawing upon a range of cognitive and language skills in producing this response. He must use his knowledge of syntax to understand the inversion in the adult's question (... are you going ...). He must retain the question in working memory while various syntactic and semantic decoding processes are being performed. Having decoded the adult's question (no mean feat for a child with specific language impairment), the child must then attempt to construct his response. Once again, this involves a range of cognitive and language processes – the retrieval of the word 'know' from semantic memory, the insertion of 'not' between the auxiliary verb 'do' and the main verb 'know', etc. Superimposed on these various processes will be knowledge that a question in conversation usually sets up an expectation of a response. My point here is not that pragmatics plays no role in the child's response in this case – awareness of and ability to respond to conversational expectations is pragmatic on many accounts. Rather, it is that the child who is able to conversationally implicate that his dad does not have a car by way of stating that he has a van is doing something considerably more sophisticated in pragmatic terms than the child who is merely addressing conversational expectations (of course, child C in 1.2 is also responding to these expectations). The former child must be capable of engaging in first-order and second-order reasoning about A's mental states. In this way, he must be able to make certain inferences about A's knowledge (first-order reasoning). Relevant to the present case is the knowledge that most people have only one mode of transport, so that if someone has a car, then that person may reasonably be taken not to have a van, and vice versa. However, in order to implicate that C's dad does not have a car, C must also have second-order knowledge. That is, C must know that A knows that C knows that most people typically operate with one mode of transport. Second-order reasoning is not involved in the exchange where the child is producing the response 'don't know' to the adult's question (to the extent that this child must be aware of the adult's expectations in order to address them – the expectation, for example, that a question should receive a response – it is clear that this exchange involves some first-order reasoning on the part of the child).

By deciding to place C's response in 1.2 in the same category as a 'don't know' response (the category 'adequate response'), Bishop *et al.*, I am arguing, have missed the true pragmatic significance of the above exchange between A and C. Their mistake is thus a variant of the third type of error discussed in section 7.3 – in failing to attribute greater pragmatic significance to C's response at 1.2, there is a clear sense in which Bishop *et al.* have missed the pragmatic point of this exchange. The question that must now be addressed is why Bishop *et al.* have failed to set C's response at 1.2 apart from other adequate, but pragmatically mundane responses. Of course, the explanation could quite simply be that this rather crude grouping of responses is an unfortunate consequence of the attempt to quantify pragmatic behaviours in conversation (it should be recalled that ALICC is a quantitative approach to conversation analysis). A more likely explanation leads us to a problem at the heart of all conversation analytic work in pragmatics.[21] These approaches are dominated by notions such as adjacency pairs, one of which is the question–response pair that is the focus of Bishop *et al.*'s investigation. The emphasis of an adjacency pair analysis is that the expectation that is set up by the asking of a question, for example, is ultimately addressed in conversation, either through the giving of a response or some account of why an answer may not be forthcoming.[22] On this approach, the child who responds 'don't know' to an adult's question and the child who implicates that his father doesn't have a car have both produced an 'adequate response' – both children have adequately addressed the expectation for a response that is set up by the adult's question. But this approach is impotent to describe, and indeed actively eschews, the particular epistemic and cognitive considerations[23] that set the response of the latter child apart from that of the former child. Yet, it is exactly these considerations that we must acknowledge if we are to appreciate the greater pragmatic sophistication of the latter child's response. It emerges that Bishop *et al.*'s investigation suffers from the same explanatory inadequacies that beset the approach of conversation analysis in general.

It has been demonstrated that a number of the errors identified in section 7.3 are committed by clinicians and researchers who use qualitative and quantitative conversation analytic procedures to assess pragmatic language skills in clients. It remains to be seen if other pragmatic language assessments can evade these same errors. In recent years, there has been growing interest amongst clinicians and researchers in the use of communication checklists and profiles for the assessment of pragmatics.[24] Two of the most influential are the Pragmatics Profile (Dewart and Summers 1995) and the Children's Communication Checklist (Bishop 2003b). These assessments were described at length in section 6.2.1 in Chapter 6. Checklists and profiles, I want to argue, are an 'exclude nothing' approach to the assessment of language pragmatics. This approach is characterised by several features. The first of these features is that the term 'pragmatics' is construed so widely that it ends up being used as a synonym for 'communication'. No aspect of an individual's verbal and nonverbal communication is deemed to be irrelevant to an assessment of pragmatics on this approach. This is clearly evident in the Pragmatics Profile, for example, where nonverbal behaviours used to express emotion and gain attention are assessed alongside items that examine a child's understanding of indirect requests and sarcasm. The problem here is that while the latter behaviours are pragmatic in nature, the former behaviours are not evidently so. The child who claps upon seeing a particular adult is certainly expressing his pleasure at being in that adult's company. To the extent that the adult will take the child's enthusiastic clapping to indicate a state of pleasure, it may even be said that the child has successfully conveyed or communicated a particular mental state. But language pragmatics, it was argued earlier, is about more than merely communicating mental states. Although we can infer a child's state of pleasure directly from his clapping behaviour, we cannot directly infer a speaker's communicative intention from his production of the utterance 'Would you like to wash your hands?' (one of the examples used in the Pragmatics Profile to examine a child's understanding of indirect requests). Indeed, to try to do so would lead us to the wrong communicative intention – that the speaker is asking a yes/no question about something we might want to do rather than requesting that we wash our hands. The point that proponents of checklists and profiles need to keep in mind can be summarised as follows: although pragmatic phenomena necessarily involve the communication of a mental state (namely, a communicative intention), not every occasion in which a mental state is communicated is an instance of a pragmatic phenomenon – clapping, for example, conveys the emotion of pleasure in a child but is not a pragmatic behaviour.

The second feature of the checklists and profiles approach to the assessment of pragmatics is its dependence on reports of the child's communication skills by parents, teachers and other carers. The rationale for this dependence is clear enough. Therapists spend relatively little time in the presence of the child compared to these other individuals. Moreover, interaction with the therapist in the setting of the clinic is unlikely to reflect how the child communicates in a range of other communication environments. In short, constraints of time and location mean that the therapist only ever receives a snapshot of the child's communication skills. There is a very real sense in which those individuals with greatest exposure to a child will be best placed to make observations about how that child communicates in a range of settings. However if, as I am arguing, pragmatics is not to be identified with communication in its entirety but is, in fact, only a subset of communication behaviours, then it is much more doubtful that parents, teachers and carers will be suitably qualified to identify these behaviours. Even in the absence of any special training or instruction, most people can accurately describe the type of gestures used by a child and the different contexts in which these gestures are employed. However, considerable knowledge and training are required to understand the difference between a direct speech act ('I want you to take off your shoes') and an indirect speech act ('Can you take off your shoes?'), especially when the grammatical form of many indirect requests is similar to that of yes/no questions – for example, 'Would you like to wash your hands?' (indirect request) and 'Would the children like to eat ice cream?' (question). Support for this view derives from a study by Bishop and Baird (2001) which found that correlations between ratings for parents and professionals on the individual pragmatic scales of the Children's Communication Checklist ranged from 0.30 to 0.58, with a correlation of 0.46 for the pragmatic composite. This correlation was found to increase significantly when professionals complete the checklist.[25] Clearly, parents and other non-professionals will always have an important role to play in the assessment of children's communication skills. However, the assumption of current checklists and profiles that pragmatics is more easily described and assessed by non-professionals than other language levels (e.g. syntax) is likely to be mistaken.

The third feature of checklists and profiles is a feature of assessments in general: they aim to provide a rational basis for intervention. It should be possible to use assessment findings to plan exactly which behaviours, skills and deficits will be targeted during a programme of intervention. However, it is hard to see how findings based on these methods can be used for this end. We have seen how many of the so-called pragmatic behaviours that are assessed by means of checklists and profiles are not related in either cognitive or conceptual terms – a cognitive capacity for complex mental state attribution is integral to the understanding of indirect requests, for example, but is not involved in the expression of emotion. Even when a developmental perspective informs a particular checklist or profile, it often does not inform the setting of targets in therapy. This occurs in the Pragmatics Profile, for example, where a strong developmental orientation to the assessment of pragmatic skills is completely overlooked at the stage of planning goals for intervention. In the absence of some unifying factor, whether this factor be cognitive, conceptual or developmental in nature, all we are left with is a set of disparate skills – a weak basis, indeed, for the planning of intervention. We discuss this issue further in the next section.

7.4.2   Pragmatic language intervention

In this section, I examine two approaches to pragmatic language intervention in children. In the first of these approaches, pragmatic language skills are targeted directly in therapy and are not treated as part of a wider programme of social communication intervention. In the second approach, pragmatics is one component in a larger intervention that targets social communication skills in children with pragmatic language impairment. The central assumptions of these interventions, I argue, reveal important misunderstandings about pragmatics in general and pragmatic language impairment in particular. In the final section, I consider a number of ways in which we can recover ourselves from the various problems that pervade clinical work in the area of pragmatics.

Richardson and Klecan-Aker (2000) are concerned to address two areas of limitation in previous research into pragmatic language intervention. First, few studies have even attempted to examine the outcome of intervention in the area of language pragmatics. Second, such studies as have been undertaken tend to confine themselves to the study of conversation: 'very little data exist on effects of teaching pragmatic language skills. Studies that have been completed tend to focus on only one aspect of pragmatics, that being conversation' (2000: 24). In addition to conversation, Richardson and Klecan-Aker targeted internal responses and qualitative and quantitative descriptions of objects in their own programme of pragmatic language intervention in children with learning disabilities. These areas were taught concurrently during six weeks of treatment. In the first ten minutes of each therapy session, subjects were instructed on how to start, maintain and end conversations. As a class, children were encouraged to think about ways in which conversations could be started and terminated. Then, in pairs, children were given time to practise a conversation on a topic chosen by the clinician before they were asked to present their rehearsed conversation to the class. The second ten minutes of each session was devoted to the receptive and expressive identification of seven emotions: happy, sad, mad, frustrated, surprised, embarrassed and bored. The children were presented with scenarios in which each of these emotions might be experienced. They were then asked to think of a situation in which they might feel these emotions. To encourage receptive identification of emotions, children were shown pictures of facial expressions corresponding to each emotion. In the final ten minutes of each session, children were taught how to describe objects according to several categories: name or label, colour, shape, size, function and material. To gain practice in using these categories, children were presented with objects which they had to describe in front of the class.

Through the techniques outlined above, Richardson and Klecan-Aker aim to improve the pragmatic language skills of the children in this study. Yet, no single technique amongst the treatment methods just described is even beginning to target language pragmatics. Consider, for example, the attempt to instruct these children in the use of greetings and farewell statements in conversation. This instructional effort may be characterised as one of trying to get subjects to learn certain rules relating to conversational practice – to begin a conversation, one says 'Hello', 'Hi', 'How are you doing?', etc. In more sophisticated instructional approaches, subjects may even be encouraged to think about the different contextual features that may influence the selection of opening utterances in conversation (it is clear that Richardson and Klecan-Aker do not even go this far). In this way, children may be taught to use opening utterances such as 'Good morning, Mr Smith' when the addressee is a schoolteacher or other person in a position of authority to the child and 'Hi, Susie' when the addressee is a friend or sibling. But here again, the child is merely learning conversational rules, for example, to begin a conversation, one says 'Good morning ...' if the addressee is an authority figure and 'Hi ...' if the addressee is a friend, etc. However, when speakers produce utterances with considerations of context in mind, they are not merely applying a number of learnt rules of conversation. Rather, they are exercising a form of reason-based judgement. The difference between the application of rules and the exercise of judgement can be clearly demonstrated by considering how one of Richardson and Klecan-Aker's subjects would respond when confronted with a scenario that is not tightly prescribed by a rule or that conflicts with a learnt rule. Such a subject will have assimilated a rule about the use of 'How are you doing?' to open a conversational exchange. And in certain contexts of use, this rule will enable the child to embark in an appropriate manner upon a conversational exchange with an addressee. But this same enquiry may be altogether less appropriate if the addressee is in evident distress or if the speaker and hearer had an extended conversation on the telephone the night before – in such cases, the same enquiry may appear conversationally obtuse and irrelevant, respectively. The child who has been taught rules of conversation will be 'blind' to the significance of these wider factors for his or her own attempts to initiate a conversation. He or she has not developed the type of reflective capacity that informs our subconscious judgements about when to use certain linguistic forms in conversation. Richardson and Klecan-Aker's instructional effort is clearly well intentioned. However, it is ultimately misguided on account of its assumption that targeting particular conversational behaviours will produce gains in language pragmatics – it is only the development of a certain rational competence that will lead to such gains.

The notion of rational competence deserves further consideration. The problem with any intervention that teaches conversational rules is that these rules require prior knowledge in order to be applied appropriately. This prior knowledge is a type of rational competence which embodies our various judgements about when a conversational rule should be applied. Also, importantly, it reflects our judgements about the conditions under which a conversational rule should no longer be presumed to hold. The child who is taught to open conversational exchanges by uttering 'How are you doing?' has really been taught very little indeed. They know a form of words that should be applied at the start of a conversation. Yet, they lack knowledge of the type of considerations that make this utterance an appropriate opening utterance in a conversation. Specifically, they lack knowledge of the vast range of conditions under which this utterance would no longer be an appropriate means of opening a conversation, conditions such as those discussed above (the addressee is in evident distress etc.). Even if the child could be taught a series of exceptions to a conversational rule, he or she would still need a form of prior knowledge to apply this 'qualified' conversational rule. Imagine, for example, that a child is taught the rule 'Open a conversational exchange by uttering "How are you doing?", unless it is clear that the addressee is distressed'. While this question may be redundant in most circumstances in which the addressee is evidently distressed, it is relatively easy to think of contexts in which the exception does not apply (i.e. the speaker should ask 'How are you doing?' when it is clear that the addressee is distressed). A reticent friend may need the prompt of this question in order to disclose the source of his or her distress. This knowledge of a friend's personality is one of the numerous judgements that form a speaker's rational competence and that influence our use of utterances in particular contexts. The mistake of approaches that aim to teach conversational rules is that of assuming that a speaker's rational competence can be fully reconstructed as a series of rules (and exceptions to those rules). What is overlooked is that there will always need to be some form of rational competence outside of these rules in order for these rules to be applied appropriately.

The second and third components in Richardson and Klecan-Aker's instructional programme fare little better as techniques for the remediation of language pragmatics. The expressive and receptive identification of emotions is now a standard part of therapeutic programmes that aim to improve the social cognition of subjects (see Adams (2005) and Adams *et al.* (2005) below). Certainly, there is clear evidence that certain populations of children and adults, particularly individuals with autistic spectrum disorder, have a specific impairment in the recognition of a range of emotional states in others.[26] However, it is not the inability of subjects to *recognise* emotional states in others that is the pragmatic impairment in this case (Richardson and Klecan-Aker's attempt to train subjects to recognise emotions would tend to suggest that they locate a pragmatic impairment at this level of recognition). Rather, the real pragmatic impairment in this case lies in the inability to use that recognition in the interpretation of an interlocutor's utterances or in the construction of one's own utterances in conversation. Consider again the case of the child who is trying to start a conversation with a friend. The decision to begin such a conversation with the enquiry 'How are you doing?' is more than a little insensitive when one's addressee is clearly upset. The mere recognition of the interlocutor's state of distress is not in itself a pragmatic language skill (although one could easily see how a failure of this recognition could have negative consequences for skills that are pragmatic in nature). Instead, the pragmatic significance of the case only truly emerges when the child uses the recognition that the interlocutor is distressed to start the conversation with the question 'What's wrong?' and not the question 'How are you doing?' Through training the children in this study to recognise a range of emotions, Richardson and Klecan-Aker are not training, I am arguing, a pragmatic language skill but a social cognitive skill. Moreover, the difference between these skills is more than merely terminological in nature. One can imagine, for example, how the children in this study could become proficient in the recognition of others' emotions – as indeed they did – and yet still fail to show any significant improvement in pragmatic language skills. Simply training emotional recognition is not sufficient in itself to produce gains in language pragmatics – the latter will only come about when subjects are trained in how to use this recognition to influence their choice of linguistic forms in conversation.

The third and final component in Richardson and Klecan-Aker's programme of intervention is even less obviously targeting pragmatic behaviours than the first two components. Subjects were taught to describe objects such as a toy telephone and a toy firetruck using a range of shape, colour and size adjectives, along with other descriptors. But this task is clearly only developing syntactic and semantic skills on the part of these children. In this respect, it is little different from the type of activity that is undertaken within conventional language therapy. Of course, in the absence of syntactic and semantic language skills, the children in this study would be unable to produce indirect speech acts, derive the implicature of a speaker's utterance and successfully execute a range of other pragmatic language functions (see section 1.6 in Chapter 1). But the necessity of these language skills to pragmatics does not thereby make these skills pragmatic. Quite apart from treating pragmatic language skills in the children in this study, Richardson and Klecan-Aker's programme of intervention is not even succeeding in targeting those skills. It remains to be seen if a treatment that targets pragmatic language skills as part of a wider programme of social communication intervention can do any better in this regard.

Two recent investigations in which a social communication framework was used to treat children with pragmatic language impairments can be used to demonstrate the features of this approach to intervention. Adams (2005) reports how this framework was used to promote 'synergistic competence' in the four areas that she deems to be the basis of social communication: social interaction, social cognition, pragmatics (verbal and nonverbal aspects) and language processing (receptive and expressive). The subject, a boy called Oliver (aged 8;01 at the start of the study), had severe language processing problems as well as difficulty with empathy and making friends at school, circumscribed interests and little appreciation of reciprocal conversational skills. Oliver met criteria for pervasive developmental disorder (he did not meet strict criteria for autism). Given Oliver's profile of difficulties, it was decided that all four areas of social communication should be targeted in his case. Intervention included adaptation work with Oliver's family and staff at his school (the social interaction component in the framework), work on empathy and inference (social cognition component), therapy on word-finding and receptive language skills (language processing component) and explicit work on pragmatics via a metapragmatic route (pragmatics component). Treatment was carried out by a specialist speech-language practitioner in twenty-four sessions over an eight-week period.

In addition to studying Oliver, Adams *et al.* (2005) examined a second child with significant social and pragmatic problems. This child displayed behaviours that were suggestive of autism, although he was not autistic. These behaviours included a lack of imagination, lack of sharing with adults and peers, a tendency to control play and insistence that peers follow his rules. His conversations displayed a lack of verbal reciprocity, problems with turn-taking, and a tendency to dominate the interaction, to be verbose and to bring conversational topics back to his own particular interests. Unlike Oliver, this child had excellent formal language skills and above average comprehension of inference. In view of the child's intact language skills, it was decided that intervention should aim to improve social interaction and nonverbal aspects of social cognition by using metapragmatic therapy techniques. This child was 9;9 years at the start of intervention.

These investigations of social communication intervention are interesting in the following respect. Notwithstanding the attempt by investigators to carve out a specific role for pragmatics within a wider framework of social communication, the view of pragmatics that emerges is as problematic as those that have been discussed so far. Consider, for example, the various behaviours that are targeted for metapragmatic therapy by Adams (2005). This therapy involved 'explicitly talking about rules and conventions and putting these into practice' (2005: 184). The specific 'aspects of pragmatics' that were addressed included 'conversational conventions, turn-taking, topic management, linguistic cohesion, speech acts, and matching style to context (e.g., politeness)' (Adams 2005: 184–5). A similar set of behaviours was targeted for treatment in the child studied by Adams *et al.* (2005).[27] Although constraints of space preclude examination of each of these aspects, discussion of one aspect – topic management – will serve to demonstrate the problems with approaches which aim to remediate conversational behaviours. The management of any conversational topic draws upon a diverse array of skills and abilities, only some of which are pragmatic in nature. A speaker must be able to establish the listener's knowledge of the topic, in order that some information may be foregrounded (explicitly stated in language), while other information may be backgrounded (presupposed by the speaker's utterances). To the extent that this speaker is constructing his utterances in accordance with his listener's knowledge state, it is clear that he is drawing upon a pragmatic competence to organise his management of a conversational topic. However, the successful management of any conversational topic requires more than a competence in language pragmatics. The speaker must also be able to think of an appropriate topic for discussion. This requires a certain imaginative capacity, which is known to be lacking in the children in these studies – it will be recalled that Oliver had circumscribed interests, while the child studied by Adams *et al.* (2005) displayed a lack of imagination. It is unremarkable, therefore, that topic management is an area of deficit in these children that requires direct therapy. In addition to imaginative and pragmatic capacities, topic management draws upon a range of formal language skills. A child such as Oliver, who has severe receptive and expressive impairments in syntax and semantics, will not have the requisite language skills to develop a topic in conversation.

It emerges that the ability to manage a topic in conversation is no more a pragmatic language skill than it is an imaginative skill or a formal language skill. The question arises, therefore, of why Adams has chosen to characterise topic management as a pragmatic behaviour when so many other competences are involved in initiating, developing and terminating a topic in conversation. Perhaps this is the competence that Adams takes to be most central to topic management. The answer, I believe, is somewhat different. Adams and her coworkers are treating topic management as pragmatic, not because they believe that a pragmatic competence is central to one's ability to manage a topic in conversation, but because they don't view pragmatics as any type of rational competence at all. Pragmatics merely describes certain surface conversational behaviours – taking turns, initiating topics, etc. It is other parts of Adams *et al.*'s social communication framework, namely social cognition, that describe the rational cognitive processes (i.e. reasoning) that permit these various conversational behaviours to come about.[28] I argued above that Richardson and Klecan-Aker had overlooked the core rational competence of pragmatics in their attempt to train children to open conversations with particular greetings – when language users select an utterance to open a conversation, it was argued, they are not merely applying a rule of conversation, but exercising a form of rational judgement or competence. In the same way, I am now claiming that Adams and her coworkers have misrepresented the notion of pragmatics. This misrepresentation takes two interrelated forms. First, these investigators are using pragmatics as a catch-all term for a range of surface conversational behaviours. Second, to the extent that these behaviours are rationally motivated or depend on cognitive processes, these rational cognitive processes are not part of a pragmatic competence, but fall within the domain of social cognition. The result is a distorted notion of pragmatics that leads investigators to believe that they can treat language pragmatics merely by instructing children in the use of surface conversational behaviours.

7.5   Overcoming problems of definition and delimitation

In section 7.4, I argued that misunderstandings about the nature and extent of pragmatics have adversely affected how clinicians and researchers assess and treat pragmatic language disorders. Some of these misunderstandings have led investigators to overlook the pragmatic significance of conversational exchanges and to attribute pragmatic impairments to subjects in areas that are not pragmatic in nature. Other misunderstandings, particularly the neglect of the rational, cognitive basis of pragmatics, have led practitioners to treat pragmatic impairments by instructing subjects in a type of conversational performance. If we are to recover ourselves from the many incorrect ways in which the term 'pragmatics' has been used in a clinical context, we must first become clear about the scope of pragmatics itself. In considering this issue of scope, I will be concerned less with providing a definition of pragmatics than with establishing a set of criteria that will help us evade the various problems demonstrated in this chapter. Some of these criteria reinforce features of standard definitions of pragmatics that have got lost in the transition between theoretical and clinical studies in pragmatics. Other criteria relate to features that have either not been acknowledged in definitions of pragmatics or that have only been acknowledged in an indirect way. All criteria, it is expected, will provide a rational basis for future enquiry in pragmatics while at the same time eliminating some of the problems that have occurred in clinical studies.

Criterion 1: language must be at the centre of an account of pragmatics   It is perhaps a sign of just how far things have gone awry in clinical pragmatics that I am beginning this list of criteria with what is, to most pragmatists, a statement of the obvious – in the absence of language, there can be no language pragmatics. Regardless of the definition of pragmatics one uses, language will be referred to in some capacity – use of language (Mey); information conveyed through language (Cruse); linguistic acts (Stalnaker). There is a widespread tendency amongst clinicians and researchers to view language as an optional component of pragmatics. In this chapter alone, we have seen several examples where investigators have set out to assess and treat language pragmatics only to end up discussing nonlinguistic behaviours such as gesture and eye contact. One reason for this neglect of language – the reason we have mentioned throughout this discussion – has been failure of workers in pragmatics to institute clear boundaries around their discipline. In the absence of limits on the domain of pragmatics, it was argued, the term 'pragmatics' had come to apply to any type of communicative behaviour whatsoever. Under this view, nonverbal behaviours that performed a communicative function were taken to reflect something about an individual's pragmatic language skills. This view quickly found favour amongst clinicians, who believed that they could study pragmatic skills in prelinguistic children or children in whom language had not emerged (e.g. autistic children) by examining nonverbal behaviours in these subjects. This position has become so firmly established amongst practitioners and researchers that it now seems as if language has never had anything to do with language pragmatics! In the same way that we wouldn't consider using terms such as 'syntax' and 'semantics' of the nonverbal communicative behaviours of the prelinguistic child or the child who has failed to develop language, I want to suggest that we shouldn't be using the term 'pragmatics' either. Pragmatics is not about the ability of the prelinguistic child to direct an adult's attention (a skill assessed by Dewart and Summers' Pragmatics Profile). Certainly, such nonlinguistic skills are important precursors to the emergence of language in general.[29] However, these behaviours have no unique significance for language pragmatics, nor are they themselves pragmatic.[30] Clearly, pragmatics involves more than language – no speaker's implicature, for example, will ever be recovered through simply decoding the linguistic forms of an utterance. Additional, nonlinguistic processes – about which we will say more below – must operate alongside language. But these additional processes should not blind us to the fact that speech acts, implicatures, presuppositions and a range of other pragmatic phenomena depend on language in order to implicate and presuppose anything at all.

Criterion 2: reasoning is integral to language pragmatics In section 7.4.2, I argued that many pragmatic language interventions had assumed that they could treat pragmatic impairments, at least those that are manifested in conversation, through training subjects in, amongst other things, the use of certain utterances to initiate and terminate conversations. This assumption was mistaken, I claimed, because pragmatics is not a type of conversational performance, but a rational competence that makes conversation possible. This competence is the basis of our ability to exercise judgement about the utterances that we use in conversation – we are not unreflectively applying rules of conversation when we open an exchange with a particular utterance, but engaging in a process of reasoning that is sensitive to features of context. It was a feature of context, the evident distress of an addressee, that led the speaker in the example discussed in section 7.4.2 to open the conversation with the question 'What's wrong?' and not 'How are you doing?' The speaker who understands the significance of the addressee's tears and cries for his choice of utterance is not merely applying conversational rules, but making a rational judgement, albeit subconsciously, about the utterance that is most appropriate to the situation in which he finds himself. In the example in section 7.4.2, this appropriateness judgement was influenced more by the speaker's purpose in speaking (for example, to understand what is wrong with a distressed friend) than by any imperative to begin a conversation with a particular greeting. This imperative is functionally equivalent to the conversational rules that some intervention approaches have attempted to impart to subjects. In other words, a prior rational competence of the type that I am proposing in relation to pragmatics is needed in order to even apply conversational rules.

To the extent that many pragmatic language interventions neglect to treat pragmatics as a rational competence, it is at least interesting to ask how this situation has come about. The answer lies, I believe, in Chomsky's famous distinction in language between competence and performance. The notion of competence captures our intuitions and judgements about the well-formedness and meaning of sentences. The reason, Chomsky argues, that we are able to tell that some sentences are well formed, while other sentences are ungrammatical or that one sentence is a paraphrase of another sentence is because we have an innate knowledge of the grammar of our language. This innate knowledge, or competence, is only one of several factors that influence how we use language on any particular occasion. Chomsky advanced the notion of performance to describe the various factors that influence our use of language. This competence–performance distinction effectively divided the study of language into two main branches of enquiry – the investigation of competence characteristics within phonology, syntax and semantics and the investigation of the performance features of language in pragmatics. Under this view of language, pragmatics is not a type of competence, nor is it even a mentalistic notion.[31] It is unsurprising, therefore, that clinicians and researchers should have tended to treat pragmatics as the study of conversational performance. It is equally unsurprising that these same investigators should have overlooked the central role of reasoning in pragmatic phenomena (if pragmatics has no rational, mentalistic core, then cognitive notions such as reasoning hold no unique significance for pragmatic phenomena). Yet, it is just this neglect of reasoning that clinicians must address if interventions in pragmatics are going to move beyond misguided efforts to train subjects in a type of conversational performance.[32]

Criterion 3: pragmatics needs a principle of charity   Throughout this discussion, we have seen several examples where conversations have been poorly interpreted and analysed by researchers and clinicians. The result has been the attribution of pragmatic impairment to conversational participants when, in reality, these participants were quite sophisticated in their use of pragmatic language skills. Pragmatics has had little difficulty in generating principles that govern interpretation – Grice's principle of cooperation is just such an interpretative principle. Pragmatics now needs a similar principle which can be applied to the various analyses that are conducted within its domain. A candidate principle is the principle of charity that has been used extensively by analysts in the field of argumentation theory. This principle applies to the formulation of missing premises during the reconstruction of argument. As Johnson and Blair (1994) characterise the principle of charity, 'your objective is to add to the stated premises the most plausible statement (consistent with the rest of the passage and likely to be believed by the arguer and used in addressing that audience) needed to make the whole set of premises relevant to the conclusion' (29). It seems clear, for example, that if something like this principle had been used by Body *et al.* (1999) during their analyses of the conversational exchanges between Pat and her therapist, then some of these investigators' more untenable interpretations of Pat's behaviour could have been avoided. These interpretations were not consistent with the rest of the conversational exchanges upon which they were based. For example, we saw how Body *et al.*'s claim that Pat had failed to grasp the underlying intention of the therapist's question in one of the exchanges examined was not consistent with a later utterance produced by Pat, in which she indicates that her daughter will not be at home for much longer. Nor are Body *et al.*'s interpretations likely to be believed by Pat (the 'arguer' in this case). It is clear, for example, that the beliefs that motivate Pat to make a telephone call are quite different from those that Body *et al.* must attribute to her in order for their interpretation to stand. It is equally unlikely that Body *et al.*'s interpretation of Pat's exchange with the therapist even accurately represents how the therapist (the 'audience') understood this exchange. One could imagine, for example, how Pat's insistence that she make a call to her daughter would be immediately comprehensible to the therapist upon learning that Pat's daughter would not be at home for much longer. In short, Body *et al.*'s interpretations of the conversational exchanges between Pat and her therapist failed to accurately reconstruct the beliefs and intentions of the participants involved in those exchanges. These interpretations are, thus, an uncharitable representation of those exchanges.

In failing to produce a charitable reconstruction of the beliefs and intentions that motivate the conversational exchange between Pat and her therapist, Body *et al.*, I am claiming, are in the same position as the argument analyst who has failed to reconstruct in a charitable way the premises that an arguer is using to support a conclusion. The failure in both these cases is related to a certain deficit of imagination, a deficit that prevents the argument analyst and Body *et al.* from putting themselves in the minds of the particular individuals whose verbal behaviour they are trying to understand (the arguer and Pat, respectively). Yet, this particular imaginative capacity is the basis of all pragmatic interpretation. For example, to understand the illocutionary force of an utterance or to recover the implicature of an utterance, we must be able to locate ourselves imaginatively inside our interlocutor's mind and grasp the particular communicative intentions that lie behind his or her use of a certain utterance. This imaginative capacity is similar to the cognitive ability to develop a theory of other minds, an ability that was described as impaired in autistic children in section 7.3. However, we saw in that section how theory of mind researchers in autism also failed to accurately reconstruct the mental states of individuals within their experimental scenarios – in a study of faux pas, for example, communicative intentions were incorrectly attributed to Lisa when, in fact, she had a false belief about the curtains in her friend Jill's house. What emerges from these various deliberations is that clinicians and researchers are failing to apply to their own analyses of language pragmatics in clinical subjects the very cognitive (imaginative) skill that is integral to all pragmatic interpretation – the ability to establish the communicative intentions and beliefs of language users. Perhaps it is in the nature of enquiry into pragmatics that we should remain detached from the imaginative skill that is the essence of pragmatic interpretation within our own interpretative practice. Whatever is the ultimate source of this detachment, it is expected that adherence to the principle of charity will go at least some way towards reducing and eliminating it.

Criterion 4: pragmatics always involves the intention to communicate Whether we are making an indirect request of someone or implicating that we don't wish to accept a speaker's invitation to a party, it is clear that pragmatic behaviours involve the intention to communicate. Notwithstanding the central role of intention in pragmatics, few definitions of pragmatics even make reference to communicative intentions – the definition by Davis (1991) is a notable exception in this regard (see note 5). This particular omission may be partly responsible for the quite widespread tendency to label as pragmatic, behaviours that are not even clearly intentional in nature. We saw this tendency in action in Baron-Cohen *et al.*'s (1999) study of faux pas in autistic subjects. This study, it was argued, could tell us nothing about the pragmatic language skills of these subjects because faux pas was, by definition, not a type of intentional communication. Body *et al.*'s analysis of Pat as variously implicating that she is head-injured or aggressive, overly familiar or impolite reveals a complete misunderstanding of the intentional character of implicature – it cannot reasonably be claimed that Pat is intentionally communicating any of these things. Other, less obvious examples of this neglect of intention were also discussed. We saw in section 7.4.1 how one of the items in Dewart and Summers' Pragmatics Profile concerns the expression of emotion. The child who enthusiastically claps his hands upon seeing an adult is almost certainly experiencing pleasure. But it is less clear that he is intending to communicate his state of pleasure to the adult – our recognition of the child's pleasure is based on his clapping behaviour and is not dependent in any way on the child having an intention to communicate his pleasure. Quite simply, the mere fact that something is communicated (e.g. the child's state of pleasure) is not enough in itself to call it pragmatic – for the term 'pragmatic' to apply, a speaker must have *intended* to communicate it.

I stated above that the omission of intention (or communicative intentions) from most definitions of pragmatics may have been at least partly responsible for the tendency to apply the term 'pragmatics' to behaviours that weren't even intentional in nature. However, there is, I believe, a more significant explanation for this omission. It is that the domain of the mental has been very actively eschewed from pragmatics. In this section alone, we have seen several examples of how mental phenomena have been driven out of pragmatics. The role of cognitive processes such as reasoning and inference has too often been overlooked (an obvious exception is Sperber and Wilson's relevance theory, which has given prominence to such processes). Analyses of pragmatic behaviours proceed, in a surprising number of cases, with little or no attention being paid to the mental states (communicative intentions, beliefs, etc.) that motivate those behaviours. Pragmatic concepts such as implicature are used when it is clear that no intentional communication is even involved in a particular case. We have also discussed in this section a possible reason for the neglect of the mental domain in pragmatics – Chomsky's competence–performance distinction, it was argued, effectively excluded pragmatics from the mentalistic concerns studied within language competence. Whatever will ultimately stand as an explanation of the problems that have been identified in this chapter, it is clear that this explanation will have as much significance for clinical pragmatics as for pragmatics itself.

7.6   Conclusion

At the start of this book, I outlined the current state of clinical pragmatics. The field was characterised as one which was beset by problems. Many clinical pragmatic studies, it was argued, misrepresented pragmatic notions. There was little consensus amongst theorists and clinicians on which linguistic features should be labelled 'pragmatic'. Clinical pragmatic studies also proceeded in a largely atheoretical fashion. The result was a large body of findings that had little explanatory value in accounts of pragmatic disorder. Each of these problems, it was argued, had adverse implications for the assessment and treatment of pragmatic disorders in clients. There was thus a compelling clinical imperative to address these difficulties and to consider ways in which future clinical pragmatic studies might avoid making them. To this end, a major revision of clinical pragmatics was envisaged. This revision sought to integrate fields of enquiry which could shed light on the nature of pragmatic disorders but which had largely been neglected by clinical investigators. A particularly promising line of investigation in this regard was the closer integration of cognitive and pragmatic theories. A likely outcome of this integration was the development of new theoretical frameworks which could explain the pragmatic skills and deficits of child and adult clients. Although the attainment of such frameworks is still some way off, several ways were suggested in which the gulf between cognitive and pragmatic theories might be narrowed. Cognitively plausible pragmatic theories and pragmatically plausible cognitive theories, it was argued, are increasingly within the grasp of clinical investigators and are a sine qua non of further progress in clinical pragmatics.

A revision of clinical pragmatics required more than a convergence of cognitive and pragmatic theories, however. It required all clinical investigators to be critical of their own analytical practice. In this chapter in particular, we have seen how pragmatic disorders were incorrectly attributed to clients and aspects of intact pragmatic performance were overlooked. Some clinical analyses, it was argued, had effectively misrepresented clients' pragmatic skills and were thus an inaccurate basis for clinical intervention. Mistaken and misleading analyses were linked to several factors – a misunderstanding of pragmatic concepts, a less than careful consideration of the performance of clients, etc. Regardless of their cause, some means needed to be found of exposing these problematic analyses when they occurred and (ideally) avoiding their occurrence in the first place. To this end, four criteria were proposed. These criteria were based upon an examination of the most frequent errors to occur in clinical pragmatic studies. The function of these criteria is a largely regulatory one – they operate by guiding investigators towards those behaviours that are properly pragmatic in nature. This regulatory function is nowhere more in evidence than in how we proceed to interpret the pragmatic skills of clients. It was argued that a pragmatic equivalent of the principle of charity was needed to regulate some of the less tenable interpretations of clients' pragmatic skills that had occurred in clinical studies. The discussions that gave rise to these criteria mark a critical turn in clinical pragmatics. It is a sign of an intellectually mature discipline that its theorists can reflect critically not just on their current state of knowledge, but also on the standards and methods by means of which this knowledge is generated. It is hoped that this book's critical examination of clinical pragmatics will contribute to the emergence of a new, mature phase in this discipline's development.

NOTES

1 Bryans (1992) succinctly captures the problem that a sprawling notion of context, such as that proposed by Stalnaker (1998), creates for a definition of pragmatics: 'Surely it is ludicrous to hold a position in which pragmatics is nothing less than a study of human life. Some aspects of the context of utterance may be relevant but *all* of them? Inextricably so?' (1992: 185; italics in original).

2 Writing in 1991, Craig states that 'pragmatic approaches have dominated research efforts in child language disorder for approximately 10 years' (1991: 163).

3 As it turns out, the dysfluency of the aphasic subjects in Prutting and Kirchner's study was related to the linguistic deficits of the nonfluent aphasics in the sample. However, these linguistic deficits were lexico-syntactic, not pragmatic in nature, so there are no grounds upon which dysfluency can be reasonably described as a pragmatic deficit.

4 Although, as I am arguing in the main text, it is incorrect to describe pause times in turn-taking as a pragmatic behaviour, this is at least an understandable error on the part of Prutting and Kirchner. In 1983, prior to the clinical investigations of these researchers, Stephen Levinson's ground-breaking book on pragmatics was published. This book attempted to demarcate the subject area of pragmatics and has had a profound influence on the development of the field, even to the present day.

The chapter entitled 'Conversational structure' in this text discusses turn-taking and pauses. However, it is now recognised amongst theorists in the field that Levinson was casting the net of pragmatics too widely in his discussion of conversation analysis: 'Levinson's book ... covers probably a little too much that is peripheral to pragmatics (see his sections on CA and ethnomethodology, for instance)' (anonymous book reviewer).

5 Communicative intentions are an explicit component of the definition of pragmatics advanced by Davis (1991): 'Pragmatics will have as its domain speakers' communicative intentions, the uses of language that require such intentions, and the strategies that hearers employ to determine what these intentions and acts are, so that they can understand what the speaker intends to communicate' (1991: 11).

6 In addition to the studies reviewed in Chapters 2 and 3, indirect speech acts, implicatures and idioms have been examined by the following investigators. Hatta *et al.* (2004) examined the ability of twenty subjects with left-hemisphere damage and twenty subjects with right-hemisphere damage to process implicatures, especially indirect request and indirect refusal. Studies have investigated the comprehension of idioms in a wide range of clinical groups. Papagno *et al.* (2004) assessed idiom comprehension in ten aphasic subjects with semantic deficits. Qualls *et al.* (2004) examined the effects of context and familiarity on the comprehension of idioms in twenty-two adolescent subjects with language-based learning disabilities. Norbury (2004) investigated the understanding of idioms in context in ninety-three children with communication disorders, who were subdivided according to the presence of autistic features and language impairment. Abrahamsen and Burke-Williams (2004) examined the ability of third- and fifth-grade children with and without learning disabilities to identify the correct idiom and to explain idiom meanings.

7 The performance of the AS/HFA subjects on this test was significantly impaired relative to the normal subjects. For subjects to pass the test, their score either had to be equal to or above eight out of ten. On the basis of this criterion, only 18% of the children with AS or HFA passed the test compared to 75% of the normal children. This difference in performance was highly significant.

8 Tests of false belief – so-called Sally-Anne experiments – and features of communication in autism are discussed at length in Chapter 9 of Cummings (2005) and in Chapter 3 of Cummings (2008).

9 As well as using notions like implicature and intention incorrectly, it is clear that on other occasions in the same study Body *et al.* (1999) use these terms appropriately to describe intentional communicative behaviours. For example, in the exchange – A: 'I'll pay you back before the weekend'; B: 'Yeah, and my mother is Genghis Khan!' – B is correctly taken to implicate 'I don't believe you' by saying something he believes to be equally false. Grice's maxim framework is also accurately applied by these investigators to the analysis of this exchange.

10 Surian *et al.*'s use of the term 'violation' is also problematic. B in the exchange in the main text is not violating any of the Gricean maxims. Rather, he is *flouting* a maxim with a view to generating an implicature. For further discussion of the distinction between flouting and violating a maxim, see Chapter 1 in Cummings (2005).

11 Kasher (1998) argues that 'some notion of context plays a major role in almost all delineations of Pragmatics. The interesting spectrum of views is divided into bands that differ from each other not in the extent to which contextual elements play major roles in their theoretical frameworks, but rather in their respective packages of

contextual elements. The smallest possible package of such elements would include just those marked by the non-pragmatic components of language, such as Syntax. The largest possible package would include the whole human context – biological, societal, cultural and what have you' (1998: 148).

12 Norbury (2005) found that all subjects displayed contextual facilitation – they responded quickly and more accurately to ambiguous words that followed a biased context. However, children with language impairment, either on its own or in combination with ASD, did not use context as efficiently as language-intact subjects. Also, the language-impaired groups displayed errors in the suppression condition that reflected poor contextual processing. Norbury remarks that 'these findings challenge the assumptions of weak central coherence theory' (2005: 142).

13 In fact, it is impossible to circumscribe the vast number of factors across a wide range of different contexts that are relevant to the calculation of implicatures. For further discussion of this point, see Chapter 4 in Cummings (2005).

14 Pragmatic interpretation, it is being claimed, is a global process. Wilson and Sperber (1991) model the global character of pragmatic interpretation on scientific enquiry: 'A global process is one in which any item of information, however remote and unrelated to the information being processed, may legitimately be used. So, for example, in creating a scientific hypothesis to account for a certain range of data it is legitimate to rely on analogies with other domains of knowledge, seemingly random association of ideas, and any other source of inspiration that comes to hand. Once a hypothesis has been formed, the extent to which it is regarded as confirmed will depend on how well it fits not only with neighbouring domains of knowledge but with one's whole overall conception of the world' (1991: 380).

15 This hypothesis was confirmed with LBLD adolescents attaining accuracy levels of 31% and 52% in the story and verification tasks, respectively. The result was explained in terms of reduced processing capabilities in the LBLD adolescents. Specifically, deficits in integration and inferencing in the LBLD adolescents prevented these subjects from using effectively the context provided in the story task to obtain idiomatic meaning.

16 This is not the same as saying that context is coextensive with life itself (see Bryans (1992) in note 1). However, it is intended to get the reader to think about context in an altogether broader way than is done by experimental psychologists in the studies reviewed in the main text.

17 Narrative assessments are increasingly being performed with a view to examining language pragmatics. Adams (2001) uses this method, amongst other forms of assessment, in a study of two children with a diagnosis of semantic-pragmatic language disorder: 'Narrative assessment is potentially a valuable instrument of assessment. In this case it was used to demonstrate aspects of progress in sequencing, inference and informativeness, i.e. in pragmatic abilities' (302).

18 Adams (2001) remarks that 'analysis of conversations has tended to be qualitative and descriptive, with adjacent turns considered in the context set up by the interlocutors' (292). Body et al.'s analysis is certainly 'qualitative and descriptive'. However, if my analysis in the main text is correct, they have done anything but consider Pat's turns 'in the context set up by the interlocutors'.

19 Adams et al. (2006) recently used Bishop's ALICC procedure in a study that was designed to generate a signal of change in pragmatic and other language behaviours for children with pragmatic language impairments. Measures of pragmatic

behaviours in conversation were made using the procedure at seven data points before and after therapy. Studies such as this one are making an important contribution in a field where investigations of the efficacy of pragmatic interventions have traditionally been lacking. Adams *et al.* (2006) remark that 'there is little systematic evidence that demonstrates the benefits of speech and language therapy for children whose difficulties lie primarily within the pragmatic domain or which indicates whether changes in pragmatic behaviours, which are a result of a specific intervention, can be measured over time' (41).

20 Adams (2002) remarks that 'ALICC has made a major contribution to the quantification of pragmatic data and allowed the characterisation of children with pragmatic language impairments to move forward. It has the benefits of providing a concrete method of measurement within controlled samples and a potential tool for evaluation of change. ALICC is the instrument of choice for quantitative analysis of conversational data provided reliability of coding for observers can be attained and there is sufficient time for training and analysis' (980). In a study that explored the effects of communication intervention in children with pragmatic language impairments, Adams *et al.* (2006) reported that ALICC 'could clearly demonstrate changes in pragmatic skills for children who were at ceiling on language tests. At present, there is no other established method of doing this' (58).

21 It should be emphasised which particular form of conversation analysis is the target of my criticism in the main text. I have in mind the CA approach that has its origins in the work of a break-away group of sociologists known as ethnomethodologists and whose pioneers were workers such as Sacks and Schegloff (the reader is referred to Chapter 6 in Levinson (1983) for an introduction to the field). This approach has had a profound influence on the subsequent development of conversation analysis in both pragmatics and clinical pragmatics. However, this is not to overlook a substantial body of work which is also a form of conversation analysis (in a mundane sense of this term) but which is so far removed from CA principles as to not be identified with it.

22 Levinson (1983: 303–8) discusses the different ways in which speakers may respond to questions and uses extracts of transcribed conversation to demonstrate some of these ways.

23 Epistemic and cognitive factors are part of the wider context in which an exchange of turns occurs in conversation. However, context receives little prominence within the analyses of CA workers. Levinson (1983) remarks that 'the data consist of tape-recordings and transcripts of naturally occurring conversation, with little attention paid to the nature of context' (295). To the extent that Bishop *et al.* have overlooked epistemic and cognitive factors in their analysis of C's response at 2.1, it could be argued that these workers have distorted the context that attends this response. As well as claiming that these theorists have missed the pragmatic significance of the exchange between A and C, it could also be argued that they have committed the further error of distorting context (the fourth category of error discussed in section 7.3).

24 This interest has been generated in large part by the fact that these assessments are not reliant on normative data, which are lacking in the area of pragmatics. Adams (2002) states that 'checklists of pragmatic behaviours circumvent the problems of lack of normative data and are more comprehensive and popular with practitioners than tests' (976).

25 In a study in which the checklist is completed by teachers and speech and language therapists, Bishop (1998) reports interrater reliability and internal consistency of around 0.80 on the five pragmatic subscales. This higher correlation between professionals can be explained by the fact that teachers and therapists, unlike parents, have knowledge of language pragmatics.

26 Downs and Smith (2004) compared cooperation, emotional understanding, personality characteristics and social behaviour in ten children with autism, sixteen children with attention deficit hyperactivity disorder and oppositional defiant disorder and ten typically developing children. The autism group was found to have worse emotion recognition and more active-but-odd behaviour than the other groups.

27 In this case, pragmatic language therapy was used to develop 'exchange structure, turn-taking, topic management, conversational skills, building sequences in narrative, referencing in discourse, cohesion and coherence' (Adams *et al.* 2005: 234).

28 The reasoning processes that are used to obtain the implied meaning of a speaker's utterances and that, I am claiming, form part of a pragmatic competence, are clearly targeted from within the social cognition component of the framework proposed by Adams *et al.* In this way, social cognition intervention aimed to 'introduce the use and understanding of metaphors and hidden meaning' (Adams 2005: 184). To this end, 'the child was supported in making deduction of the likely meaning from the social context'. I am arguing in the main text that it is only a weakened notion of pragmatics that has been drained of its rational cognitive content that leads Adams *et al.* to view this aspect of intervention as social cognitive in nature rather than pragmatic.

29 One of the most significant nonverbal behaviours in the prelinguistic period to be linked to language development is joint attention. Bruinsma *et al.* (2004) remark that 'the construct of joint attention has been noted as an early developing area prior to the transition to symbolic communication' (169). There has now been extensive validation of the link between nonverbal behaviours and language development in both typically developing and disordered children. In a study of thirteen normally developing children, D'Odorico *et al.* (1997) found that gaze directed towards an interlocutor at the start of vocal turns at age 1;0 was related to language production at age 1;8. Paavola *et al.* (2005) found that maternal responsiveness and infant intentional communicative acts at ten months predicted comprehensive skills in twenty-seven healthy Finnish infants at twelve months, while only intentional communicative acts predicted expressive skills. Calandrella and Wilcox (2000) examined the relationship between prelinguistic communication behaviours at the start of a twelve-month period and expressive and receptive language outcomes at the end of this period in twenty-five toddlers with developmental delay. Prelinguistic communication behaviours included intentional nonverbal communication acts, all of which involved coordinated or joint attention between the communication referent and an adult, and gestural indicating behaviour and social interaction signals, which did not involve coordinated attention to an adult. It was found that the rate of intentional nonverbal communication at the start of the study predicted spontaneous word productions at the end of the study. Also, the rate of intentional communication and rate of gestural-indicating behaviour at six months into the study predicted language outcomes at the end of the study. In a study of eighteen children with developmental disabilities, Brady *et al.* (2004) found that the level of gestural attainment by the children, rate of communication and parent response contingency were significant

predictors of language outcome. Kane *et al.* (2004) found positive, though weak, correlations between prelinguistic communication skills and language learning in eighteen prelingually deaf children who underwent unilateral cochlear implantation at an average age of fifteen months.

30 If anything, early nonverbal behaviours have more significance for the development of lexical-semantic abilities. Bruinsma *et al.* (2004) state that 'preverbal communication and joint attention have long been of interest to researchers and practitioners. Both attending to social partners and sharing attentional focus between objects or events and others precede the onset of a child's first lexicon' (169). Clinical studies have found significant relationships between prelinguistic behaviour and vocabulary development in disordered children. McCathren *et al.* (1999) examined the relationship between prelinguistic vocalisation and expressive vocabulary one year later in fifty-eight toddlers with developmental delay. It was found that rate of vocalisation, rate of vocalisations with consonants and rate of vocalisations used interactively all positively related to later expressive vocabulary. McDuffie *et al.* (2005) examined four prelinguistic behaviours (attention-following, motor imitation, commenting and requesting) in twenty-nine two- and three-year-olds with autism spectrum disorders. It was found that commenting and motor imitation of actions without objects were unique predictors of vocabulary production six months later.

31 Searle makes the very same point that I am developing here when he charges Chomsky with having a 'residual suspicion' that treating speech acts as our basic unit of meaning inevitably involves making 'a retreat to behaviorism'. Chomsky's suspicion is unfounded, Searle contends, because human action is inherently a mentalistic notion: 'It is one of the ironies of the history of behaviorism that behaviorists should have failed to see that the notion of a human action must be a "mentalistic" and "introspective" notion since it essentially involves the notion of human *intentions*' (1974: 31). It is perhaps fitting that we should conclude this study of clinical pragmatics by invoking the same Searlean insights on language use from which we set out in Chapter 1: that our knowledge of how to use language to perform a range of speech acts is part of our linguistic competence and, as such, has the same mentalistic character that Chomsky affords to his notion of grammar.

32 Of course, it should not be overlooked that some clinicians and researchers are taking a cognitive approach to pragmatics. Such an approach is advocated by Body *et al.* (1999) who believe that pragmatics is too rooted in disciplines such as philosophy to be of service in its current form in the treatment of subjects with traumatic brain injury. Although this study has been shown to be lacking in many respects, these authors should at least be congratulated on their emphasis of the cognitive character of pragmatic phenomena.

Bibliography

Abbeduto, L. and Hesketh, L. J. 1997. 'Pragmatic development in individuals with mental retardation: learning to use language in social interactions', *Mental Retardation and Developmental Disabilities Research Reviews* **3**:4, 323–33.

Abbeduto, L., Brady, N. and Kover, S. T. 2007. 'Language development and fragile X syndrome: profiles, syndrome-specificity, and within-syndrome differences', *Mental Retardation and Developmental Disabilities Research Reviews* **13**:1, 36–46.

Abbeduto, L., Davies, B. and Furman, L. 1988. 'The development of speech act comprehension in mentally retarded individuals and nonretarded children', *Child Development* **59**:6, 1460–72.

Abbeduto, L., Short-Meyerson, K., Benson, G. and Dolish, J. 2004. 'Relationship between theory of mind and language ability in children and adolescents with intellectual disability', *Journal of Intellectual Disability Research* **48**:2, 150–9.

Abbeduto, L., Short-Meyerson, K., Benson, G., Dolish, J. and Weissman, M. 1998. 'Understanding referential expressions in context: use of common ground by children and adolescents with mental retardation', *Journal of Speech, Language, and Hearing Research* **41**:6, 1348–62.

Abbeduto, L., Pavetto, M., Kesin, E., Weissman, M. D., Karadottir, S., O'Brien, A. and Cawthon, S. 2001. 'The linguistic and cognitive profile of Down syndrome: evidence from a comparison with fragile X syndrome', *Down's Syndrome, Research and Practice* **7**:1, 9–15.

Abbeduto, L., Murphy, M. M., Richmond, E. K., Amman, A., Beth, P., Weissman, M. D., Kim, J., Cawthon, S. W. and Karadottir, S. 2006. 'Collaboration in referential communication: comparison of youth with Down syndrome or fragile X syndrome', *American Journal on Mental Retardation* **111**:3, 170–83.

Abkarian, G. G. 1992. 'Communication effects of prenatal alcohol exposure', *Journal of Communication Disorders* **25**:4, 221–40.

Abrahamsen, E. P. and Burke-Williams, D. 2004. 'Comprehension of idioms by children with learning disabilities: metaphoric transparency and syntactic frozenness', *Journal of Psycholinguistic Research* **33**:3, 203–15.

Adams, C. 2001. 'Clinical diagnostic and intervention studies of children with semantic-pragmatic language disorder', *International Journal of Language and Communication Disorders* **36**:3, 289–305.

  2002. 'Practitioner review: the assessment of language pragmatics', *Journal of Child Psychology and Psychiatry* **43**:8, 973–87.

  2005. 'Social communication intervention for school-age children: rationale and description', *Seminars in Speech and Language* **26**:3, 181–8.

Adams, C. and Bishop, D.V. 1989. 'Conversational characteristics of children with semantic-pragmatic disorder. 1: exchange structure, turntaking, repairs and cohesion', *British Journal of Disorders of Communication* **24**:3, 211–39.

Adams, C., Baxendale, J., Lloyd, J. and Aldred, C. 2005. 'Pragmatic language impairment: case studies of social and pragmatic language therapy', *Child Language Teaching and Therapy* **21**:3, 227–50.

Adams, C., Green, J., Gilchrist, A. and Cox, A. 2002. 'Conversational behaviour of children with Asperger syndrome and conduct disorder', *Journal of Child Psychology and Psychiatry* **43**:5, 679–90.

Adams, C., Lloyd, J., Aldred, C. and Baxendale, J. 2006. 'Exploring the effects of communication intervention for developmental pragmatic language impairments: a signal-generation study', *International Journal of Language and Communication Disorders* **41**:1, 41–65.

Adlam, A.L., Bozeat, S., Arnold, R., Watson, P. and Hodges, J.R. 2006. 'Semantic knowledge in mild cognitive impairment and mild Alzheimer's disease', *Cortex* **42**:5, 675–84.

Aguilar-Mediavilla, E.M., Sanz-Torrent, M. and Serra-Raventos, M. 2002. 'A comparative study of the phonology of pre-school children with specific language impairment (SLI), language delay (LD) and normal acquisition', *Clinical Linguistics & Phonetics* **16**:8, 573–96.

Airenti, G., Bara, B.G. and Colombetti, M. 1993a. 'Conversation and behaviour games in the pragmatics of dialogue', *Cognitive Science* **17**, 197–256.

1993b. 'Failures, exploitations and deceits in communication', *Journal of Pragmatics* **20**:4, 303–26.

Al-Haidar, F.A. 2003. 'Co-morbidity and treatment of attention deficit hyperactivity disorder in Saudi Arabia', *Eastern Mediterranean Health Journal* **9**:(5–6), 988–95.

Alt, M., Plante, E. and Creusere, M. 2004. 'Semantic features in fast mapping: performance of preschoolers with specific language impairment versus preschoolers with normal language', *Journal of Speech, Language, and Hearing Research* **47**:2, 407–20.

American Heart Association 2006. *Heart disease and stroke statistics – 2006 update*, Dallas: American Heart Association.

American Psychiatric Association 1994, 2000. *Diagnostic and statistical manual of mental disorders*, Washington, DC: American Psychiatric Association.

Andersen-Wood, L. and Smith, B.R. 1997. *Working with pragmatics*, Bicester: Winslow Press.

Andersson, C.B. and Thomsen, P.H. 1998. 'Electively mute children: an analysis of 37 Danish cases', *Nordic Journal of Psychiatry* **52**:3, 231–8.

Angeleri, R., Bosco, F.M., Zettin, M., Sacco, K., Colle, L. and Bara, B.G. 2008. 'Communicative impairment in traumatic brain injury: a complete pragmatic assessment', *Brain and Language* **107**:3, 229–45.

Archibald, L.M.D. and Gathercole, S.E. 2006a. 'Short-term and working memory in specific language impairment', *International Journal of Language & Communication Disorders* **41**:6, 675–93.

2006b. 'Visuospatial immediate memory in specific language impairment', *Journal of Speech, Language, and Hearing Research* **49**:2, 265–77.

258   Bibliography

Armstrong, L., Brady, M., Mackenzie, C. and Norrie, J. 2007. 'Transcription-less analysis of aphasic discourse: a clinician's dream or a possibility?', *Aphasiology* **21**:(3–4), 355–74.

Astington, J.W. 1988. 'Children's understanding of the speech act of promising', *Journal of Child Language* **15**:1, 157–73.

Aubert, S., Barat, M., Campan, M., Dehail, P., Joseph, P.A. and Mazaux, J.M. 2004. '[Non verbal communication abilities in severe traumatic brain injury]', *Annales de Réadaptation et de Médecine Physique* **47**:4, 135–41.

Austin, J.L. 1962. *How to do things with words*, Oxford: Clarendon Press.

Avent, J.R., Wertz, R.T. and Auther, L.L. 1998. 'Relationship between language impairment and pragmatic behavior in aphasic adults', *Journal of Neurolinguistics* **11**:(1–2), 207–21.

Bach, L.J., Happe, F., Fleminger, S. and Powell, J. 2000. 'Theory of mind: independence of executive function and the role of the frontal cortex in acquired brain injury', *Cognitive Neuropsychiatry* **5**:3, 175–92.

Bailey, A., Le Couteur, A., Gottesman, I., Bolton, P., Simonoff, E., Yuzda, E. and Rutter, M. 1995. 'Autism as a strongly genetic disorder: evidence from a British twin study', *Psychological Medicine* **25**:1, 63–77.

Bara, B.G. and Tirassa, M. 2000. 'Neuropragmatics: brain and communication', *Brain and Language* **71**:1, 10–14.

Bara, B.G., Bosco, F.M. and Bucciarelli, M. 1999. 'Developmental pragmatics in normal and abnormal children', *Brain and Language* **68**:3, 507–28.

Bara, B.G., Bucciarelli, M. and Geminiani, G.C. 2000. 'Development and decay of extralinguistic communication', *Brain and Cognition* **43**:1–3, 21–7.

Bara, B.G., Cutica, I. and Tirassa, M. 2001. 'Neuropragmatics: extralinguistic communication after closed head injury', *Brain and Language* **77**:1, 72–94.

Bara, B.G., Tirassa, M. and Zettin, M. 1997. 'Neuropragmatics: neuropsychological constraints on formal theories of dialogue', *Brain and Language* **59**:1, 7–49.

Baraff, L.J., Lee, S.I. and Schriger, D.L. 1993. 'Outcomes of bacterial meningitis in children: a meta-analysis', *The Pediatric Infectious Disease Journal* **12**:5, 389–94.

Barnes, M.A. and Dennis, M. 1998. 'Discourse after early-onset hydrocephalus: core deficits in children of average intelligence', *Brain and Language* **61**:3, 309–34.

Barnes, M.A., Faulkner, H., Wilkinson, M. and Dennis, M. 2004. 'Meaning construction and integration in children with hydrocephalus', *Brain and Language* **89**:1, 47–56.

Baron-Cohen, S. 1991. 'The development of a theory of mind in autism: deviance and delay?', *Psychiatric Clinics of North America* **14**:1, 33–51.

  2000. 'Theory of mind and autism: a fifteen year review', in S. Baron-Cohen, H. Tager-Flusberg and D.J. Cohen (eds.), *Understanding other minds: perspectives from developmental cognitive neuroscience*, New York: Oxford University Press, 3–20.

Baron-Cohen, S. and Howlin, P. 1993. 'The theory of mind deficit in autism: some questions for teaching and diagnosis', in S. Baron-Cohen, H. Tager-Flusberg and D.J. Cohen (eds.), *Understanding other minds: perspectives from autism*, New York: Oxford University Press, 466–80.

Baron-Cohen, S., Leslie, A.M. and Frith, U. 1985. 'Does the autistic child have a "theory of mind"?', *Cognition* **21**:1, 37–46.

Baron-Cohen, S., Tager-Flusberg, H. and Cohen, D.J. 2000. 'A note on nosology', in S. Baron-Cohen, H. Tager-Flusberg and D.J. Cohen (eds.), *Understanding other minds: perspectives from developmental cognitive neuroscience*, New York: Oxford University Press, viii–xiii.

Baron-Cohen, S., O'Riordan, M., Stone, V., Jones, R. and Plaisted, K. 1999. 'Recognition of faux pas by normally developing children and children with Asperger syndrome or high-functioning autism', *Journal of Autism and Developmental Disorders* **29**:5, 407–18.

Barry, T.D., Klinger, L.G., Lee, J.M., Palardy, N., Gilmore, T. and Bodin, S.D. 2003. 'Examining the effectiveness of an outpatient clinic-based social skills group for high-functioning children with autism', *Journal of Autism and Developmental Disorders* **33**:6, 685–701.

Bartak, L., Rutter, M. and Cox, A. 1975. 'A comparative study of infantile autism and specific developmental receptive language disorder: I. The children', *British Journal of Psychiatry* **126**:2, 127–45.

Bartels-Tobin, L.R. and Hinckley, J.J. 2005. 'Cognition and discourse production in right hemisphere disorder', *Journal of Neurolinguistics* **18**:6, 461–77.

Bartha, L., Mariën, P., Poewe, W. and Benke, T. 2004. 'Linguistic and neuropsychological deficits in crossed conduction aphasia: report of three cases', *Brain and Language* **88**:1, 83–95.

Barton, M. and Volkmar, F. 1998. 'How commonly are known medical conditions associated with autism?', *Journal of Autism and Developmental Disorders* **28**:4, 273–8.

Bay, E., Hagerty, B.M. and Williams, R.A. 2007. 'Depressive symptomatology after mild-to-moderate traumatic brain injury: a comparison of three measures', *Archives of Psychiatric Nursing* **21**:1, 2–11.

Bazin, N., Perruchet, P., Hardy-Bayle, M.C. and Feline, A. 2000. 'Context-dependent information processing in patients with schizophrenia', *Schizophrenia Research* **45**:1–2, 93 101.

Becker, M., Warr-Leeper, G.A. and Leeper, H.A. 1990. 'Fetal alcohol syndrome: a description of oral motor, articulatory, short-term memory, grammatical, and semantic abilities', *Journal of Communication Disorders* **23**:2, 97–124.

Bedore, L.M. and Leonard, L.B. 1998. 'Specific language impairment and grammatical morphology: a discriminant function analysis', *Journal of Speech, Language, and Hearing Research* **41**:5, 1185–92.

Beeke, S. 2003. '"I suppose" as a resource for the construction of turns at talk in agrammatic aphasia', *Clinical Linguistics & Phonetics* **17**:4–5, 291–8.

Beeke, S., Maxim, J. and Wilkinson, R. 2007. 'Using conversation analysis to assess and treat people with aphasia', *Seminars in Speech and Language* **28**:2, 136–47.

Beeke, S., Wilkinson, R. and Maxim, J. 2003a. 'Exploring aphasic grammar. 1: a single case analysis of conversation', *Clinical Linguistics & Phonetics* **17**:2, 81–107.

2003b. 'Exploring aphasic grammar. 2: do language testing and conversation tell a similar story?', *Clinical Linguistics & Phonetics* **17**:2, 109–34.

Beeson, P.M., Bayles, K.A., Rubens, A.B. and Kaszniak, A.W. 1993. 'Memory impairment and executive control in individuals with stroke-induced aphasia', *Brain and Language* **45**:2, 253–75.

Befi-Lopes, D.M., Rodrigues, A. and Rocha, L.C. 2004. 'Pragmatic abilities in the discourse of children with and without specific language impairment', *Pró-fono: Revista de Atualização Científica* **16**:1, 57–66.

Bell, B., Dow, C., Watson, E.R., Woodard, A., Hermann, B. and Seidenberg, M. 2003. 'Narrative and procedural discourse in temporal lobe epilepsy', *Journal of the International Neuropsychological Society* **9**:5, 733–9.

Bellgrove, M.A., Chambers, C.D., Vance, A., Hall, N., Karamitsios, M. and Bradshaw, J.L. 2006. 'Lateralized deficit of response inhibition in early-onset schizophrenia', *Psychological Medicine* **36**:4, 495–505.

Benasich, A.A. and Tallal, P. 2002. 'Infant discrimination of rapid auditory cues predicts later language impairment', *Behavioural Brain Research* **136**:1, 31–49.

Benner, G.J., Nelson, J.R. and Epstein, M.H. 2002. 'Language skills of children with EBD: a literature review', *Journal of Emotional and Behavioral Disorders* **10**:1, 43–56.

Bennetto, L., Pennington, B.F., Porter, D., Taylor, A.K. and Hagerman, R.J. 2001. 'Profile of cognitive functioning in women with the fragile X mutation', *Neuropsychology* **15**:2, 290–9.

Benson, G., Abbeduto, L., Short, K., Nuccio, J.B. and Maas, F. 1993. 'Development of a theory of mind in individuals with mental retardation', *American Journal of Mental Retardation* **98**:3, 427–33.

Benton, A.L., Hamsher, K. deS., Varney, N.R. and Spreen, O. 1983. *Contributions to neuropsychological assessment: a clinical manual*, New York: Oxford University Press.

Berg, D. 2006. 'Marker for a preclinical diagnosis of Parkinson's disease as a basis for neuroprotection', *Journal of Neural Transmission* Supplementum **71**, 123–32.

Berg, E., Björnram, C., Hartelius, L., Laakso, K. and Johnels, B. 2003. 'High-level language difficulties in Parkinson's disease', *Clinical Linguistics & Phonetics* **17**:1, 63–80.

Beverly, B.L. and Williams, C.C. 2004. 'Present tense *be* use in young children with specific language impairment: less is more', *Journal of Speech, Language, and Hearing Research* **47**:4, 944–56.

Bibby, H. and McDonald, S. 2005. 'Theory of mind after traumatic brain injury', *Neuropsychologia* **43**:1, 99–114.

Biederman, J., Wilens, T.E., Spencer, T.J. and Adler, L.A. 2007. 'Diagnosis and treatment of adults with attention-deficit/hyperactivity disorder', *CNS Spectrums* **12**:4 Supplement 6, 1–15.

Bignell, S. and Cain, K. 2007. 'Pragmatic aspects of communication and language comprehension in groups of children differentiated by teacher ratings of inattention and hyperactivity', *British Journal of Developmental Psychology* **25**:4, 499–512.

Bishop, D.V.M. 1983. *Test for reception of grammar*. Published by the author and available from the Age and Cognitive Performance Research Centre, University of Manchester, M13 9PL.

   1998. 'Development of the children's communication checklist (CCC): a method for assessing qualitative aspects of communicative impairment in children', *Journal of Child Psychology and Psychiatry* **39**:6, 879–91.

   2000a. 'Pragmatic language impairment: a correlate of SLI, a distinct subgroup, or part of the autistic continuum?', in D.V.M. Bishop and L.B. Leonard (eds.),

Speech and language impairments in children: causes, characteristics, interven-tion and outcome, Hove, East Sussex: Psychology Press Ltd, 99–113.

2000b. 'What's so special about Asperger syndrome? The need for further explor-ation of the borderlands of autism', in A. Klin, F.R. Volkmar and S.S. Sparrow (eds.), *Asperger syndrome,* New York: The Guilford Press, 254–77.

2003a. 'Autism and specific language impairment: categorical distinction or con-tinuum?', *Novartis Foundation Symposium* **251**, 213–26.

2003b. *The children's communication checklist, version 2 (CCC-2),* London: Psychological Corporation.

Bishop, D.V.M. and Adams, C. 1989. 'Conversational characteristics of children with semantic-pragmatic disorder. II: what features lead to a judgement of inappro-priacy?', *British Journal of Disorders of Communication* **24**:3, 241–63.

1992. 'Comprehension problems in children with specific language impairment: literal and inferential meaning', *Journal of Speech and Hearing Research* **35**:1, 119–29.

Bishop, D.V.M. and Baird, G. 2001. 'Parent and teacher report of pragmatic aspects of communication: use of the Children's Communication Checklist in a clinical set-ting', *Developmental Medicine & Child Neurology* **43**:12, 809–18.

Bishop, D.V.M. and Norbury, C.F. 2002. 'Exploring the borderlands of autistic dis-order and specific language impairment: a study using standardised diagnostic instruments', *Journal of Child Psychology and Psychiatry* **43**:7, 917–29.

Bishop, D.V.M. and Rosenbloom, L. 1987. 'Classification of childhood language dis-orders', in W. Yule and M. Rutter (eds.), *Language development and disorders,* London: MacKeith Press, 16–41.

Bishop, D.V.M., North, T. and Donlan, C. 1995. 'Genetic basis of specific language impairment: evidence from a twin study', *Developmental Medicine and Child Neurology* **37**:1, 56–71.

Bishop, D.V.M., Laws, G., Adams, C. and Norbury, C.F. 2006a. 'High heritability of speech and language impairments in 6-year-old twins demonstrated using parent and teacher report', *Behavior Genetics* **36**:2, 173–84.

Bishop, D.V.M., Chan, J., Adams, C., Hartley, J. and Weir, F. 2000. 'Conversational responsiveness in specific language impairment: evidence of disproportionate pragmatic difficulties in a subset of children', *Development and Psychopathology* **12**:2, 177–99.

Bishop, D.V.M., Maybery, M., Wong, D., Maley, A. and Hallmayer, J. 2006b. 'Characteristics of the broader phenotype in autism: a study of siblings using the children's communication checklist-2', *American Journal of Medical Genetics. Part B, Neuropsychiatric Genetics* **141**:2, 117–22.

Bisset, J. and Novak, A. 1995. 'Drawing inferences from emotional situations: left ver-sus right hemisphere deficit', *Clinical Aphasiology* **23**, 217–25.

Black, B. and Uhde, T.W. 1995. 'Psychiatric characteristics of children with selective mutism: a pilot study', *Journal of the American Academy of Child and Adolescent Psychiatry* **34**:7, 847–56.

Blair, M., Marczinski, C.A., Davis-Faroque, N. and Kertesz, A. 2007. 'A longitudinal study of language decline in Alzheimer's disease and frontotemporal dementia', *Journal of the International Neuropsychological Society* **13**:2, 237–45.

Bliss, L.S. 1993. *Pragmatic language intervention: interactive activities,* USA: Thinking Publications.

Blonder, L., Burns, A., Bowers, D., Moore, R. and Heilman, K. 1993. 'Right hemisphere facial expressivity during natural conversation', *Brain and Cognition* **21**:1, 44–56.

Bock, J. K. 1977. 'The effect of a pragmatic presupposition on syntactic structure in question answering', *Journal of Verbal Learning and Verbal Behavior* **16**:6, 723–34.

Body, R. and Parker, M. 2005. 'Topic repetitiveness after traumatic brain injury: an emergent, jointly managed behaviour', *Clinical Linguistics & Phonetics* **19**:5, 379–92.

Body, R., Perkins, M. and McDonald, S. 1999. 'Pragmatics, cognition, and communication in traumatic brain injury', in S. McDonald, L. Togher and C. Code (eds.), *Communication disorders following traumatic brain injury*, East Sussex: Psychology Press Ltd, 81–112.

Boles, L. 1998. 'Conversational discourse analysis as a method for evaluating progress in aphasia: a case report', *Journal of Communication Disorders* **31**:3, 261–73.

Booth, S. and Perkins, L. 1999. 'The use of conversation analysis to guide individualized advice to carers and evaluate change in aphasia: a case study', *Aphasiology* **13**:(4–5), 283–303.

Booth, S. and Swabey, D. 1999. 'Group training in communication skills for carers of adults with aphasia', *International Journal of Language and Communication Disorders* **34**:3, 291–309.

Borg, E. 2004. *Minimal semantics*, Oxford: Clarendon Press.

Borod, J., Rorie, K., Pick, L., Bloom, R., Andelman, F., Campbell, A., Obler, L., Tweedy, J., Welkowitz, J. and Sliwinski, M. 2000. 'Verbal pragmatics following unilateral stroke: emotional content and valence', *Neuropsychology* **14**:1, 112–24.

Boscolo, B., Ratner, N. B. and Rescorla, L. 2002. 'Fluency of school-aged children with a history of specific expressive language impairment: an exploratory study', *American Journal of Speech-Language Pathology* **11**:1, 41–9.

Botting, N. 2004. 'Children's communication checklist (CCC) scores in 11-year-old children with communication impairments', *International Journal of Language & Communication Disorders* **39**:2, 215–27.

  2005. 'Non-verbal cognitive development and language impairment', *Journal of Child Psychology and Psychiatry* **46**:3, 317–26.

Botting, N. and Adams, C. 2005. 'Semantic and inferencing abilities in children with communication disorders', *International Journal of Language & Communication Disorders* **40**:1, 49–66.

Botting, N. and Conti-Ramsden, G. 1999. 'Pragmatic language impairment without autism: the children in question', *Autism* **3**:4, 371–96.

Boudreau, D. M. and Chapman, R. S. 2000. 'The relationship between event representation and linguistic skill in narratives of children and adolescents with Down syndrome', *Journal of Speech, Language, and Hearing Research* **43**:5, 1146–59.

Boudreau, D. M. and Hedberg, N. L. 1999. 'A comparison of early literacy skills in children with specific language impairment and their typically developing peers', *American Journal of Speech-Language Pathology* **8**:3, 249–60.

Bózzola, F. G., Gorelick, P. B. and Freels, S. 1992. 'Personality changes in Alzheimer's disease', *Archives of Neurology* **49**:3, 297–300.

Brady, N. C., Marquis, J., Fleming, K. and McLean, L. 2004. 'Prelinguistic predictors of language growth in children with developmental disabilities', *Journal of Speech, Language, and Hearing Research* **47**:3, 663–77.

Brenneise-Sarshad, R., Nicholas, L. E. and Brookshire, R. H. 1991. 'Effects of apparent listener knowledge and picture stimuli on aphasic and non-brain-damaged speakers' narrative discourse', *Journal of Speech and Hearing Research* **34**:1, 168–76.

Briscoe, J., Bishop, D. V. M. and Norbury, C. F. 2001. 'Phonological processing, language and literacy: a comparison of children with mild-to-moderate sensorineural hearing loss and those with specific language impairment', *Journal of Child Psychology and Psychiatry* **42**:3, 329–40.

Brown, W. S., Paul, L. K., Symington, M. and Dietrich, R. 2005. 'Comprehension of humor in primary agenesis of the corpus callosum', *Neuropsychologia* **43**:6, 906–16.

Brownell, H., Pincus, D., Blum, A., Rehak, A. and Winner, E. 1997. 'The effects of right-hemisphere brain damage on patients' use of terms of personal reference', *Brain and Language* **57**:1, 60–79.

Brownlie, E. B., Beitchman, J. H., Escobar, M., Young, A., Atkinson, L., Johnson, C., Wilson, B. and Douglas, L. 2004. 'Early language impairment and young adult delinquent and aggressive behavior', *Journal of Abnormal Child Psychology*, **32**:4, 453–67.

Bruce, B., Thernlund, G. and Nettelbladt, U. 2006. 'ADHD and language impairment: a study of the parent questionnaire FTF (five to fifteen)', *European Child & Adolescent Psychiatry* **15**:1, 52–60.

Bruinsma, Y., Koegel, R. L. and Koegel, L. K. 2004. 'Joint attention and children with autism: a review of the literature', *Mental Retardation and Developmental Disabilities Research Reviews* **10**:3, 169–75.

Brundage, S. 1996. 'Comparison of proverb interpretations provided by right-hemisphere-damaged adults and adults with probable dementia of the Alzheimer type', *Clinical Aphasiology* **24**, 215–31.

Brüne, M. and Bodenstein, L. 2005. 'Proverb comprehension reconsidered – "theory of mind" and the pragmatic use of language in schizophrenia', *Schizophrenia Research* **75**: (2–3), 233–9.

Bryan, K. L. 1988. 'Assessment of language disorders after right hemisphere damage', *British Journal of Disorders of Communication* **23**:2, 111–25.

1995. *The right hemisphere language battery*, London: Whurr Publishers.

Bryans, J. 1992. 'Review of Davis (1991)', *Canadian Philosophical Reviews* **12**, 184–6.

Bucciarelli, M., Colle, L. and Bara, B. G. 2003. 'How children comprehend speech acts and communicative gestures', *Journal of Pragmatics* **35**:2, 207–41.

Buckley, S. and Le Prèvost, P. 2002. 'Speech and language therapy for children with Down syndrome', *Down Syndrome News and Update* **2**:2, 70–6.

Buitelaar, J. K., van der Wees, M., Swaab-Barneveld, H. and van der Gaag, R. J. 1999. 'Theory of mind and emotion-recognition functioning in autistic spectrum disorders and in psychiatric control and normal children', *Development and Psychopathology* **11**:1, 39–58.

Burch, K., Wilkinson, R. and Lock, S. 2002. 'A single case study of conversation-focused therapy for a couple where one partner has aphasia', *Proceedings of the therapy symposium*, British Aphasiology Society, Hayes Conference Centre, Swanwick, Derbyshire, 11–12 September, 2002, 1–12.

Burns, M., Halper, A. S. and Mogil, S. I. 1985. *Clinical management of right hemisphere dysfunction*, Rockville: Aspen.

Burt, S. A., McGue, M., DeMarte, J. A., Krueger, R. F. and Iacono, W. G. 2006. 'Timing of menarche and the origins of conduct disorder', *Archives of General Psychiatry* **63**:8, 890–6.

Calandrella, A. M. and Wilcox, M. J. 2000. 'Predicting language outcomes for young prelinguistic children with developmental delay', *Journal of Speech, Language and Hearing Research* **43**:5, 1061–71.

Cannito, M. P., Jarecki, J. M. and Pierce, R. S. 1986. 'Effects of thematic structure on syntactic comprehension in aphasia', *Brain and Language* **27**:1, 38–49.

Capps, L., Kehres, J. and Sigman, M. 1998. 'Conversational abilities among children with autism and children with developmental delays', *Autism* **2**:4, 325–44.

Capps, L., Losh, M. and Thurber, C. 2000. '"The frog ate the bug and made his mouth sad": narrative competence in children with autism', *Journal of Abnormal Child Psychology* **28**:2, 193–204.

Carlomagno, S., Santoro, A., Menditti, A., Pandolfi, M. and Marini, A. 2005. 'Referential communication in Alzheimer's type dementia', *Cortex* **41**:4, 520–34.

Carroll, K., Murad, S., Eliahoo, J. and Majeed, A. 2001. 'Stroke incidence and risk factors in a population-based prospective cohort study', *Health Statistics Quarterly* **12**, 18–26.

Carruthers, P. and Smith, P. K. 1996. 'Introduction', in P. Carruthers and P. K. Smith (eds.), *Theories of theories of mind*, Cambridge: Cambridge University Press, 1–8.

Carston, R. 2002. 'Linguistic meaning, communicated meaning and cognitive pragmatics', *Mind & Language* **17**: (1–2), 127–48.

Carston, R., Guttenplan, S. and Wilson, D. 2002. 'Introduction: special issue on pragmatics and cognitive science', *Mind & Language* **17**: (1–2), 1–2.

Catts, H. W., Adlof, S. M., Hogan, T. P. and Weismer, S. E. 2005. 'Are specific language impairment and dyslexia distinct disorders', *Journal of Speech, Language, and Hearing Research* **48**:6, 1378–96.

CBTRUS. 2005. *Statistical report: primary brain tumors in the United States, 1998–2002*, Hinsdale: Central Brain Tumor Registry of the United States.

Centers for Disease Control and Prevention (CDC). 2007. 'Rates of hospitalization related to traumatic brain injury – nine states, 2003', *Morbidity and Mortality Weekly Report* **56**:8, 167–70.

Chaika, E. 1990. *Understanding psychotic speech: beyond Freud and Chomsky*, Springfield: Charles C. Thomas.

Champagne-Lavau, M., Stip, E. and Joanette, Y. 2006. 'Social cognition deficit in schizophrenia: accounting for pragmatic deficits in communication abilities?', *Current Psychiatry Reviews* **2**:3, 309–15.

Chandler, S., Christie, P., Newson, E. and Prevezer, W. 2002. 'Developing a diagnostic and intervention package for 2- to 3-year olds with autism', *Autism* **6**:1, 47–69.

Channon, S. and Crawford, S. 2000. 'The effects of anterior lesions on performance on a story comprehension test: left anterior impairment on a theory of mind-type task', *Neuropsychologia* **38**:7, 1006–17.

Chapman, R. S. 2006. 'Language learning in Down syndrome: the speech and language profile compared to adolescents with cognitive impairment of unknown origin', *Down's Syndrome, Research and Practice* **10**:2, 61–6.

Chapman, R. S., Hesketh, L. J. and Kistler, D. J. 2002. 'Predicting longitudinal change in language production and comprehension in individuals with Down syndrome: hierarchical linear modeling', *Journal of Speech, Language, and Hearing Research* **45**:5, 902–15.

Chapman, S. B. and Ulatowska, H. K. 1989. 'Discourse in aphasia: integration deficits in processing reference', *Brain and Language* **36**:4, 651–68.

Chapman, S. B., Ulatowska, H., King, K., Johnson, J. and McIntire, D. 1995. 'Discourse in early Alzheimer's disease versus normal advanced aging', *American Journal of Speech-Language Pathology* **4**:4, 124–9.

Chapman, S. B., Ulatowska, H. K., Franklin, L. R., Shobe, A. E., Thompson, J. L. and McIntire, D. D. 1997. 'Proverb interpretation in fluent aphasia and Alzheimer's disease: implications beyond abstract thinking', *Aphasiology* **11**: (4–5), 337–50.

Charlop, M. H. and Milstein, J. P. 1989. 'Teaching autistic children conversational speech using video modeling', *Journal of Applied Behavior Analysis* **22**:3, 275–85.

Charman, T. and Campell, A. 1997. 'Reliability of theory of mind task performance by individuals with a learning disability: a research note', *Journal of Child Psychology and Psychiatry* **38**:6, 725–30.

Charman, T., Carroll, F. and Sturge, C. 2001. 'Theory of mind, executive function and social competence in boys with ADHD', *Emotional and Behavioural Difficulties* **6**:1, 31–49.

Cheang, H. and Pell, M. 2006. 'A study of humour and communicative intention following right hemisphere stroke', *Clinical Linguistics & Phonetics* **20**:6, 447–62.

Cherney, L. and Canter, G. 1992. 'Informational content in the discourse of patients with probable Alzheimer's disease and patients with right brain damage', *Clinical Aphasiology* **21**, 123–34.

Cheuk, D. K., Wong, V. and Leung, G. M. 2005. 'Multilingual home environment and specific language impairment: a case-control study in Chinese children', *Paediatric and Perinatal Epidemiology* **19**:4, 303–14.

Chien, H. C., Ku, C. H., Lu, R. B., Chu, H., Tao, Y. H. and Chou, K. R. 2003. 'Effects of social skills training on improving social skills of patients with schizophrenia', *Archives of Psychiatric Nursing* **17**:5, 228–36.

Chin, H. Y. and Bernard-Opitz, V. 2000. 'Teaching conversational skills to children with autism: effect on the development of a theory of mind', *Journal of Autism and Developmental Disorders* **30**:6, 569–83.

Choudhury, N., Leppanen, P. H., Leevers, H. J. and Benasich, A. A. 2007. 'Infant information processing and family history of specific language impairment: converging evidence for RAP deficits from two paradigms', *Developmental Science* **10**:2, 213–36.

Church, M. W., Eldis, F., Blakley, B. W. and Bawle. E. V. 1997. 'Hearing, language, speech, vestibular, and dentofacial disorders in fetal alcohol syndrome', *Alcoholism: Clinical and Experimental Research* **21**:2, 227–37.

Clark, H. H. and Schaefer, E. F. 1987. 'Collaborating on contributions to conversation', *Language and Cognitive Processes* **2**:1, 1–23.

 1989. 'Contributing to discourse', *Cognitive Science* **13**:2, 259–94.

Clegg, J., Brumfitt, S., Parks, R. W. and Woodruff, P. W. R. 2007. 'Speech and language therapy intervention in schizophrenia: a case study', *International Journal of Language and Communication Disorders* **42**:S1, 81–101.

Clem, K. and Morgenlander, J.C. 2006. *Amyotrophic Lateral Sclerosis*, USA: eMedicine.com, Inc. (online, available at: www.emedicine.com/emerg/topic24.htm).

Clough, C.G., Chaudhuri, K.R. and Sethi, K.D. 2003. *Parkinson's disease*, Oxford: Health Press.

Cobble, M. 1998. 'Language impairment in motor neurone disease', *Journal of the Neurological Sciences* **160**: Supplement 1, 47–52.

Coelho, C.A. 2002. 'Story narratives of adults with closed head injury and non-brain-injured adults: influence of socioeconomic status, elicitation task, and executive functioning', *Journal of Speech, Language, and Hearing Research* **45**:6, 1232–48.

2007. 'Management of discourse deficits following traumatic brain injury: progress, caveats, and needs', *Seminars in Speech and Language* **8**:2, 122–35.

Coelho, C.A. and Flewellyn, L. 2003. 'Longitudinal assessment of coherence in an adult with fluent aphasia', *Aphasiology* **17**:2, 173–82.

Coelho, C.A., Liles, B.Z. and Duffy, R.J. 1991. 'Discourse analyses with closed head injured adults: evidence for differing patterns of deficits', *Archives of Physical Medicine and Rehabilitation* **72**:7, 465–8.

1995. 'Impairments of discourse abilities and executive functions in traumatically brain-injured adults', *Brain Injury* **9**:5, 471–7.

Coelho, C., Youse, K. and Le, K. 2002. 'Conversational discourse in closed-head-injured and non-brain-injured adults', *Aphasiology* **16**: (4–6), 659–72.

Coelho, C.A., Grela, B., Corso, M., Gamble, A. and Feinn, R. 2005. 'Microlinguistic deficits in the narrative discourse of adults with traumatic brain injury', *Brain Injury* **19**:13, 1139–45.

Cohen, N.J., Barwick, M.A., Horodezky, N.B., Vallance, D.D. and Im, N. 1998. 'Language, achievement, and cognitive processing in psychiatrically disturbed children with previously identified and unsuspected language impairments', *Journal of Child Psychology and Psychiatry* **39**:6, 865–77.

Colle, L., Baron-Cohen, S., Wheelwright, S. and van der Lely, H.K. 2008. 'Narrative discourse in adults with high-functioning autism or Asperger syndrome', *Journal of Autism and Developmental Disorders* **38**:1, 28–40.

Cone-Wesson, B. 2005. 'Prenatal alcohol and cocaine exposure: influences on cognition, speech, language, and hearing', *Journal of Communication Disorders* **38**:4, 279–302.

Conti-Ramsden, G. and Botting, N. 2004. 'Social difficulties and victimization in children with SLI at 11 years of age', *Journal of Speech, Language, and Hearing Research* **47**:1, 145–61.

Conti-Ramsden, G. and Durkin, K. 2007. 'Phonological short-term memory, language and literacy: developmental relationships in early adolescence in young people with SLI', *Journal of Child Psychology and Psychiatry* **48**:2, 147–56.

Conti-Ramsden, G., Simkin, Z. and Botting, N. 2006. 'The prevalence of autistic spectrum disorders in adolescents with a history of specific language impairment (SLI)', *Journal of Child Psychology and Psychiatry* **47**:6, 621–8.

Corcoran, R. 2003. 'Inductive reasoning and the understanding of intention in schizophrenia', *Cognitive Neuropsychiatry* **8**:3, 223–35.

Corcoran, R. and Frith, C.D. 1996. 'Conversational conduct and the symptoms of schizophrenia', *Cognitive Neuropsychiatry* **1**:4, 305–18.

Cornish, K.M., Munir, F. and Cross, G. 2001. 'Differential impact of the FMR-1 full mutation on memory and attention functioning: a neuropsychological perspective', *Journal of Cognitive Neuroscience* **1**:13, 144–50.

Cornish, K. M., Burack, J. A., Rahman, A., Munir, F., Russo, N. and Grant, C. 2005. 'Theory of mind deficits in children with fragile X syndrome', *Journal of Intellectual Disability Research* **49**:5, 372–8.

Coulthard, R. 1985. *An introduction to discourse analysis*, London: Longman.

Covington, M. A., He, C., Brown, C., Naçi, L., McClain, J. T., Fjordbak, B. S., Semple, J. and Brown, J. 2005. 'Schizophrenia and the structure of language: the linguist's view', *Schizophrenia Research* **77**:1, 85–98.

Craig, H. K. 1991. 'Pragmatic characteristics of the child with specific language impairment: an interactionist perspective', in T. M. Gallagher (ed.), *Pragmatics of language: clinical practice issues*, San Diego: Singular Publishing Group, 163–98.

Cram, D. and Hedley, P. 2005. 'Pronouns and procedural meaning: the relevance of spaghetti code and paranoid delusion', *Oxford Working Papers in Linguistics, Philology and Phonetics* **10**, 187–210.

Crespo-Eguilaz, N. and Narbona, J. 2006. 'Subtypes of specific language impairment in Spanish-speaking children: a cluster analysis of linguistic features', *Revista de Neurologia* **10**:43, Supplement 1, 193–200.

Crosson, J. and Geers, A. 2001. 'Analysis of narrative ability in children with cochlear implants', *Ear and Hearing* **22**:5, 381–94.

Cruse, D. A. 2000. *Meaning in language: an introduction to semantics and pragmatics*, Oxford: Oxford University Press.

Crystal, D. and Varley, R. 1998. *Introduction to language pathology*, London: Whurr Publishers.

Cuerva, A. G., Sabe, L., Kuzis, G., Tiberti, C., Dorrego, F. and Starkstein, S. E. 2001. 'Theory of mind and pragmatic abilities in dementia', *Neuropsychiatry, Neuropsychology, and Behavioural Neurology* **14**:3, 153–8.

Cummings, L. 2005. *Pragmatics: a multidisciplinary perspective*, Edinburgh: Edinburgh University Press.

2007a. 'Pragmatics and adult language disorders: past achievements and future directions', *Seminars in Speech and Language* **28**:2, 98–112.

2007b. 'Clinical pragmatics: a field in search of phenomena?', *Language and Communication* **27**:4, 396–432.

2008. *Clinical linguistics*, Edinburgh: Edinburgh University Press.

Cummings, L. (ed.) 2009. *The pragmatics encyclopedia*, London: Routledge.

Currie, G. 1996. 'Simulation-theory, theory-theory and the evidence from autism', in P. Carruthers and P. K. Smith (eds.), *Theories of theories of mind*, Cambridge: Cambridge University Press, 242–56.

Cutica, I., Bucciarelli, M. and Bara, B. 2006. 'Neuropragmatics: extralinguistic pragmatic ability is better preserved in left-hemisphere-damaged patients than in right-hemisphere-damaged patients', *Brain and Language* **98**:1, 12–25.

D'Odorico, L., Cassibba, R. and Salerni, N. 1997. 'Temporal relationships between gaze and vocal behavior in prelinguistic and linguistic communication', *Journal of Psycholinguistic Research* **26**:5, 539–56.

Damico, J. S. 1985. 'Clinical discourse analysis: a functional approach to language assessment', in C. S. Simon (ed.), *Communication skills and classroom success: assessment of language-learning disabled students*, London: Taylor & Francis, 165–203.

Damico, J. S. and Nelson, R. L. 2005. 'Interpreting problematic behavior: systematic compensatory adaptations as emergent phenomena in autism', *Clinical Linguistics & Phonetics* **19**:5, 405–17.

Damico, J. S., Oelschlaeger, M. and Simmons-Mackie, N. 1999. 'Qualitative methods in aphasia research: conversation analysis', *Aphasiology* **13**:(9–11), 667–79.

Damico, J. S., Simmons-Mackie, N. and Wilson, B. 2006. 'The negotiation of intelligibility in an aphasic dyad', *Clinical Linguistics & Phonetics* **20**: (7–8), 599–605.

David, A. S. 1993. 'Cognitive neuropsychiatry', *Psychological Medicine* **23**:1, 1–5.

Davis, A. D., Sanger, D. D. and Morris-Friehe, M. 1991. 'Language skills of delinquent and nondelinquent adolescent males', *Journal of Communication Disorders* **24**:4, 251–66.

Davis, G. A. and Coelho, C. A. 2004. 'Referential cohesion and logical coherence of narration after closed head injury', *Brain and Language* **89**:3, 508–23.

Davis, G. A., O'Neill-Pirozzi, T. M. and Coon, M. 1997. 'Referential cohesion and logical coherence of narration after right hemisphere stroke', *Brain and Language* **56**:2, 183–210.

Davis, S. 1991. *Pragmatics: a reader*, New York: Oxford University Press.

Dawson, D. R. and Chipman, M. 1995. 'The disablement experienced by traumatically brain-injured adults living in the community', *Brain Injury* **9**:4, 339–53.

de Guise, E., Feyz, M., LeBlanc, J., Richard, S. L. and Lamoureux, J. 2005. 'Overview of traumatic brain injury patients at a tertiary trauma centre', *Canadian Journal of Neurological Sciences* **32**:2, 186–93.

de Neys, W. and Schaeken, W. 2007. 'When people are more logical under cognitive load: dual task impact on scalar implicature', *Experimental Psychology* **54**:2, 128–33.

de Villiers, J. G. and de Villiers, P. A. 2000. 'Linguistic determinism and the understanding of false belief', in P. Mitchell and K. J. Riggs (eds.), *Children's reasoning and the mind*, Hove, East Sussex: Psychology Press, 191–228.

de Villiers, J. G. and Pyers, J. E. 2002. 'Complements to cognition: a longitudinal study of the relationship between complex syntax and false-belief-understanding', *Cognitive Development* **17**:1, 1037–60.

DeLisi, L. E. 2001. 'Speech disorder in schizophrenia: review of the literature and exploration of its relation to the uniquely human capacity for language', *Schizophrenia Bulletin* **27**:3, 481–96.

Demir, S. O., Görgülü, G. and Köseoglu, F. 2006. 'Comparison of rehabilitation outcome in patients with aphasic and non-aphasic traumatic brain injury', *Journal of Rehabilitation Medicine* **38**:1, 68–71.

Dennis, M. and Barnes, M. A. 1993. 'Oral discourse after early-onset hydrocephalus: linguistic ambiguity, figurative language, speech acts, and script-based inferences', *Journal of Pediatric Psychology* **18**:5, 639–52.

Dennis, M., Jacennik, B. and Barnes, M. A. 1994. 'The content of narrative discourse in children and adolescents after early-onset hydrocephalus and in normally developing age peers', *Brain and Language* **46**:1, 129–65.

Dennis, M., Lazenby, A. L. and Lockyer, L. 2001. 'Inferential language in high-function children with autism', *Journal of Autism and Developmental Disorders* **31**:1, 47–54.

Department of Health 2001. *Valuing people: a new strategy for learning disability for the 21st century*, London: Department of Health.

Dewart, H. and Summers, S. 1988. *The pragmatics profile of early communication skills*, Windsor: NFER Nelson.

  1995. *Pragmatics profile of everyday communication skills in children*, Windsor: NFER Nelson.

Di Legge, S., Fang, J., Saposnik, G. and Hachinski, V. 2005. 'The impact of lesion side on acute stroke treatment', *Neurology* **65**:1, 81–6.

Diehl, J.J., Bennetto, L. and Young, E.C. 2006. 'Story recall and narrative coherence of high-functioning children with autism spectrum disorders', *Journal of Abnormal Child Psychology* **34**:1, 87–102.

Dipper, L.T., Bryan, K.L. and Tyson, J. 1997. 'Bridging inference and relevance theory: an account of right hemisphere damage', *Clinical Linguistics & Phonetics* **11**:3, 213–28.

Dobbinson, S., Perkins, M.R. and Boucher, J. 1998. 'Structural patterns in conversations with a woman who has autism', *Journal of Communication Disorders* **31**:2, 113–33.

2003. 'The interactional significance of formulas in autistic language', *Clinical Linguistics & Phonetics* **17**:(4–5), 299–307.

Docherty, N.M., Cohen, A.S., Nienow, T.M., Dinzeo, T.J. and Dangelmaier, R.E. 2003. 'Stability of formal thought disorder and referential communication disturbances in schizophrenia', *Journal of Abnormal Psychology* **112**:3, 469–75.

Douglas, J.M. and Bracy, C.A. 2006. 'The nature of impaired conversational skill following severe traumatic brain injury', International Aphasia Rehabilitation Conference: Sheffield UK, 4–6 June 2006.

Douglas, J.M., O'Flaherty, C.A. and Snow, P.C. 2000. 'Measuring perception of communicative ability: the development and evaluation of the La Trobe communication questionnaire', *Aphasiology* **14**:3, 251–68.

Downs, A. and Smith, T. 2004. 'Emotional understanding, cooperation, and social behaviour in high-functioning children with autism', *Journal of Autism and Developmental Disorders* **34**:6, 625–35.

Drabick, D.A., Beauchaine, T.P., Gadow, K.D., Carlson, G.A. and Bromet, E.J. 2006. 'Risk factors for conduct problems and depressive symptoms in a cohort of Ukrainian children', *Journal of Clinical Child and Adolescent Psychology* **35**:2, 244–52.

Dunn, L.M., Dunn, L.M. and Whetton, C. 1982. *British picture vocabulary scale*, Windsor: NFER Nelson.

Duong, A., Whitehead, V., Hanratty, K. and Chertkow, H. 2006. 'The nature of lexico-semantic processing deficits in mild cognitive impairment', *Neuropsychologia* **44**:10, 1928–35.

Eadie, P.A., Fey, M.E., Douglas, J.M. and Parsons, C.L. 2002. 'Profiles of grammatical morphology and sentence imitation in children with specific language impairment and Down syndrome', *Journal of Speech, Language, and Hearing Research* **45**:4, 720–32.

Edwards, J. and Lahey, M. 1996. 'Auditory lexical decisions of children with specific language impairment', *Journal of Speech and Hearing Research* **39**:6, 1263–73.

Ehrlich, J.S. and Sipes, A.L. 1985. 'Group treatment of communication skills for head trauma patients', *Cognitive Rehabilitation* **3**:1, 32–8.

Eisele, J.A., Lust, B. and Aram, D.M. 1998. 'Presupposition and implication of truth: linguistic deficits following early brain lesions', *Brain and Language* **61**:3, 376–94.

Elizur, Y. and Perednik, R. 2003. 'Prevalence and description of selective mutism in immigrant and native families: a controlled study', *Journal of the American Academy of Child and Adolescent Psychiatry* **42**:12, 1451–9.

Ellis, C., Rosenbek, J. C., Rittman, M. R. and Boylstein, C. A. 2005. 'Recovery of cohesion in narrative discourse after left-hemisphere stroke', *Journal of Rehabilitation Research & Development* **42**:6, 737–46.

Ely, R. and Gleason, J. B. 2006. 'I'm sorry I said that: apologies in young children's discourse', *Journal of Child Language* **33**:3, 599–620.

Emerich, D. M., Creaghead, N. A., Grether, S. M., Murray, D. and Grasha, C. 2003. 'The comprehension of humorous materials by adolescents with high-functioning autism and Asperger's syndrome', *Journal of Autism and Developmental Disorders* **33**:3, 253–7.

Engelter, S. T., Gostynski, M., Papa, S., Frei, M., Born, C., Ajdacic-Gross, V., Gutzwiller, F. and Lyrer, P. A. 2006. 'Epidemiology of aphasia attributable to first ischemic stroke: incidence, severity, fluency, etiology, and thrombolysis', *Stroke* **37**:6, 1379–84.

Enticott, P. G., Ogloff, J. R. P. and Bradshaw, J. L. 2008. 'Response inhibition and impulsivity in schizophrenia', *Psychiatry Research* **157**: (1–3), 251–54.

Farmer, M. and Oliver, A. 2005. 'Assessment of pragmatic difficulties and socio-emotional adjustment in practice', *International Journal of Language and Communication Disorders* **40**:4, 403–29.

Fazio, B. B. 1998. 'The effect of presentation rate on serial memory in young children with specific language impairment', *Journal of Speech, Language, and Hearing Research* **41**:6, 1375–83.

Feeney, A., Scrafton, S., Duckworth, A. and Handley, S. J. 2004. 'The story of some: everyday pragmatic inference by children and adults', *Canadian Journal of Experimental Psychology* **58**:2, 121–32.

Feuerstein, R. 1980. *Instrumental enrichment*, Baltimore: University Park Press.

Feyereisen, P., Berrewaerts, J. and Hupet, M. 2007. 'Pragmatic skills in the early stages of Alzheimer's disease: an analysis by means of a referential communication task', *International Journal of Language and Communication Disorders* **42**:1, 1–17.

Fiddick, L., Cosmides, L. and Tooby, J. 2000. 'No interpretation without representation: the role of domain-specific representations and inferences in the Wason selection task', *Cognition* **77**:1, 1–79.

Fine, C., Lumsden, J. and Blair, R. J. R. 2001. 'Dissociation between "theory of mind" and executive functions in a patient with early left amygdala damage', *Brain* **124**:2, 287–98.

Fink, J. N. 2005. 'Underdiagnosis of right-brain stroke', *Lancet* **366**:9483, 349–51.

Flaada, J. T., Leibson, C. L., Mandrekar, J. N., Diehl, N., Perkins, P. K., Brown, A. W. and Malec, J. F. 2007. 'Relative risk of mortality after traumatic brain injury: a population-based study of the role of age and injury severity', *Journal of Neurotrauma* **24**:3, 435–45.

Flax, J. F., Realpe-Bonilla, T., Hirsch, L. S., Brzustowicz, L. M., Bartlett, C. W. and Tallal, P. 2003. 'Specific language impairment in families: evidence for co-occurrence with reading impairments', *Journal of Speech, Language, and Hearing Research* **46**:3, 530–43.

Fodor, J. A. 1983. *The modularity of mind: an essay on faculty psychology*, Cambridge, MA: The MIT Press.

1992. 'A theory of the child's theory of mind', *Cognition* **44**:3, 283–96.

Foerch, C., Misselwitz, B., Sitzer, M., Berger, K., Steinmetz, H. and Neumann-Haefelin, T. 2005. 'Difference in recognition of right and left hemispheric stroke', *Lancet* **366**:9483, 392–3.

Fombonne, E. 2002. 'Prevalence of childhood disintegrative disorder', *Autism* **6**:2, 149–57.

2003. 'Epidemiology of pervasive developmental disorders', *Trends in Evidence-Based Neuropsychiatry* **5**:1, 29–36.

Foster-Cohen, S. H. 1994. 'Exploring the boundary between syntax and pragmatics: relevance and the binding of pronouns', *Journal of Child Language* **21**:1, 237–55.

Frattali, C. M., Thompson, C. K., Holland, A. L., Wohl, C. B. and Ferketic, M. M. 1995. *Functional assessment of communication skills for adults (ASHA FACS)*, Rockville: American Speech-Language-Hearing Association.

Fridriksson, J., Nettles, C., Davis, M., Morrow, L. and Montgomery, A. 2006. 'Functional communication and executive function in aphasia', *Clinical Linguistics & Phonetics* **20**:6, 401–10.

Friedland, D. and Miller, N. 1998. 'Conversation analysis of communication breakdown after closed head injury', *Brain Injury* **12**:1, 1–14.

Friend, K. B., Rabin, B. M., Groninger, L., Deluty, R. H., Bever, C. and Grattan, L. 1999. 'Language functions in patients with multiple sclerosis', *The Clinical Neuropsychologist* **13**:1, 78–94.

Frith, C. D. 1992. *The cognitive neuropsychology of schizophrenia*, Hove: Lawrence Erlbaum Associates.

Frye, D. 2000. 'Theory of mind, domain specificity, and reasoning', in P. Mitchell and K. J. Riggs (eds.), *Children's reasoning and the mind*, East Sussex: Psychology Press, 149–67.

Fuller, G. 1995. 'Simulation and psychological concepts', in M. Davies and T. Stone (eds.), *Mental simulation: evaluations and applications*, Oxford: Blackwell, 19–32.

Fyrberg, A., Marchioni, M. and Emanuelson, I. 2007. 'Severe acquired brain injury: rehabilitation of communicative skills in children and adolescents', *International Journal of Rehabilitation Research* **30**:2, 153–7.

Gallagher, T. M. and Darnton, B. A. 1978. 'Conversational aspects of the speech of language-disordered children: revision behaviors', *Journal of Speech and Hearing Research* **21**:1, 118–35.

Gardner, H. and Brownell, H. H. 1986. *Right hemisphere communication battery*, Boston: Psychology Service, Veterans Administration Medical Center.

Garner, C., Callias, M. and Turk, J. 1999. 'Executive function and theory of mind performance of boys with fragile-X syndrome', *Journal of Intellectual Disability Research* **43**:6, 466–74.

Gaulin, C. and Campbell, T. 1994. 'Procedure for assessing verbal working memory in normal school-age children: some preliminary data', *Perceptual and Motor Skills* **79**:1, 55–64.

Geurts, H. M., Verte, S., Oosterlaan, J., Roeyers, H. and Sergeant, J. A. 2004. 'How specific are executive functioning deficits in attention deficit hyperactivity disorder and autism?', *Journal of Child Psychology and Psychiatry* **45**:4, 836–54.

Gibbon, F., McCann, J., Peppé, S., O'Hare, A. and Rutherford, M. 2004. 'Articulation abilities of children with high-functioning autism', in B. Murdoch, J. Goozee, B. Whelan and K. Docking (eds.), *Proceedings of the 26th World Congress of the International Association of Logopedics and Phoniatrics*, Brisbane, Australia: IALP.

Gibbs, R. W. 2002. 'A new look at literal meaning in understanding what is said and implicated', *Journal of Pragmatics* **34**:4, 457–86.

Gil, M., Cohen, M., Korn, C. and Groswasser, Z. 1996. 'Vocational outcome of aphasic patients following severe traumatic brain injury', *Brain Injury* **10**:1, 39–45.

Gillam, R. B., Cowan, N. and Marler, J. A. 1998. 'Information processing by school-age children with specific language impairment: evidence from a modality effect paradigm', *Journal of Speech, Language, and Hearing Research* **41**:4, 913–26.

Gillberg, C. 1989. 'Asperger's syndrome in 23 Swedish children', *Developmental Medicine & Child Neurology* **31**:4, 520–31.

Gilmour, J., Hill, B., Place, M. and Skuse, D. H. 2004. 'Social communication deficits in conduct disorder: a clinical and community survey', *Journal of Child Psychology and Psychiatry* **45**:5, 967–78.

Gimpel, G. A. and Holland, M. L. 2003. *Emotional and behavioral problems of young children*, New York: The Guilford Press.

Glennen, S. and Bright, B. J. 2005. 'Five years later: language in school-age internationally adopted children', *Seminars in Speech and Language* **26**:1, 86–101.

Glosser, G. and Deser, T. 1991. 'Patterns of discourse production among neurological patients with fluent language disorders', *Brain and Language* **40**:1, 67–88.

Glosser, G. and Goodglass, H. 1990. 'Disorders in executive control functions among aphasic and other brain-damaged patients', *Journal of Clinical and Experimental Neuropsychology* **12**:4, 485–502.

Gonzalez de Dios, J. and Moya, M. 1996. 'Perinatal asphyxia, hypoxic-ischemic encephalopathy and neurological sequelae in full-term newborns: II. Description and interrelation', *Revista de Neurologia* **24**:132, 969–76.

Goodglass, H., Kaplan, E. and Barresi, B. 2001. *Boston diagnostic aphasia examination*, Baltimore: Lippincott Williams & Wilkins.

Gopnik, A. 1996. 'Theories and modules: creation myths, developmental realities and Neurath's boat', in P. Carruthers and P. K. Smith (eds.), *Theories of theories of mind*, Cambridge: Cambridge University Press, 169–83.

Gopnik, A. and Meltzoff, A. N. 1997. *Words, thoughts, and theories*, Cambridge, MA: MIT Press.

Gordon, R. M. 1986. 'Folk psychology as simulation', *Mind & Language* **1**:2, 158–71.
    1995. 'Reply to Stich and Nichols', in M. Davies and T. Stone (eds.), *Folk psychology: the theory of mind debate*, Oxford and Cambridge, MA: Blackwell, 174–84.
    1996. '"Radical" simulationism', in P. Carruthers and P. K. Smith (eds.), *Theories of theories of mind*, Cambridge: Cambridge University Press, 11–21.

Gorwood, P., Leboyer, M., Jay, M., Payan, C. and Feingold, J. 1995. 'Gender and age at onset in schizophrenia: impact of family history', *American Journal of Psychiatry* **152**:2, 208–12.

Gray, R. M., Jordan, C. M., Zeigler, R. S. and Livingston, R. B. 2002. 'Two sets of twins with selective mutism: neuropsychological findings', *Child Neuropsychology* **8**:1, 41–51.

Grela, B. G. and Leonard, L. B. 2000. 'The influence of argument-structure complexity on the use of auxiliary verbs by children with SLI', *Journal of Speech, Language, and Hearing Research* **43**:5, 1115–25.

Gresham, F. M. and Elliott, S. N. 1990. *Social skills rating system*, Circle Pines: American Guidance Service.

Grice, H. P. 1975. 'Logic and conversation', in P. Cole and J. Morgan (eds.), *Syntax and semantics 3: speech acts*, New York: Academic Press, 41–58.

1981. 'Presupposition and conversational implicature', in P. Cole (ed.), *Radical pragmatics*, New York: Academic Press, 183–98.

Griffin, R., Friedman, O., Ween, J., Winner, E., Happé, F. G. E. and Brownell, H. 2006. 'Theory of mind and the right cerebral hemisphere: refining the scope of impairment', *Laterality* **11**:3, 195–225.

Hadwin, J., Baron-Cohen, S., Howlin, P. and Hill, K. 1997. 'Does teaching theory of mind have an effect on the ability to develop conversation in children with autism?', *Journal of Autism and Developmental Disorders* **27**:5, 519–37.

Hale, C. M. and Tager-Flusberg, H. 2005. 'Social communication in children with autism: the relationship between theory of mind and discourse development', *Autism* **9**:2, 157–78.

Halliday, M. A. K. and Hasan, R. 1976. *Cohesion in English*, London: Longman.

Hammill, D. D., Brown, V. L., Larsen, S. C. and Wiederholt, J. L. 1987. *Test of adolescent language-2*, Austin: Pro-Ed.

Happé, F. G. E. 1993. 'Communicative competence and theory of mind in autism: a test of relevance theory', *Cognition* **48**:2, 101–19.

Happé, F. G. E., Briskman, J. and Frith, U. 2001. 'Exploring the cognitive phenotype of autism: weak "central coherence" in parents and siblings of children with autism: I. experimental tests', *Journal of Child Psychology and Psychiatry* **42**:3, 299–307.

Happé, F. G. E., Brownell, H. and Winner, E. 1999. 'Acquired "theory of mind" impairments following stroke', *Cognition* **70**:3, 211–40.

Hartley, L. L. and Jensen, P. J. 1991. 'Narrative and procedural discourse after closed head injury', *Brain Injury* **5**:3, 267–85.

Hatta, T., Hasegawa, J. and Wanner, P. J. 2004. 'Differential processing of implicature in individuals with left and right brain damage', *Journal of Clinical Experimental Neuropsychology* **26**:5, 667–76.

Havet-Thomassin, V., Allain, P., Etcharry-Bouyx, F. and Le Gall, D. 2006. 'What about theory of mind after severe brain injury?', *Brain Injury* **20**:1, 83–91.

Hayiou-Thomas, M. E., Bishop, D. V. and Plunkett, K. 2004. 'Simulating SLI: general cognitive processing stressors can produce a specific linguistic profile', *Journal of Speech, Language, and Hearing Research* **47**:6, 1347–62.

Hays, S. J., Niven, B. E., Godfrey, H. P. D. and Linscott, R. J. 2004. 'Clinical assessment of pragmatic language impairment: a generalisability study of older people with Alzheimer's disease', *Aphasiology* **18**:8, 693–714.

Heath, R. L. and Blonder, L. X. 2005. 'Spontaneous humor among right hemisphere stroke survivors', *Brain and Language* **93**:3, 267–76.

Heerey, E. A., Capps, L. M., Keltner, D. and Kring, A. M. 2005. 'Understanding teasing: lessons from children with autism', *Journal of Abnormal Child Psychology* **33**:1, 55–68.

Helland, W. A. and Heimann, M. 2007. 'Assessment of pragmatic language impairment in children referred to psychiatric services: a pilot study of the children's communication checklist in a Norwegian sample', *Logopedics, Phoniatrics, Vocology* **32**:1, 23–30.

Helm-Estabrooks, N. 2002. 'Cognition and aphasia: a discussion and a study', *Journal of Communication Disorders* **35**:2, 171–86.

Henry, J. D., Phillips, L. H., Crawford, J. R., Ietswaart, M. and Summers, F. 2006. 'Theory of mind following traumatic brain injury: the role of emotion recognition and executive dysfunction', *Neuropsychologia* **44**:10, 1623–8.

Henshilwood, L. and Ogilvy, D. 1999. 'Narrative discourse productions in older language impaired learning disabled children: employing stricter reliability measures', *South African Journal of Communication Disorders* **46**, 45–53.

Heyer, J. L. 1995. 'The responsibilities of speech-language pathologists toward children with ADHD', *Seminars in Speech and Language* **16**:4, 275–88.

Hick, R., Botting, N. and Conti-Ramsden, G. 2005. 'Cognitive abilities in children with specific language impairment: consideration of visuo-spatial skills', *International Journal of Language & Communication Disorders* **40**:2, 137–49.

Hill, D. A., Gridley, G., Cnattingius, S., Mellemkjaer, L., Linet, M., Adami, H. O., Olsen, J. H., Nyren, O. and Fraumeni, J. F. Jr. 2003. 'Mortality and cancer incidence among individuals with Down syndrome', *Archives of Internal Medicine* **163**:6, 705–11.

Hird, K. and Kirsner, K. 2003. 'The effect of right hemisphere damage on collaborative planning in conversation: an analysis of intentional structure', *Clinical Linguistics & Phonetics* **17**: (4–5), 309–15.

Hirtz, D., Thurman, D. J., Gwinn-Hardy, K., Mohamed, M., Chaudhuri, A. R. and Zalustsky, R. 2007. 'How common are the "common" neurologic disorders?', *Neurology* **68**:5, 326–37.

Hoffman, L. M. and Gillam, R. B. 2004. 'Verbal and spatial information processing constraints in children with specific language impairment', *Journal of Speech, Language, and Hearing Research* **47**:1, 114–25.

Hooper, H. E. 1983. *The Hooper visual organisation test manual*, Los Angeles: Western Psychological Services.

Hoy, J. A., Hatton, C. and Hare, D. 2004. 'Weak central coherence: a cross-domain phenomenon specific to autism?', *Autism* **8**:3, 267–81.

Hu, H., Tellez-Rojo, M. M., Bellinger, D., Smith, D., Ettinger, A. S., Lamadrid-Figueroa, H., Schwartz, J., Schnaas, L., Mercado-Garcia, A. and Hernandez-Avila, M. 2006. 'Fetal lead exposure at each stage of pregnancy as a predictor of infant mental development', *Environmental Health Perspectives* **114**:11, 1730–5.

Hubbell, R. D. 1977. 'On facilitating spontaneous talking in young children', *Journal of Speech and Hearing Disorders* **42**:2, 216–31.

Huber-Okrainec, J., Blaser, S. E. and Dennis, M. 2005. 'Idiom comprehension deficits in relation to corpus callosum agenesis and hypoplasia in children with spina bifida meningomyelocele', *Brain and Language* **93**:3, 349–68.

Hultman, C. M., Torrang, A., Tuvblad, C., Cnattingius, S., Larsson, J. O. and Lichtenstein, P. 2007. 'Birth weight and attention-deficit/hyperactivity symptoms in childhood and early adolescence: a prospective Swedish twin study', *Journal of the American Academy of Child and Adolescent Psychiatry* **46**:3, 370–7.

Hummel, L. J. and Prizant, B. M. 1993. 'Language and social skills in the school-age population: a socioemotional perspective for understanding social difficulties of school-age children with language disorders', *Language, Speech, and Hearing Services in Schools* **24**:4, 216–24.

Humphries, T., Koltun, H., Malone, M. and Roberts, W. 1994. 'Teacher-identified oral language difficulties among boys with attention problems', *Journal of Developmental and Behavioural Pediatrics* **15**:2, 92–8.

Hunt, K. W. 1965. *Grammatical structures written at three grade levels (NCTE research report no. 3)*, Urbana: National Council of Teachers of English.

Hux, K., Sanger, D., Reid, R. and Maschka, A. 1997. 'Discourse analysis procedures: reliability issues', *Journal of Communication Disorders* **30**:2, 133–50.

Hyter, Y. D., Rogers-Adkinson, D. L., Self, T. L., Simmons, B. F. and Jantz, J. 2001. 'Pragmatic language intervention for children with language and emotional/behavioural disorders', *Communication Disorders* **23**:1, 4–16.

Iakimova, G., Passerieux, C. and Hardy-Baylé, M. C. 2006. 'Interpretation of ambiguous idiomatic statements in schizophrenic and depressive patients. Evidence for common and differential cognitive patterns', *Psychopathology* **39**:6, 277–85.

Ilomaki, E., Viilo, K., Hakko, H., Marttunen, M., Makikyro, T., Rasanen, P. and STUDY-70 Workgroup. 2006. 'Familial risks, conduct disorder and violence: a Finnish study of 278 adolescent boys and girls', *European Child & Adolescent Psychiatry* **15**:1, 46–51.

James, D. M. and Stojanovik, V. 2007. 'Communication skills in blind children: a preliminary investigation', *Child: Care, Health and Development* **33**:1, 4–10.

Jaszczolt, K. M. 2008. 'Semantics and pragmatics: the boundary issue', in K. von Heusinger, P. Portner and C. Maienborn (eds.), *Semantics: an international handbook of natural language meaning*, Berlin: Mouton de Gruyter.

Jensen, A. M., Chenery, H. J. and Copland, D. A. 2006. 'A comparison of picture description abilities in individuals with vascular subcortical lesions and Huntington's disease', *Journal of Communication Disorders* **39**:1, 62–77.

John, S. F., Lui, M. and Tannock, R. 2003. 'Children's story retelling and comprehension using a narrative resource', *Canadian Journal of School Psychology* **18**:(1–2), 91–113.

Johnson, R. H. and Blair, J. A. 1994. *Logical self-defense*, New York: McGraw-Hill.

Johnston, E. B., Weinrich, B. D. and Glaser, A. J. 1991. *A sourcebook of pragmatic activities, revised*, San Antonio: Communication Skills Builders.

Johnston, F. and Stansfield, J. 1997. 'Expressive pragmatic skills in pre-school children with and without Down's syndrome: parental perceptions', *Journal of Intellectual Disability Research* **41**:1, 19–29.

Johnston, J. R., Miller, J. and Tallal, P. 2001. 'Use of cognitive state predicates by language-impaired children', *International Journal of Language & Communication Disorders* **36**:3, 349–70.

Johnstone, N., Hexum, C. L. and Ashkanazi, G. 1995. 'Extent of cognitive decline in traumatic brain injury based on estimates of premorbid intelligence', *Brain Injury* **9**:4, 377–84.

Jolliffe, T. and Baron-Cohen, S. 1999. 'A test of central coherence theory: linguistic processing in high-functioning adults with autism or Asperger syndrome: is local coherence impaired?', *Cognition* **71**:2, 149–85.

  2000. 'Linguistic processing in high-functioning adults with autism or Asperger's syndrome: is global coherence impaired?', *Psychological Medicine* **30**:5, 1169–87.

  2001. 'A test of central coherence theory: can adults with high-functioning autism or Asperger syndrome integrate fragments of an object?', *Cognitive Neuropsychiatry* **6**:3, 193–216.

Jordan, F. M., Murdoch, B. E. and Buttsworth, D. L. 1991. 'Closed-head-injured children's performance on narrative tasks', *Journal of Speech and Hearing Research* **34**:3, 572–82.

Jordan, R. R. 1989. 'An experimental comparison of the understanding and use of speaker-addressee personal pronouns in autistic children', *British Journal of Disorders of Communication* **24**:2, 169–79.

Joseph, R. M., McGrath, L. M. and Tager-Flusberg, H. 2005. 'Executive dysfunction and its relation to language ability in verbal school-age children with autism', *Developmental Neuropsychology* **27**:3, 361–78.

Kagan, A., Black, S. E., Duchan, J. F., Simmons-Mackie, N. and Square, P. 2001. 'Training volunteers as conversation partners using "supported conversation for adults with aphasia" (SCA): a controlled trial', *Journal of Speech, Language, and Hearing Research* **44**:3, 624–38.

Kane, M. O., Schopmeyer, B., Mellon, N. K., Wang, N. Y. and Niparko, J. K. 2004. 'Prelinguistic communication and subsequent language acquisition in children with cochlear implants', *Archives of Otolaryngology – Head & Neck Surgery* **130**:5, 619–23.

Kasher, A. 1991a. 'Pragmatics and the modularity of mind', in S. Davies (ed.), *Pragmatics: a reader*, New York: Oxford University Press, 567–82.

1991b. 'On the pragmatic modules: a lecture', *Journal of Pragmatics* **16**:5, 381–97.

1998. 'Postscript', in A. Kasher (ed.), *Pragmatics: critical concepts*, London: Routledge, 144–54.

Kasher, A., Batori, G., Soroker, N., Graves, D. and Zaidel, E. 1999. 'Effects of right- and left-hemisphere damage on understanding conversational implicatures', *Brain and Language* **68**:3, 566–90.

Kaye, J. A., Del Mar Melero-Montes, M. and Jick, H. 2001. 'Mumps, measles and rubella vaccine and the incidence of autism recorded by general practitioners: a time trend analysis', *British Medical Journal* **322**:7284, 460–3.

Kempson, R. M. 1988. 'The relation between language, mind, and reality', in R. M. Kempson (ed.), *Mental representations: the interface between language and reality*, Cambridge: Cambridge University Press, 3–25.

Kerns, K. A., Don, A., Mateer, C. A. and Streissguth, A. P. 1997. 'Cognitive deficits in nonretarded adults with fetal alcohol syndrome', *Journal of Learning Disabilities* **30**:6, 685–93.

Kertesz, A. 2006. *Western aphasia battery-revised*, San Antonio: Harcourt Assessment.

Kiang, M., Light, G. A., Prugh, J., Coulson, S., Braff, D. L. and Kutas, M. 2007. 'Cognitive, neurophysiological, and functional correlates of proverb interpretation abnormalities in schizophrenia', *Journal of the International Neuropsychological Society* **13**:4, 653–63.

Kim, Y. T. and Lombardino, L. J. 1991. 'The efficacy of script contexts in language comprehension intervention with children who have mental retardation', *Journal of Speech and Hearing Research* **34**:4, 845–57.

Kircher, T. T. J., Leube, D. T., Erb, M., Grodd, W. and Rapp, A. M. 2007. 'Neural correlates of metaphor processing in schizophrenia', *NeuroImage* **34**:1, 281–9.

Kircher, T. T. J., Bulimore, E. T., Brammer, M. J., Williams, S. C., Broome, M. R., Murray, R. M. and McGuire, P. K. 2001. 'Differential activation of temporal cortex during sentence completion in schizophrenic patients with and without formal thought disorder', *Schizophrenia Research* **50**: (1–2), 27–40.

Kirk, J. W., Mazzocco, M. M. and Kover, S. T. 2005. 'Assessing executive dysfunction in girls with fragile X or Turner syndrome using the Contingency Naming Test (CNT)', *Developmental Neuropsychology* **28**:3, 755–77.

Kjelgaard, M. M. and Tager-Flusberg, H. 2001. 'An investigation of language impairment in autism: implications for genetic subgroups', *Language and Cognitive Processes* **16**: (2–3), 287–308.

Kleiman, L.I. 2003. *Functional communication profile – revised*, East Moline: LinguiSystems.

Kleinhans, N., Akshoomoff, N. and Delis, D.C. 2005. 'Executive functions in autism and Asperger's disorder: flexibility, fluency, and inhibition', *Developmental Neuropsychology* **27**:3, 379–401.

Klin, A. and Volkmar, F.R. 1995. *Asperger's syndrome: guidelines for assessment and diagnosis*, Pittsburgh: Learning Disabilities Association of America.

Klugman, T.M. and Ross, E. 2002. 'Perceptions of the impact of speech, language, swallowing, and hearing difficulties on quality of life of a group of South African persons with multiple sclerosis', *Folia Phoniatrica et Logopaedica* **54**:4, 201–21.

Knapp, M. and Prince, M. 2007. *Dementia UK: the full report*, London: Alzheimer's Society.

Koskiniemi, M., Kyykka, T., Nybo, T. and Jarho, L. 1995. 'Long-term outcome after severe brain injury in preschoolers is worse than expected', *Archives of Pediatrics & Adolescent Medicine* **149**:3, 249–54.

Kozinetz, C.A., Skender, M.L., MacNaughton, N., Almes, M.J., Schultz, R.J., Percy, A.K. and Glaze, D.G. 1993. 'Epidemiology of Rett syndrome: a population-based registry', *Pediatrics* **91**:2, 445–50.

Kraus, J.F. and McArthur, D.L. 1996. 'Epidemiologic aspects of brain injury', *Neurologic Clinics* **14**:2, 435–50.

Lahey, M. and Edwards, J. 1996. 'Why do children with specific language impairment name pictures more slowly than their peers?', *Journal of Speech and Hearing Research* **39**:5, 1081–98.

1999. 'Naming errors of children with specific language impairment', *Journal of Speech, Language, and Hearing Research* **42**:1, 195–205.

Lalonde, J., Turgay, A. and Hudson, J.I. 1998. 'Attention-deficit hyperactivity disorder subtypes and comorbid disruptive behaviour disorders in a child and adolescent mental health clinic', *Canadian Journal of Psychiatry* **43**:6, 623–8.

Landa, R., Piven, J., Wzorek, M.M., Gayle, J.O., Chase, G.A. and Folstein, S.E. 1992. 'Social language use in parents of autistic individuals', *Psychological Medicine* **22**:1, 245–54.

Langdon, R. and Coltheart, M. 1999. 'Mentalising, schizotypy, and schizophrenia', *Cognition* **71**:1, 43–71.

Langdon, R., Davies, M. and Coltheart, M. 2002. 'Understanding minds and understanding communicated meanings in schizophrenia', *Mind & Language* **17**: (1–2), 68–104.

Laws, G. 2004. 'Contributions of phonological memory, language comprehension and hearing to the expressive language of adolescents and young adults with Down syndrome', *Journal of Child Psychology and Psychiatry* **45**:6, 1085–95.

Laws, G. and Bishop, D.V.M. 2004. 'Pragmatic language impairment and social deficits in Williams syndrome: a comparison with Down's syndrome and specific language impairment', *International Journal of Language & Communication Disorders* **39**:1, 45–64.

Laws, K.R., Crawford, J.R., Gnoato, F. and Sartori, G. 2007. 'A predominance of category deficits for living things in Alzheimer's disease and Lewy body dementia', *Journal of the International Neuropsychological Society* **13**:3, 401–9.

Lee, A., Hobson, R.P. and Chiat, S. 1994. 'I, you, me, and autism: an experimental study', *Journal of Autism and Developmental Disorders* **24**:2, 155–76.

Leech, G. N. 1983. *Principles of pragmatics*, London: Longman.

Lehman, B. 2006. 'Clinical relevance of discourse characteristics after right hemisphere brain damage', *American Journal of Speech-Language Pathology* **15**:3, 255–67.

Leinonen, E. and Kerbel, D. 1999. 'Relevance theory and pragmatic impairment', *International Journal of Language and Communication Disorders* **34**:4, 367–90.

Leinonen, E., Letts, C. and Smith, B. R. 2000. *Children's pragmatic communication difficulties*, London: Whurr Publishers.

Leonard, L. B. 1995. 'Functional categories in the grammars of children with specific language impairment', *Journal of Speech and Hearing Research* **38**:6, 1270–83.

1998. *Children with specific language impairment*, Cambridge, MA: The MIT Press.

Leonard, L. B., Deevy, P., Miller, C. A., Rauf, L., Charest, M. and Kurtz, R. 2003. 'Surface forms and grammatical functions: past tense and passive participle use by children with specific language impairment', *Journal of Speech, Language, and Hearing Research* **46**:1, 43–55.

Lessa Mansur, L., Radanovic, M., Santos Penha, S., Iracema Zanotto de Mendonça, L. and Cristina Adda, C. 2006. 'Language and visuospatial impairment in a case of crossed aphasia', *Laterality* **11**:6, 525–39.

Levinson, S. C. 1983. *Pragmatics*, Cambridge: Cambridge University Press.

2000. *Presumptive meanings: the theory of generalized conversational implicature*, Cambridge, MA: The MIT Press.

Levorato, M. C. and Cacciari, C. 1995. 'The effects of different tasks on the comprehension and production of idioms in children', *Journal of Experimental Child Psychology* **60**:2, 261–83.

2002. 'The creation of new figurative expressions: psycholinguistic evidence in Italian children, adolescents and adults', *Journal of Child Language* **29**:1, 127–50.

Lewine, J. D., Davis, J. T., Bigler, E. D., Thoma, R., Hill, D., Funke, M., Sloan, J. H., Hall, S. and Orrison, W. W. 2007. 'Objective documentation of traumatic brain injury subsequent to mild head trauma: multimodal brain imaging with MEG, SPECT, and MRI', *Journal of Head Trauma Rehabilitation* **22**:3, 141–55.

Li, E. C., Williams, S. E. and Della Volpe, A. 1995. 'The effects of topic and listener familiarity on discourse variables in procedural and narrative discourse tasks', *Journal of Communication Disorders* **28**:1, 39–55.

Liberman, R. P., Wallace, C. J., Blackwell, G., Kopelowicz, A., Vaccaro, J. V. and Mintz, J. 1998. 'Skills training versus psychosocial occupational therapy for persons with persistent schizophrenia', *American Journal of Psychiatry* **155**:8, 1087–91.

Lind, M. 2005. 'Conversation – more than words: a Norwegian case study of the establishment of a contribution in aphasic interaction', *International Journal of Applied Linguistics* **15**:2, 213–39.

Linscott, R. J. 1996. 'The profile of functional impairment in communication: a measure of communication impairment for clinical use', *Brain Injury* **10**:6, 397–412.

2005. 'Thought disorder, pragmatic language impairment, and generalized cognitive decline in schizophrenia', *Schizophrenia Research* **75**: (2–3), 225–32.

Lippert-Grüner, M., Kuchta, J., Hellmich, M. and Klug, N. 2006. 'Neurobehavioural deficits after severe traumatic brain injury (TBI)', *Brian Injury* **20**:6, 569–74.

Lloyd-Richmond, H. and Starczewski, H. 2008. *SNAP-Dragons: stories/narratives assessment procedure*, Milton Keynes: Speechmark Publishing.

Loban, W. 1976. *Language development: kindergarten through grade 12*, Urbana: National Council of Teachers of English.

Lock, S., Wilkinson, R. and Bryan, K. 2001a. *SPPARC: supporting partners of people with aphasia in relationships and conversations*, Bicester: Winslow Press.

Lock, S., Wilkinson, R., Bryan, K., Maxim, J., Edmundson, A., Bruce, C. and Moir, D. 2001b. 'Supporting partners of people with aphasia in relationships and conversation (SPPARC)', *International Journal of Language and Communication Disorders* **36**:Supplement, 25–30.

Lopez, B.R., Lincoln, A.J., Ozonoff, S. and Lai, Z. 2005. 'Examining the relationship between executive functions and restricted, repetitive symptoms of autistic disorder', *Journal of Autism and Developmental Disorders* **35**:4, 445–60.

Lorch, E.P., Sanchez, R.P., Van den Broek, P., Milich, R., Murphy, E.L., Lorch, R.F. and Welsh, R. 1999. 'The relation of story structure properties to recall of television stories in young children with attention-deficit hyperactivity disorder and nonreferred peers', *Journal of Abnormal Child Psychology* **27**:4, 293–309.

Lorusso, M.L., Galli, R., Libera, L., Gagliardi, C., Borgatti, R. and Hollebrandse, B. 2007. 'Indicators of theory of mind in narrative production: a comparison between individuals with genetic syndromes and typically developing children', *Clinical Linguistics & Phonetics* **21**:1, 37–53.

Losh, M. and Capps, L. 2003. 'Narrative ability in high-functioning children with autism or Asperger's syndrome', *Journal of Autism and Developmental Disorders* **33**:3, 239–51.

Loukusa, S., Leinonen, E., Jussila, K., Mattila, M.L., Ryder, N., Ebeling, H. and Moilanen, I. 2007b. 'Answering contextually demanding questions: pragmatic errors produced by children with Asperger syndrome or high-functioning autism', *Journal of Communication Disorders* **40**:5, 357–81.

Loukusa, S., Leinonen, E., Kuusikko, S., Jussila, K., Mattila, M.L., Ryder, N., Ebeling, H. and Moilanen, I. 2007a. 'Use of context in pragmatic language comprehension by children with Asperger syndrome or high-functioning autism', *Journal of Autism and Developmental Disorders* **37**:6, 1049–59.

Loveland, K.A. and Tunali, B. 1991. 'Social scripts for conversational interactions in autism and Down syndrome', *Journal of Autism and Developmental Disorders* **21**:2, 177–86.

Loveland, K.A., Landry, S.H., Hughes, S.O., Hall, S.K. and McEvoy, R.E. 1988. 'Speech acts and the pragmatic deficits of autism', *Journal of Speech and Hearing Research* **31**:4, 593–604.

Luckasson, R., Borthwick-Duffy, S., Buntinx, W.H.E., Coulter, D.L., Craig, E.M., Reeve, A., Schalock, R.L., Snell, M.E., Spitalnik, D.M., Spreat, S. and Tassé, M.J. 2002. *Mental retardation: definition, classification, and systems of supports*, 10th edn., Washington, DC: American Association on Mental Retardation.

Lum, J.A., Conti-Ramsden, G. and Lindell, A.K. 2007. 'The attentional blink reveals sluggish attentional shifting in adolescents with specific language impairment', *Brain & Development* **63**:3, 287–95.

Mackie, C. and Dockrell, J.E. 2004. 'The nature of written language deficits in children with SLI', *Journal of Speech, Language, and Hearing Research* **47**:6, 1469–83.

MacLennan, D.L., Cornis-Pop, M., Picon-Nieto, L. and Sigford, B. 2002. 'The prevalence of pragmatic communication impairments in traumatic brain injury', *Premier Outlook* **3**:4, 38–45.

MacWhinney, B. 2000. *The CHILDES project: tools for analyzing talk*, Mahwah: Lawrence Erlbaum.

Manassis, K., Fung, D., Tannock, R., Sloman, L., Fiksenbaum, L. and McInnes, A. 2003. 'Characterizing selective mutism: is it more than social anxiety?', *Depression and Anxiety* **18**:3, 153–61.

Marini, A., Carlomagno, S., Caltagirone, C. and Nocentini, U. 2005. 'The role played by the right hemisphere in the organization of complex textual structures', *Brain and Language* **93**:1, 46–54.

Marshall, J., Chiat, S., Robson, J. and Pring, T. 1996b. 'Calling a salad a federation: an investigation of semantic jargon. part 2 – verbs', *Journal of Neurolinguistics* **9**:4, 251–60.

Marshall, J., Pring, T., Chiat, S. and Robson, J. 1996a. 'Calling a salad a federation: an investigation of semantic jargon. part 1 – nouns', *Journal of Neurolinguistics* **9**:4, 237–50.

  2001. 'When ottoman is easier than chair: an inverse frequency effect in jargon aphasia', *Cortex* **37**:1, 33–53.

Martin, I. and McDonald, S. 2003. 'Weak coherence, no theory of mind, or executive dysfunction? Solving the puzzle of pragmatic language disorders', *Brain and Language* **85**:3, 451–66.

  2004. 'An exploration of causes of non-literal language problems in individuals with Asperger syndrome', *Journal of Autism and Developmental Disorders* **34**:3, 311–28.

Marton, K. and Schwartz, R. G. 2003. 'Working memory capacity and language processes in children with specific language impairment', *Journal of Speech, Language, and Hearing Research* **46**:5, 1138–53.

Mathers, M. 2005. 'Some evidence for distinctive language use by children with attention deficit hyperactivity disorder', *Clinical Linguistics & Phonetics* **19**:3, 215–25.

Mattson, S. N., Goodman, A. M., Caine, C., Delis, D. C. and Riley, E. P. 1999. 'Executive functioning in children with heavy prenatal alcohol exposure', *Alcoholism, Clinical and Experimental Research* **23**:11, 1808–15.

Mazzocco, M. M., Pennington, B. F. and Hagerman, R. J. 1993. 'The neurocognitive phenotype of female carriers of fragile X: additional evidence for specificity', *Journal of Developmental and Behavioral Pediatrics* **14**:5, 328–35.

McCabe, P., Sheard, C. and Code, C. 2007. 'Pragmatic skills in people with HIV/AIDS', *Disability and Rehabilitation* **29**:16, 1251–60.

McCaleb, P. and Prizant, B. M. 1985. 'Encoding of new versus old information by autistic children', *Journal of Speech and Hearing Disorders* **50**:3, 230–40.

McCathren, R. B., Yoder, P. J. and Warren, S. F. 1999. 'The relationship between prelinguistic vocalization and later expressive vocabulary in young children with developmental delay', *Journal of Speech, Language, and Hearing Research* **42**:4, 915–24.

McDonald, B. C., Flashman, L. A. and Saykin, A. J. 2002. 'Executive dysfunction following traumatic brain injury: neural substrates and treatment strategies', *NeuroRehabilitation* **17**:4, 333–44.

McDonald, S. 1992. 'Communication disorders following closed head injury: new approaches to assessment and rehabilitation', *Brain Injury* **6**:3, 293–8.

  2000a. 'Neuropsychological studies of sarcasm', *Metaphor and Symbol* **15**: (1–2), 85–98.

  2000b. 'Exploring the cognitive basis of right-hemisphere pragmatic language disorders', *Brain and Language* **75**:1, 82–107.

McDonald, S. and Flanagan, S. 2004. 'Social perception deficits after traumatic brain injury: interaction between emotion recognition, mentalizing ability, and social communication', *Neuropsychology* **18**:3, 572–9.

McDuffie, A., Yoder, P. and Stone, W. 2005. 'Prelinguistic predictors of vocabulary in young children with autism spectrum disorders', *Journal of Speech, Language, and Hearing Research* **48**:5, 1080–97.

McEvoy, R. E., Loveland, K. A. and Landry, S. H. 1988. 'The functions of immediate echolalia in autistic children: a developmental perspective', *Journal of Autism and Developmental Disorders* **18**:4, 657–68.

McGrath, J. J. 2006. 'Variations in the incidence of schizophrenia: data versus dogma', *Schizophrenia Bulletin* **32**:1, 195–7.

McGregor, K. K., Newman, R. M., Reilly, R. M. and Capone, N. C. 2002. 'Semantic representation and naming in children with specific language impairment', *Journal of Speech, Language, and Hearing Research* **45**:5, 998–1014.

McInnes, A., Humphries, T., Hogg-Johnson, S. and Tannock, R. 2003. 'Listening comprehension and working memory are impaired in attention-deficit hyperactivity disorder irrespective of language impairment', *Journal of Abnormal Child Psychology*, **31**:4, 427–43.

McInnes, A., Fung, D., Manassis, K., Fiksenbaum, L. and Tannock, R. 2004. 'Narrative skills in children with selective mutism: an exploratory study', *American Journal of Speech-Language Pathology* **13**:4, 304–15.

McNamara, P. and Durso, R. 2003. 'Pragmatic communication skills in patients with Parkinson's disease', *Brain and Language* **84**:3, 414–23.

McTear, M. 1985. *Children's conversation*, Oxford: Blackwell.

Medical Research Council 2001. *MRC Review of autism research: epidemiology and causes*, London: Medical Research Council.

Meilijson, S. R., Kasher, A. and Elizur, A. 2004. 'Language performance in chronic schizophrenia: a pragmatic approach', *Journal of Speech, Language, and Hearing Research* **47**:3, 695–713.

Melinder, M. R. and Barch, D. M. 2003. 'The influence of a working memory load manipulation on language production in schizophrenia', *Schizophrenia Bulletin* **29**:3, 473–85.

Mentis, M. and Lundgren, K. 1995. 'Effects of prenatal exposure to cocaine and associated risk factors on language development', *Journal of Speech and Hearing Research* **38**:6, 1303–18.

Mentis, M., Briggs-Whittaker, J. and Gramigna, G. D. 1995. 'Discourse topic management in senile dementia of the Alzheimer's type', *Journal of Speech and Hearing Research* **38**:5, 1054–66.

Merritt, D. D. and Liles, B. Z. 1989. 'Narrative analysis: clinical applications of story generation and story retelling', *Journal of Speech and Hearing Disorders* **54**:3, 438–47.

Merson, R. M. and Rolnick, M. I. 1998. 'Speech-language pathology and dysphagia in multiple sclerosis', *Physical Medicine and Rehabilitation Clinics of North America* **9**:3, 631–41.

Mey, J. 2001. *Pragmatics: an introduction*, Oxford: Blackwell.

Michelotti, J., Charman, T., Slonims, V. and Baird, G. 2002. 'Follow-up of children with language delay and features of autism from preschool years to middle childhood', *Developmental Medicine and Child Neurology* **44**:12, 812–19.

Milders, M., Ietswaart, M. and Crawford, J.R. 2006. 'Impairments in theory of mind shortly after traumatic brain injury and at 1-year follow-up', *Neuropsychology* **20**:4, 400–8.

Miles, S. and Chapman, R.S. 2002. 'Narrative content as described by individuals with Down syndrome and typically developing children', *Journal of Speech, Language, and Hearing Research* **45**:1, 175–89.

Miller, C.A. 2001. 'False belief understanding in children with specific language impairment', *Journal of Communication Disorders* **34**: (1–2), 73–86.

   2004. 'False belief and sentence complement performance in children with specific language impairment', *International Journal of Language & Communication Disorders* **39**:2, 191–213.

Miller, C.A., Kail, R., Leonard, L.B. and Tomblin, J.B. 2001. 'Speed of processing in children with specific language impairment', *Journal of Speech, Language, and Hearing Research* **44**:2, 416–33.

Miller, C.A., Leonard, L.B., Kail, R.V., Zhang, X., Tomblin, J.B. and Francis, D.J. 2006. 'Response time in 14-year-olds with language impairment', *Journal of Speech, Language, and Hearing Research* **49**:4, 712–28.

Miller, J.F. and Chapman, R.S. 2006. *Systematic analysis of language transcripts (SALT), version 9*, Madison: Waisman Research Center.

Mitchell, R.L.C. and Crow, T.J. 2005. 'Right hemisphere language functions and schizophrenia: the forgotten hemisphere', *Brain* **128**:5, 963–78.

Monetta, L. and Pell, M. 2007. 'Effects of verbal working memory deficits on metaphor comprehension in patients with Parkinson's disease', *Brain and Language* **101**:1, 80–9.

Montague, M., Maddux, C.D. and Dereshiwsky, M.I. 1990. 'Story grammar and comprehension and production of narrative prose by students with learning disabilities', *Journal of Learning Disabilities* **23**:3, 190–7.

Montgomery, J.W. 1995. 'Sentence comprehension in children with specific language impairment: the role of phonological working memory', *Journal of Speech and Hearing Research* **38**:1, 187–99.

   2000. 'Verbal working memory and sentence comprehension in children with specific language impairment', *Journal of Speech, Language, and Hearing Research* **43**:2, 293–308.

Monuteaux, M.C., Blacker, D., Biederman, J., Fitzmaurice, G. and Buka, S.L. 2006. 'Maternal smoking during pregnancy and offspring overt and covert conduct problems: a longitudinal study', *Journal of Child Psychology and Psychiatry* **47**:9, 883–90.

Moore, C.J., Daly, E.M., Schmitz, N., Tassone, F., Tysoe, C., Hagerman, R.J., Hagerman, P.J., Morris, R.G., Murphy, K.C. and Murphy, D.G. 2004. 'A neuropsychological investigation of male premutation carriers of fragile X syndrome', *Neuropsychologia* **42**:14, 1934–47.

Müller, N. (ed.) 2000. *Pragmatics in speech and language pathology*, Amsterdam: John Benjamins.

Munir, F., Cornish, K.M. and Wilding, J. 2000a. 'Nature of the working memory deficit in fragile-X syndrome', *Brain and Cognition* **44**:3, 387–401.

   2000b. 'A neuropsychological profile of attention deficits in young males with fragile X syndrome', *Neuropsychologia* **38**:9, 1261–70.

Murdoch, B. E., Hudson, L. J. and Boon, D. L. 1999. 'Effects of treatment for paediatric cancer on brain structure and function', in B. Murdoch (ed.), *Communication disorders in childhood cancer*, London: Whurr Publishers, 21–54.

Murdoch, B. E., Chenery, H. J., Wilks, V. and Boyle, R. S. 1987. 'Language disorders in dementia of the Alzheimer type', *Brain and Language* **31**:1, 122–37.

Murphy, M. M. and Abbeduto, L. 2007. 'Gender differences in repetitive language in fragile X syndrome', *Journal of Intellectual Disability Research* **51**:5, 387–400.

Myers, P. S. 1979. 'Profiles of communication deficits in patients with right cerebral hemisphere damage: implications for diagnosis and treatment', *Clinical Aphasiology Conference*, Phoenix: BRK Publishers, 38–46.

  1991. 'Inference failure: the underlying impairment in right-hemisphere communication disorders', *Clinical Aphasiology Conference*, Santa Fe: Pro-Ed, 167–80.

  2005. 'Profiles of communication deficits in patients with right cerebral hemisphere damage: implications for diagnosis and treatment', *Aphasiology* **19**:12, 1147–60.

Myers, P. S. and Brookshire, R. 1994. 'The effects of visual and inferential complexity on the picture descriptions of non-brain-damaged and right-hemisphere-damaged adults', *Clinical Aphasiology* **22**, 25–34.

Naarding, P., Kremer, H. P. H. and Zitman, F. G. 2001. 'Huntington's disease: a review of the literature on prevalence and treatment of neuropsychiatric phenomena', *European Psychiatry* **16**:8, 439–45.

Naremore, R. C., Densmore, A. E. and Harman, D. R. 1995. *Language intervention with school-aged children: conversation, narrative and text*, San Diego: Singular Publishing Group.

Nelson, L. D., Orme, D., Osann, K. and Lott, I. T. 2001. 'Neurological changes and emotional functioning in adults with Down syndrome', *Journal of Intellectual Disability Research* **45**:5, 450–6.

Nelson, J. R., Benner, G. J., Neill, S. and Stage, S. A. 2006. 'Interrelationships among language skills, externalizing behavior, and academic fluency and their impact on the academic skills of students with ED', *Journal of Emotional and Behavioral Disorders* **14**:4, 209–16.

Newbury, D. F., Bishop, D. V. and Monaco, A. P. 2005. 'Genetic influences on language impairment and phonological short-term memory', *Trends in Cognitive Sciences* **9**:11, 528–34.

Newman, R. M. and McGregor, K. K. 2006. 'Teachers and laypersons discern quality differences between narratives produced by children with or without SLI', *Journal of Speech, Language, and Hearing Research* **49**:5, 1022–36.

Nicholas, L. E. and Brookshire, R. H. 1993. 'A system for quantifying the informativeness and efficiency of the connected speech of adults with aphasia', *Journal of Speech and Hearing Research* **36**:2, 338–50.

Nicolle, S. and Clark, B. 1999. 'Experimental pragmatics and what is said: a response to Gibbs and Moise', *Cognition* **69**:3, 337–54.

Niemi, J., Gundersen, H., Leppasaari, T. and Hugdahl, K. 2003. 'Speech lateralization and attention/executive functions in a Finnish family with specific language impairment (SLI)', *Journal of Clinical and Experimental Neuropsychology* **25**:4, 457–64.

Nikolopoulos, T. P., Lloyd, H., Starczewski, H. and Gallaway, C. 2003. 'Using SNAP dragons to monitor narrative abilities in young deaf children following cochlear implantation', *Journal of Pediatric Otorhinolaryngology* **67**:5, 535–41.

Ninio, A. and Snow, E. C. 1996. *Pragmatic development*, Boulder: Westview Press.

Nippold, M. A. 1998. *Later language development: the school-age and adolescent years*, Austin: Pro-Ed.

Nippold, M. A., Ward-Lonergan, J. M. and Fanning, J. L. 2005. 'Persuasive writing in children, adolescents, and adults: a study of syntactic, semantic, and pragmatic development', *Language, Speech, and Hearing Services in Schools* **36**:2, 125–38.

Noens, I. L. J. and van Berckelaer-Onnes, I. A. 2005. 'Captured by details: sense-making, language and communication in autism', *Journal of Communication Disorders* **38**:2, 123–41.

Norbury, C. F. 2004. 'Factors supporting idiom comprehension in children with communication disorders', *Journal of Speech, Language, and Hearing Research* **47**:5, 1179–93.

  2005. 'Barking up the wrong tree? Lexical ambiguity resolution in children with language impairments and autistic spectrum disorders', *Journal of Experimental Child Psychology* **90**:2, 142–71.

Norbury, C. F. and Bishop, D. V. M. 2002. 'Inferential processing and story recall in children with communication problems: a comparison of specific language impairment, pragmatic language impairment and high-functioning autism', *International Journal of Language & Communication Disorders* **37**:3, 227–51.

  2003. 'Narrative skills of children with communication impairments', *International Journal of Language and Communication Disorders* **38**:3, 287–313.

Norbury, C. F., Nash, M., Baird, G. and Bishop, D. 2004. 'Using a parental checklist to identify diagnostic groups in children with communication impairment: a validation of the children's communication checklist-2', *International Journal of Language and Communication Disorders* **39**:3, 345–64.

Noveck, I. A. 2001. 'When children are more logical than adults: experimental investigations of scalar implicature', *Cognition* **78**:2, 165–88.

Noveck, I. A. and Posada, A. 2003. 'Characterizing the time course of an implicature: an evoked potentials study', *Brain and Language* **85**:2, 203–10.

Numminen, H., Lehto, J. E. and Ruoppila, I. 2001. 'Tower of Hanoi and working memory in adult persons with intellectual disability', *Research in Developmental Disabilities* **22**:5, 373–87.

Nys, G. M., van Zandvoort, M. J., de Kort, P. L., Jansen, B. P., de Haan, E. H. and Kappelle, L. J. 2007. 'Cognitive disorders in acute stroke: prevalence and clinical determinants', *Cerebrovascular Diseases* **23**: (5–6), 408–16.

Oelschlaeger, M. L. and Damico, J. S. 2000. 'Partnership in conversation: a study of word search strategies', *Journal of Communication Disorders* **33**:3, 205–23.

Oelschlaeger, M. L. and Thorne, J. C. 1999. 'Application of the correct information unit analysis to the naturally occurring conversation of a person with aphasia', *Journal of Speech, Language, and Hearing Research* **42**:3, 636–48.

Oetting, J. B., Rice, M. L. and Swank, L. K. 1995. 'Quick incidental learning (QUIL) of words by school-age children with and without SLI', *Journal of Speech and Hearing Research* **38**:2, 434–45.

Oosterlaan, J., Scheres, A. and Sergeant, J. A. 2005. 'Which executive functioning deficits are associated with AD/HD, ODD/CD and comorbid AD/HD+ODD/CD?', *Journal of Abnormal Child Psychology* **33**:1, 69–85.

Orange, J. B., Lubinski, R. B. and Higginbotham, D. J. 1996. 'Conversational repair by individuals with dementia of the Alzheimer's type', *Journal of Speech and Hearing Research* **39**:4, 881–95.

Osuji, I. J., McGarrahan, A., Mihalakos, P., Garver, D., Kingsbury, S. and Cullum, C. M. 2007. 'Neuropsychological functioning in MRI-derived subgroups of schizophrenia', *Schizophrenia Research* **92**: (1–3), 189–96.

Ozonoff, S. and Miller, J. N. 1995. 'Teaching theory of mind: a new approach to social skills training for individuals with autism', *Journal of Autism and Developmental Disorders* **25**:4, 415–33.

Ozonoff, S., Williams, B. J., Rauch, A. M. and Opitz, J. M. 2000. 'Behavior phenotype of FG syndrome: cognition, personality, and behavior in eleven affected boys', *American Journal of Medical Genetics* **97**:2, 112–18.

Ozonoff, S., Cook, I., Coon, H., Dawson, G., Joseph, R. M., Klin, A., McMahon, W. M., Minshew, N., Munson, J. A., Pennington, B. F., Rogers, S. J., Spence, M. A., Tager-Flusberg, H., Volkmar, F. R. and Wrathall, D. 2004. 'Performance on Cambridge neuropsychological test automated battery subtests sensitive to frontal lobe function in people with autistic disorder: evidence from the collaborative programs of excellence in autism network', *Journal of Autism and Developmental Disorders* **34**:2, 139–50.

Paavola, L., Kunnari, S. and Moilanen, I. 2005. 'Maternal responsiveness and infant intentional communication: implications for the early communicative and linguistic development', *Child: Care, Health and Development* **31**:6, 727–35.

Paneth, N. and Stark, R. I. 1983. 'Cerebral palsy and mental retardation in relation to indicators of perinatal asphyxia: an epidemiologic overview', *American Journal of Obstetrics and Gynecology* **147**:8, 960–6.

Papagno, C. 2001. 'Comprehension of metaphors and idioms in patients with Alzheimer's disease: a longitudinal study', *Brain* **124**:7, 1450–60.

Papagno, C. and Caporali, A. 2007. 'Testing idiom comprehension in aphasic patients: the effects of task and idiom type', *Brain and Language* **100**:2, 208–20.

Papagno, C. and Vallar, G. 2001. 'Understanding metaphors and idioms: a single-case neuropsychological study in a person with Down syndrome', *Journal of the International Neuropsychological Society* **7**:4, 516–28.

Papagno, C., Lucchelli, F., Muggia, S. and Rizzo, S. 2003. 'Idiom comprehension in Alzheimer's disease: the role of the central executive', *Brain* **126**:11, 2419–30.

Papagno, C., Tabossi, P., Colombo, M. R. and Zampetti, P. 2004. 'Idiom comprehension in aphasic patients', *Brain and Language* **89**:1, 226–34.

Papagno, C., Curti, R., Rizzo, S., Crippa, F. and Colombo, M. 2006. 'Is the right hemisphere involved in idiom comprehension? A neuropsychological study', *Neuropsychology* **20**:5, 598–606.

Papagno, C., Cappa, S. F., Forelli, A., Laiacona, M., Vallar, G., Garavaglia, G. and Capitani, E. 1995. 'La comprensione non letterale del linguaggio: taratura di un test di comprensione di metafore e di espressioni idiomatiche', *Archivio di Psicologia, Neurologia e Psichiatria*, **56**:4, 402–20.

Paradis, M. (ed.) 1998a. *Pragmatics in neurogenic communication disorders*, Oxford and Tarrytown: Pergamon.

  1998b. 'The other side of language: pragmatic competence', *Journal of Neurolinguistics* **11**: (1–2), 1–10.

Parkinson, G. M. 2006. 'Pragmatic difficulties in children with autism associated with childhood epilepsy', *Pediatric Rehabilitation* **9**:3, 229–46.

Parsons, S. and Mitchell, P. 2002. 'The potential of virtual reality in social skills training for people with autistic spectrum disorders', *Journal of Intellectual Disability
Research* **46**:5, 430–43.

Passafiume, D., Di Giacomo, D. and Carolei, A. 2006. 'Word-stem completion task
to investigate semantic network in patients with Alzheimer's disease', *European
Journal of Neurology* **13**:5, 460–4.

Paul, R. 1992. *Pragmatic activities for language intervention: semantics, syntax and
emerging literacy*, San Antonio: Communication Skills Builders.

Paul, R., Augustyn, A., Klin, A. and Volkmar, F. R. 2005. 'Perception and production
of prosody by speakers with autism spectrum disorders', *Journal of Autism and
Developmental Disorders* **35**:2, 205–20.

Pearce, W. M., McCormack, P. F. and James, D. G. 2003. 'Exploring the boundaries
of SLI: findings from morphosyntactic and story grammar analyses', *Clinical
Linguistics & Phonetics* **17**: (4–5), 325–34.

Peña, E. D., Gillam, R. B., Malek, M., Ruiz-Felter, R., Resendiz, M., Fiestas, C. and
Sabel, T. 2006. 'Dynamic assessment of school-age children's narrative abil-
ity: an experimental investigation of classification accuracy', *Journal of Speech,
Language, and Hearing Research* **49**:5, 1037–57.

Penn, C. 1988. 'The profiling of syntax and pragmatics in aphasia', *Clinical Linguistics &
Phonetics* **2**:3, 179–207.

    1999. 'Pragmatic assessment and therapy for persons with brain damage: what have
clinicians gleaned in two decades?', *Brain and Language* **68**:3, 535–52.

Pennington, B. F., Rogers, S. J., Bennetto, L., Griffith, E. M., Reed, D. T. and Shyu,
V. 1997. 'Validity tests of the executive dysfunction hypothesis of autism', in
J. Russell (ed.), *Autism as an executive disorder*, New York: Oxford University
Press, 143–78.

Perkins, L. 1995. 'Applying conversation analysis to aphasia: clinical implications and
analytic issues', *European Journal of Disorders of Communication* **30**:3, 372–83.

Perkins, L., Crisp, J. and Walshaw, D. 1999. 'Exploring conversation analysis as an assessment tool for aphasia: the issue of reliability', *Aphasiology* **13**: (4–5), 259–81.

Perkins, L., Whitworth, A. and Lesser, R. 1997. *Conversation analysis profile for people
with cognitive impairment*, London: Whurr Publishers.

Perkins, M. R. (ed.) 2005. 'Clinical pragmatics: an emergentist perspective', *Clinical
Linguistics & Phonetics* **19**:5, 363–451.

    2008. *Pragmatic impairment*, Cambridge: Cambridge University Press.

Perner, J. and Lang, B. 2000. 'Theory of mind and executive function: is there a developmental relationship?', in S. Baron-Cohen, H. Tager-Flusberg and D. J. Cohen
(eds.), *Understanding other minds: perspectives from developmental cognitive
neuroscience*, New York: Oxford University Press, 150–81.

Perovic, A. 2006. 'Syntactic deficit in Down syndrome: more evidence for the modular
organisation of language', *Lingua* **116**:10, 1616–30.

Persson, C., Niklasson, L., Oskarsdottir, S., Johansson, S., Jonsson, R. and Soderpalm,
E. 2006. 'Language skills in 5–8-year-old children with 22q11 deletion syndrome',
International Journal of Language & Communication Disorders **41**:3, 313–33.

Phelps-Terasaki, D. and Phelps-Gunn, T. 1992. *Test of pragmatic language*, San
Antonio: The Psychological Corporation.

Plaisted, K. C. 2000. 'Aspects of autism that theory of mind cannot explain', in
S. Baron-Cohen, H. Tager-Flusberg and D. J. Cohen (eds.), *Understanding other*

minds: perspectives from developmental cognitive neuroscience, New York: Oxford University Press, 222–50.

Powell, J. E., Edwards, A., Edwards, M., Pandit, B. S., Sungum-Paliwal, S. R. and Whitehouse, W. 2000. 'Changes in the incidence of childhood autism and other autistic spectrum disorders in preschool children from two areas of the West Midlands, UK', *Developmental Medicine & Child Neurology* **42**:9, 624–8.

Premack, D. and Woodruff, G. 1978. 'Does the chimpanzee have a "theory of mind"?', *Behavioral and Brain Sciences* **1**:4, 515–26.

Prinz, P. M. 1982. 'An investigation of the comprehension and production of requests in normal and language-disordered children', *Journal of Communication Disorders* **15**:2, 75–93.

Prinz, P. M. and Ferrier, L. J. 1983. '"Can you give me that one?": the comprehension, production and judgment of directives in language-impaired children', *Journal of Speech and Hearing Research* **48**:1, 44–54.

Prizant, B. M. and Duchan, J. F. 1981. 'The functions of immediate echolalia in autistic children', *Journal of Speech and Hearing Disorders* **46**:3, 241–9.

Prutting, C. A. and Kirchner, D. M. 1987. 'A clinical appraisal of the pragmatic aspects of language', *Journal of Speech and Hearing Disorders* **52**:2, 105–19.

Purdy, M., Belanger, S. and Liles, B. 1992. 'Right-hemisphere-damaged subjects' ability to use context in inferencing', *Clinical Aphasiology* **21**, 135–43.

Putnam, H. 1990. *Realism with a human face*, Cambridge, MA: Harvard University Press.

1992. *Renewing philosophy*, Cambridge, MA: Harvard University Press.

1994a. *Words and life*, Cambridge, MA: Harvard University Press.

1994b. 'The Dewey Lectures 1994. Sense, nonsense, and the senses: an inquiry into the powers of the human mind', *The Journal of Philosophy* **91**, 445–517.

Qualls, C. D. and Harris, J. 1999. 'Effects of familiarity on idiom comprehension in African American and European American fifth graders', *Language, Speech, and Hearing Services in Schools* **30**:2, 141–51.

Qualls, C. D., Lantz, J. M., Pietrzyk, R. M., Blood, G. W. and Hammer, C. S. 2004. 'Comprehension of idioms in adolescents with language-based learning disabilities compared to their typically developing peers', *Journal of Communication Disorders* **37**:4, 295–311.

Rainville, C., Giroire, J. M., Periot, M., Cuny, E. and Mazaux, J. M. 2003. 'The impact of right subcortical lesions on executive functions and spatio-cognitive abilities: a case study', *Neurocase* **9**:4, 356–67.

Rakowicz, W. P. and Hodges, J. R. 1998. 'Dementia and aphasia in motor neuron disease: an underrecognised association?', *Journal of Neurology, Neurosurgery and Psychiatry* **65**:6, 881–9.

Rapin, I. 1996. 'Developmental language disorders: a clinical update', *Journal of Child Psychology and Psychiatry* **37**:6, 643–55.

Rapin, I. and Allen, D. A. 1983. 'Developmental language disorders: nosologic considerations', in U. Kirk (ed.), *Neuropsychology of language, reading, and spelling*, New York: Academic Press, 155–84.

Rapin, I. and Dunn, M. 2003. 'Update on the language disorders of individuals on the autistic spectrum', *Brain & Development* **25**:3, 166–72.

Raven, J. C. 1965. *The coloured progressive matrices*, New York: The Psychological Corporation.

Rayner, H. and Marshall, J. 2003. 'Training volunteers as conversation partners for people with aphasia', *International Journal of Language and Communication Disorders* **38**:2, 149–64.

Redmond, S. M. 2004. 'Conversational profiles of children with ADHD, SLI and typical development', *Clinical Linguistics & Phonetics* **18**:2, 107–25.

Redmond, S. M. and Rice, M. L. 2001. 'Detection of irregular verb violations by children with and without SLI', *Journal of Speech, Language, and Hearing Research* **44**:3, 655–69.

Rees, N. S. and Shulman, M. 1978. 'I don't understand what you mean by comprehension', *Journal of Speech and Hearing Disorders* **43**:2, 208–19.

Rehak, A., Kaplan, J. and Gardner, H. 1992. 'Sensitivity to conversational deviance in right-hemisphere-damaged patients', *Brain and Language* **42**:2, 203–17.

Ribeiro, B. T. 1994. *Coherence in psychotic discourse*, New York: Oxford University Press.

Ribeiro, B. T. and Pinto, D. S. 2009. 'Psychotic discourse', in L. Cummings (ed.), *The pragmatics encyclopedia*, London: Routledge.

Rice, M. L. and Wexler, K. 1996. 'Toward tense as a clinical marker of specific language impairment in English-speaking children', *Journal of Speech and Hearing Research* **39**:6, 1239–57.

Rice, M. L., Haney, K. R. and Wexler, K. 1998a. 'Family histories of children with SLI who show extended optional infinitives', *Journal of Speech, Language, and Hearing Research* **41**:2, 419–32.

Rice, M. L., Wexler, K. and Cleave, P. L. 1995. 'Specific language impairment as a period of extended optional infinitive', *Journal of Speech and Hearing Research* **38**:4, 850–63.

Rice, M. L., Wexler, K. and Hershberger, S. 1998b. 'Tense over time: the longitudinal course of tense acquisition in children with specific language impairment', *Journal of Speech, Language, and Hearing Research* **41**:6, 1412–31.

Rice, M. L., Wexler, K., Marquis, J. and Hershberger, S. 2000. 'Acquisition of irregular past tense by children with specific language impairment', *Journal of Speech, Language, and Hearing Research* **43**:5, 1126–45.

Richards, R. G., Sampson, F. C., Beard, S. M. and Tappenden, P. 2002. 'A review of the natural history and epidemiology of multiple sclerosis: implications for resource allocation and health economic models', *Health Technology Assessment* **6**:10, 1–73.

Richardson, K. and Klecan-Aker, J. S. 2000. 'Teaching pragmatics to language-learning disabled children: a treatment outcome study', *Child Language Teaching and Therapy* **16**:1, 23–42.

Ricker, J. H. and Millis, S. R. 1996. 'Differential visuospatial dysfunction following striatal, frontal white matter, or posterior thalamic infarction', *International Journal of Neuroscience* **84**: (1–4), 75–85.

Rinaldi, M. C., Marangolo, P. and Baldassarri, F. 2004. 'Metaphor comprehension in right brain-damaged patients with visuo-verbal and verbal material: a dissociation (re)considered', *Cortex* **40**:3, 479–90.

Rinaldi, W. 2000. 'Pragmatic comprehension in secondary school-aged students with specific developmental language disorder', *International Journal of Language & Communication Disorders* **35**:1, 1–29.

    2001. *Social use of language programme – revised*, Windsor: NFER Nelson.

Ripich, D. N., Carpenter, B. D. and Ziol, E. W. 2000. 'Conversational cohesion patterns in men and women with Alzheimer's disease: a longitudinal study', *International Journal of Language and Communication Disorders* **35**:1, 49–64.

Ripich, D. N., Vertes, D., Whitehouse, P., Fulton, S. and Ekelman, B. 1991. 'Turn-taking and speech act patterns in the discourse of senile dementia of the Alzheimer's type patients', *Brain and Language* **40**:3, 330–43.

Robbins, T. W. 1997. 'Integrating the neurobiological and neuropsychological dimensions of autism', in J. Russell (ed.), *Autism as an executive disorder*, New York: Oxford University Press, 21–53.

Robert, P. H., Darcourt, G., Koulibaly, M. P., Clairet, S., Benoit, M., Garcia, R., Dechaux, O. and Darcourt, J. 2006. 'Lack of initiative and interest in Alzheimer's disease: a single photon emission computed tomography study', *European Journal of Neurology* **13**:7, 729–35.

Roberts, J. E., Price, J. and Malkin, C. 2007b. 'Language and communication development in Down syndrome', *Mental Retardation and Developmental Disabilities Research Reviews* **13**:1, 26–35.

Roberts, J. E., Hennon, E. A., Price, J. R., Dear, E., Anderson, K. and Vandergrift, N. A. 2007a. 'Expressive language during conversational speech in boys with fragile X syndrome', *American Journal of Mental Retardation* **112**:1, 1–17.

Roberts, J. M. 1989. 'Echolalia and comprehension in autistic children', *Journal of Autism and Developmental Disorders* **19**:2, 271–81.

Robson, J., Pring, T., Marshall, J. and Chiat, S. 2003. 'Phoneme frequency effects in jargon aphasia: a phonological investigation of nonword errors', *Brain and Language* **85**:1, 109–24.

Rocha, L. C. and Befi-Lopes, D. M. 2006. 'Analyses of answers presented by children with and without specific language impairment', *Pró-fono: Revista de Atualização Científica* **18**:3, 229–38.

Rom, A. and Bliss, L. S. 1981. 'A comparison of verbal communicative skills of language impaired and normal speaking children', *Journal of Communication Disorders* **14**:2, 133–40.

1983. 'The use of nonverbal pragmatic behaviors by language-impaired and normal-speaking children', *Journal of Communication Disorders* **16**:4, 251–6.

Roncone, R., Mazza, M., Frangou, I., De Risio, A., Ussorio, D., Tozzini, C. and Casacchia, M. 2004. 'Rehabilitation of theory of mind deficit in schizophrenia: a pilot study of metacognitive strategies in group treatment', *Neuropsychological Rehabilitation* **14**:4, 421–35.

Rönnberg, J., Larsson, C., Fogelsjöö, A., Nilsson, L. G., Lindberg, M. and Angquist, K. A. 1996. 'Memory dysfunction in mild aphasics', *Scandinavian Journal of Psychology* **37**:1, 46–61.

Roth, F. P. and Spekman, N. J. 1984. 'Assessing the pragmatic abilities of children: part 1. Organizational framework and assessment parameters', *Journal of Speech and Hearing Disorders* **49**:1, 2–11.

Rowan, L. E., Leonard, L. B., Chapman, K. and Weiss, A. L. 1983. 'Performative and presuppositional skills in language-disordered and normal children', *Journal of Speech and Hearing Research* **26**:1, 97–106.

Rowe, J., Lavender, A. and Turk, V. 2006. 'Cognitive executive function in Down's syndrome', *British Journal of Clinical Psychology* **45**:1, 5–17.

Royal College of Speech and Language Therapists. 2005. *Clinical guidelines*, Oxon: Speechmark Publishing.

Ruser, T. F., Arin, D., Dowd, M., Putnam, S., Winklosky, B., Rosen-Sheidley, B., Piven, J., Tomblin, B., Tager-Flusberg, H. and Folstein, S. 2007. 'Communicative competence in parents of children with autism and parents of children with specific language impairment', *Journal of Autism and Developmental Disorders* **37**:7, 1323–36.

Russell, J. 1997a. 'How executive disorders can bring about an inadequate "theory of mind"', in J. Russell (ed.), *Autism as an executive disorder*, New York: Oxford University Press, 256–304.

1997b. 'Introduction', in J. Russell (ed.), *Autism as an executive disorder*, New York: Oxford University Press, 1–17.

Ryder, N. and Leinonen, E. 2003. 'Use of context in question answering by 3-, 4- and 5-year-old children', *Journal of Psycholinguistic Research* **32**:4, 397–415.

Schelletter, C. and Leinonen, E. 2003. 'Normal and language-impaired children's use of reference: syntactic versus pragmatic processing', *Clinical Linguistics & Phonetics* **17**: (4–5), 335–43.

Scherz, J. W., Edwards, H. T. and Kallail, K. J. 1995. 'Communicative effectiveness of doctor–patient interactions', *Health Communication* **7**:2, 163–77.

Schmitzer, A., Strauss, M. and DeMarco, S. 1997. 'Contextual influences on comprehension of multiple-meaning words by right hemisphere brain-damaged and non-brain-damaged adults', *Aphasiology* **11**: (4–5), 447–59.

Schodorf, J. K. and Edwards, H. T. 1983. 'Comparative analysis of parent–child interactions with language-disordered and linguistically normal children', *Journal of Communication Disorders* **16**:2, 71–83.

Scholl, B. J. and Leslie, A. M. 1999. 'Modularity, development and "theory of mind"', *Mind & Language* **14**:1, 131–53.

Schuele, C. M. and Hadley, P. A. 1999. 'Potential advantages of introducing specific language impairment to families', *American Journal of Speech-Language Pathology* **8**:1, 11–22.

Schul, R., Stiles, J., Wulfeck, B. and Townsend, J. 2004. 'How "generalized" is the "slowed processing" in SLI? The case of visuospatial attentional orienting', *Neuropsychologia* **42**:5, 661–71.

Schultz, R. T., Grelotti, D. J. and Pober, B. 2001. 'Genetics of childhood disorders: XXVI. Williams syndrome and brain-behavior relationships', *Journal of the American Academy of Child and Adolescent Psychiatry* **40**:5, 606–9.

Scott, C. M. and Windsor, J. 2000. 'General language performance measures in spoken and written narrative and expository discourse of school-age children with language learning disabilities', *Journal of Speech, Language, and Hearing Research* **43**:2, 324–39.

Searle, J. R. 1969. *Speech acts: an essay in the philosophy of language*, Cambridge: Cambridge University Press.

1974. 'Chomsky's revolution in linguistics', in G. Harman (ed.), *On Noam Chomsky: criticial essays*, New York: Anchor Press/ Doubleday, 2–33.

Sebastian, C. S. 2002. *Mental retardation*, USA: eMedicine.com (online, available at: www.emedicine.com/med/topic3095.htm).

Segal, G. 1996. 'The modularity of theory of mind', in P. Carruthers and P. K. Smith (eds.), *Theories of theories of mind*, Cambridge: Cambridge University Press, 141–57.

Segerdahl, P. 1996. *Language use: a philosophical investigation into the basic notions of pragmatics*, Suffolk: Macmillan Press.

Selman, R. L., Beardslee, W., Hickey Schultz, L., Krupa, M. and Podorefsky, D. 1986. 'Assessing adolescent interpersonal negotiation strategies: toward the integration of structural and functional models', *Developmental Psychology* **22**:4, 450–9.

Semel, E., Wiig, E. H. and Secord, W. A. 2003. *Clinical evaluation of language fundamentals, fourth edition (CELF-4)*, Toronto, Canada: The Psychological Corporation.

Sergeant, J. A., Geurts, H. and Oosterlaan, J. 2002. 'How specific is a deficit of executive functioning for attention-deficit/hyperactivity disorder?', *Behavioural Brain Research* **130**: (1–2), 3–28.

Shah, A. and Frith, U. 1993. 'Why do autistic individuals show superior performance on the block design task?', *Journal of Child Psychology and Psychiatry* **34**:8, 1351–64.

Shamay-Tsoory, S. G., Tomer, R. and Aharon-Peretz, J. 2005a. 'The neuroanatomical basis of understanding sarcasm and its relationship to social cognition', *Neuropsychology* **19**:3, 288–300.

Shamay-Tsoory, S. G., Tomer, R., Berger, B. D., Goldsher, D. and Aharon-Peretz, J. 2005b. 'Impaired "affective theory of mind" is associated with right ventromedial prefrontal damage', *Cognitive and Behavioural Neurology* **18**:1, 55–67.

Shammi, P. and Stuss, D. 1999. 'Humour appreciation: a role of the right frontal lobe', *Brain* **122**:4, 657–66.

Shea, S. E. 2006. 'Mental retardation in children ages 6 to 16', *Seminars in Pediatric Neurology* **13**:4, 262–70.

Sheinkopf, S. J., Mundy, P., Oller, D. K. and Steffens, M. 2000. 'Vocal atypicalities of preverbal autistic children', *Journal of Autism and Developmental Disorders* **30**:4, 345–54.

Sheldon, L. and Turk, J. 2000. 'Monozygotic boys with fragile X syndrome', *Developmental Medicine & Child Neurology* **42**:11, 768–74.

Shriberg, L. D., Tomblin, J. B. and McSweeny, J. L. 1999. 'Prevalence of speech delay in 6-year-old children and comorbidity with language impairment', *Journal of Speech, Language, and Hearing Research* **42**:6, 1461–81.

Shriberg, L. D., Paul, R., McSweeny, J. L., Klin, A., Cohen, D. J. and Volkmar, F. R. 2001. 'Speech and prosody characteristics of adolescents and adults with high-functioning autism and Asperger syndrome', *Journal of Speech, Language, and Hearing Research* **44**:5, 1097–1115.

Siegal, M., Carrington, J. and Radel, M. 1996. 'Theory of mind and pragmatic understanding following right hemisphere damage', *Brain and Language* **53**:1, 40–50.

Simmons-Mackie, N., Threats, T. T. and Kagan, A. 2005. 'Outcome assessment in aphasia: a survey', *Journal of Communication Disorders* **38**:1, 1–27.

Simon, J. A., Keenan, J. M., Pennington, B. F., Taylor, A. K. and Hagerman, R. J. 2001. 'Discourse processing in women with fragile X syndrome: evidence for a deficit establishing coherence', *Cognitive Neuropsychology* **18**:1, 1–18.

Sitnikova, T., Salisbury, D. F., Kuperberg, G. and Holcomb, P. J. 2002. 'Electrophysiological insights into language processing in schizophrenia', *Psychophysiology* **39**:6, 851–60.

Skarakis, E. and Greenfield, P. M. 1982. 'The role of new and old information in the verbal expression of language-disordered children', *Journal of Speech and Hearing Research* **25**:3, 462–7.

Skuse, D. H. 2000. 'Imprinting, the X-chromosome, and the male brain: explaining sex differences in the liability to autism', *Pediatric Research* **47**:1, 9–16.

Smith, B. R. and Leinonen, E. 1992. *Clinical pragmatics: unravelling the complexities of communicative failure*, London: Chapman & Hall.

Smith, S. D. 2007. 'Genes, language development, and language disorders', *Mental Retardation and Developmental Disabilities Research Reviews* **13**:1, 96–105.

Snow, P., Douglas, J. and Ponsford, J. 1998. 'Conversational discourse abilities following severe traumatic brain injury: a follow-up study', *Brain Injury* **12**:11, 911–35.

Sobesky, W. E., Pennington, B. F., Porter, D., Hull, C. E. and Hagerman, R. J. 1994. 'Emotional and neurocognitive deficits in fragile X', *American Journal of Medical Genetics* **51**:4, 378–85.

Sodian, B. and Frith, U. 1992. 'Deception and sabotage in autistic, retarded and normal children', *Journal of Child Psychology and Psychiatry* **33**:3, 591–605.

Sohlberg, M. M., Perlewitz, P. G., Johansen, A., Schultz, J., Johnson, L. and Hartry, A. 1992. *Improving pragmatic skills in persons with head injury*, Tucson: Communication Skill Builders.

Soroker, N., Kasher, A., Giora, R., Batori, G., Corn, C., Gil, M. and Zaidel, E. 2005. 'Processing of basic speech acts following localized brain damage: a new light on the neuroanatomy of language', *Brain and Cognition* **57**:2, 214–17.

Sosin, D. M., Sniezek, J. E. and Thurman, D. J. 1996. 'Incidence of mild and moderate brain injury in the United States, 1991', *Brain Injury* **10**:1, 47–54.

Spanoudis, G., Natsopoulos, D. and Panayiotou, G. 2007. 'Mental verbs and pragmatic language difficulties', *International Journal of Language and Communication Disorders* **42**:4, 487–504.

Sperber, D. and Wilson, D. 1986, 1995. *Relevance: communication and cognition*, Oxford: Blackwell.
    2002. 'Pragmatics, modularity and mind-reading', *Mind & Language* **17**: (1–2), 3–23.

Sperber, D., Cara, F. and Girotto, V. 1995. 'Relevance theory explains the selection task', *Cognition* **57**:1, 31–95.

Sprich, S., Biederman, J., Crawford, M. H., Mundy, E. and Faraone, S. V. 2000. 'Adoptive and biological families of children and adolescents with ADHD', *Journal of the American Academy of Child and Adolescent Psychiatry* **39**:11, 1432–7.

Stalnaker, R. C. 1998. 'Pragmatics', in A. Kasher (ed.), *Pragmatics: critical concepts*, London: Routledge, 55–69.

Stein, N. L. and Glenn, C. G. 1979. 'An analysis of story comprehension in elementary school children', in R. O. Freedle (ed.), *New directions in discourse processing*, Norwood: Ablex, 53–120.

Steinhausen, H. C. and Juzi, C. 1996. 'Elective mutism: an analysis of 100 cases', *Journal of the American Academy of Child and Adolescent Psychiatry* **35**:5, 606–14.

Stemmer, B. (ed.) 1999. 'Pragmatics: theoretical and clinical issues', *Brain and Language* **68**:3, 389–594.

Stojanovik, V. and James, D. 2006. 'Short-term longitudinal study of a child with Williams syndrome', *International Journal of Language and Communication Disorders* **41**:2, 213–23.

Stone, V. E., Baron-Cohen, S. and Knight, R. T. 1998. 'Frontal lobe contributions to theory of mind', *Journal of Cognitive Neuroscience* **10**:5, 640–56.

Stribling, P., Rae, J. and Dickerson, P. 2007. 'Two forms of spoken repetition in a girl with autism', *International Journal of Language and Communication Disorders* **42**:4, 427–44.

Strong, C. 1998. *The Strong narrative assessment procedure*, Eau Claire: Thinking Publications.

Stroop, J. R. 1935. 'Studies of interference in serial verbal reaction', *Journal of Experimental Psychology*, **18**, 643–62.

Sudhalter, V. and Belser, R. C. 2001. 'Conversational characteristics of children with fragile X syndrome: tangential language', *American Journal on Mental Retardation* **106**:5, 389–400.

Sullivan, K. and Tager-Flusberg, H. 1999. 'Second-order belief attribution in Williams syndrome: intact or impaired?', *American Journal of Mental Retardation* **104**:6, 523–32

Sullivan, K., Winner, E. and Tager-Flusberg, H. 2003. 'Can adolescents with Williams syndrome tell the difference between lies and jokes?', *Developmental Neuropsychology* **23**: (1–2), 85–103.

Sumiyoshi, C., Matsui, M., Sumiyoshi, T., Yamashita, I., Sumiyoshi, S. and Kurachi, M. 2001. 'Semantic structure in schizophrenia as assessed by the category fluency test: effect of verbal intelligence and age of onset', *Psychiatry Research* **105**:3, 187–99.

Surian, L. 1996. 'Are children with autism deaf to gricean maxims?', *Cognitive Neuropsychiatry* **1**:1, 55–72.

Surian, L. and Siegal, M. 2001. 'Sources of performance on theory of mind tasks in right hemisphere-damaged patients', *Brain and Language* **78**:2, 224–32.

Surian, L., Baron-Cohen, S. and Van der Lely, H. 1996. 'Are children with autism deaf to gricean maxims?', *Cognitive Neuropsychiatry* **1**:1, 55–71.

Svenson, L. W., Cwik, V. A. and Martin, W. R. 1999. 'The prevalence of motor neurone disease in the province of Alberta', *Canadian Journal of Neurological Sciences* **26**:2, 119–22.

Szatmari, P., Jones, M. B., Zwaigenbaum, L. and MacLean, J. E. 1998. 'Genetics of autism: overview and new directions', *Journal of Autism and Developmental Disorders* **28**:5, 351–68.

Tager-Flusberg, H. and Sullivan, K. 2000. 'A componential view of theory of mind: evidence from Williams syndrome', *Cognition* **76**:1, 59–90.

Tallal, P., Hirsch, L. S., Realpe-Bonilla, T., Miller, S., Brzustowicz, L. M., Bartlett, C. and Flax, J. F. 2001. 'Familial aggregation in specific language impairment', *Journal of Speech, Language, and Hearing Research* **44**:5, 1172–82.

Tanguay, P. E., Robertson, J. and Derrick, A. 1998. 'A dimensional classification of autism spectrum disorder by social communication domains', *Journal of the American Academy of Child and Adolescent Psychiatry* **37**:3, 271–7.

Tarling, K., Perkins, M. R. and Stojanovik, V. 2006. 'Conversational success in Williams syndrome: communication in the face of cognitive and linguistic limitations', *Clinical Linguistics & Phonetics* **20**: (7–8), 583–90.

Tényi, T., Herold, R., Szili, I. M. and Trixler, M. 2002. 'Schizophrenics show a failure in the decoding of violations of conversational implicatures', *Psychopathology* **35**:1, 25–7.

Thomas, P. 1997. 'What can linguistics tell us about thought disorder?', in J. France and N. Muir (eds.), *Communication and the mentally ill patient: developmental and linguistic approaches to schizophrenia*, London: Jessica Kingsley Publishers, 30–42.

Thompson, S., Herrmann, N., Rapoport, M. J. and Lanctôt, K. L. 2007. 'Efficacy and safety of antidepressants for treatment of depression in Alzheimer's disease: a metaanalysis', *Canadian Journal of Psychiatry* **52**:4, 248–55.

Thomson, A. M., Taylor, R. and Whittle, I. R. 1998. 'Assessment of communication impairment and the effects of resective surgery in solitary, right-sided supratentorial intracranial tumours: a prospective study', *British Journal of Neurosurgery* **12**:5, 423–9.

Thordardottir, E. T., Chapman, R. S. and Wagner, L. 2002. 'Complex sentence production by adolescents with Down syndrome', *Applied Psycholinguistics* **23**:2, 163–83.

Timler, G. R., Olswang, L. B. and Coggins, T. E. 2005. '"Do I know what I need to do?" A social communication intervention for children with complex clinical profiles', *Language, Speech, and Hearing Services in Schools* **36**:1, 73–85.

Tirosh, E. and Cohen, A. 1998. 'Language deficit with attention-deficit disorder: a prevalent comorbidity', *Journal of Child Neurology* **13**:10, 493–7.

Togher, L. and Hand, L. 1998. 'Use of politeness markers with different communication partners: an investigation of five subjects with traumatic brain injury', *Aphasiology* **12**: (7–8), 755–70.

Tomblin, J. B., Zhang, X., Buckwalter, P. and Catts, H. 2000. 'The association of reading disability, behavioural disorders, and language impairment among second-grade children', *Journal of Child Psychology and Psychiatry* **41**:4, 473–82.

Tomblin, J. B., Records, N. L., Buckwalter, P., Zhang, X., Smith, E. and O'Brien, M. 1997. 'Prevalence of specific language impairment in kindergarten children', *Journal of Speech, Language, and Hearing Research* **40**:6, 1245–60.

Tompkins, C., Lehman, M. and Baumgaertner, A. 1999. 'Suppression and inference revision in right brain-damaged and non-brain-damaged adults', *Aphasiology* **13**: (9–11), 725–42.

Tompkins, C. A., Baumgaertner, A., Lehman, M. T. and Fassbinder, W. 2000. 'Mechanisms of discourse comprehension impairment after right hemisphere brain damage: suppression in lexical ambiguity resolution', *Journal of Speech, Language, and Hearing Research* **43**:1, 62–78.

Tompkins, C., Baumgaertner, A., Lehman, M. and Fossett, T. 1997. 'Suppression and discourse comprehension in right brain-damaged adults: a preliminary report', *Aphasiology* **11**: (4–5), 505–19.

Tompkins, C. A., Fassbinder, W., Lehman Blake, M., Baumgaertner, A. and Javaram, N. 2004. 'Inference generation during text comprehension by adults with right hemisphere brain damage: activation failure versus multiple activation', *Journal of Speech, Language, and Hearing Research* **47**:6, 1380–95.

Tompkins, C., Boada, R., McGarry, K., Jones, J., Rahn, A. and Ranier, S. 1992. 'Connected speech characteristics of right-hemisphere-damaged adults: a re-examination', *Clinical Aphasiology* **21**, 113–22.

Towbin, K. E., Pradella, A., Gorrindo, T., Pine, D. S. and Leibenluft, E. 2005. 'Autism spectrum traits in children with mood and anxiety disorders', *Journal of Child and Adolescent Psychopharmacology* **15**:3, 452–64.

Tractenberg, R. E., Weiner, M. F., Patterson, M. B., Gamst, A. and Thal, L. J. 2002. 'Emergent psychopathology in Alzheimer's disease patients over 12 months associated with functional, not cognitive, changes', *Journal of Geriatric Psychiatry and Neurology* **15**:2, 110–17.

Tsuang, M. 2000. 'Schizophrenia: genes and environment', *Biological Psychiatry* **47**:3, 210–20.

Turkstra, L. S., Dixon, T. M. and Baker, K. K. 2004. 'Theory of mind and social beliefs in adolescents with traumatic brain injury', *NeuroRehabilitation* **19**:3, 245–56.

Turkstra, L. S., McDonald, S. and Kaufmann, P. M. 1995. 'Assessment of pragmatic communication skills in adolescents after traumatic brain injury', *Brain Injury* **10**:5, 329–45.

Turner, S. and Whitworth, A. 2006. 'Clinicians' perceptions of candidacy for conversation partner training in aphasia: how do we select candidates for therapy and do we get it right?', *Aphasiology* **20**:7, 616–43.

Uchiyama, H., Seki, A., Kageyama, H., Saito, D. N., Koeda, T., Ohno, K. and Sadato, N. 2006. 'Neural substrates of sarcasm: a functional magnetic-resonance imaging study', *Brain Research* **1124**:1, 100–10.

Ulatowska, H. K. and Olness, G. S. 2007. 'Pragmatics in discourse performance: insights from aphasiology', *Seminars in Speech and Language* **28**:2, 148–58.

van der Henst, J. B. 1999. 'The mental model theory of spatial reasoning re-examined: the role of relevance in premise order', *British Journal of Psychology* **90**:1, 73–84.

van der Lely, H. K., Rosen, S. and Adlard, A. 2004. 'Grammatical language impairment and the specificity of cognitive domains: relations between auditory and language abilities', *Cognition* **94**:2, 167–83.

van Leer, E. and Turkstra, L. 1999. 'The effect of elicitation task on discourse coherence and cohesion in adolescents with brain injury', *Journal of Communication Disorders* **32**:5, 327–49.

Varley, R. 1993. 'Deictic terms, lexical retrieval and utterance length in aphasia: an investigation of inter-relations', *European Journal of Disorders of Communication* **28**:1, 23–41.

Varley, R. and Siegal, M. 2000. 'Evidence for cognition without grammar from causal reasoning and "theory of mind" in an agrammatic aphasic patient', *Current Biology* **10**:12, 723–6.

Varley, R., Siegal, M. and Want, S. C. 2001. 'Severe impairment in grammar does not preclude theory of mind', *Neurocase* **7**:6, 489–93.

Verschueren, J. and Östman, J.-O. (eds.) 2006. *Handbook of pragmatics: 2006 installment*, Amsterdam: John Benjamins.

Verté, S., Geurts, H. M., Roeyers, H., Rosseel, Y., Oosterlaan, J. and Sergeant, J. A. 2006. 'Can the children's communication checklist differentiate autism spectrum subtypes?', *Autism* **10**:3, 266–87.

Volden, J. 2004. 'Conversational repair in speakers with autism spectrum disorder', *International Journal of Language & Communication Disorders* **39**:2, 171–89.

Volkmar, F. R., Klin, A., Siegel, B., Szatmari, P., Lord, C., Campbell, M., Freeman, B. J., Cicchetti, D. V., Rutter, M., Kline, W., Buitelaar, J., Hattab, Y., Fombonne, E., Fuentes, J., Werry, J., Stone, W., Kerbershian, J., Hoshino, Y., Bregman, J., Loveland, K., Szymanski, L. and Towbin, K. 1994. 'Field trial for autistic disorder in DSM-IV', *American Journal of Psychiatry* **151**:9, 1361–7.

Vostanis, P., Graves, A., Meltzer, H., Goodman, R., Jenkins, R. and Brugha, T. 2006. 'Relationship between parental psychopathology, parenting strategies and child mental health-findings from the GB national study', *Social Psychiatry and Psychiatric Epidemiology* **41**:7, 509–14.

Wacker, A., Holder, M., Will, B. E., Winkler, P. A. and Ilmberger, J. 2002. 'Comparison of the Aachen aphasia test, clinical study and Aachen aphasia bedside test in brain tumor patients', *Der Nervenarzt* **73**:8, 765–9.

Walder, D. J., Seidman, L. J., Cullen, N., Su, J., Tsuang, M. T. and Goldstein, J. M. 2006. 'Sex differences in language dysfunction in schizophrenia', *American Journal of Psychiatry* **163**:3, 470–7.

Wang, A. T., Lee, S. S., Sigman, M. and Dapretto, M. 2006. 'Neural basis of irony comprehension in children with autism: the role of prosody and context', *Brain* **129**:4, 932–43.

Ward-Lonergan, J. M., Liles, B. Z. and Anderson, A. M. 1999. 'Verbal retelling abilities in adolescents with and without language-learning disabilities for social studies lectures', *Journal of Learning Disabilities* **32**:3, 213–23.

Wechsler, D. 1981. *Wechsler adult intelligence scale – revised*, New York: The Psychological Corporation.

   1987. *Wechsler memory scale – revised*, New York: The Psychological Corporation.

Weinrich, M., McCall, D., Boser, K. I. and Virata, T. 2002. 'Narrative and procedural discourse production by severely aphasic patients', *Neurorehabilitation and Neural Repair* **16**:3, 249–74.

Weismer, S. E. and Hesketh, L. J. 1996. 'Lexical learning by children with specific language impairment: effects of linguistic input presented at varying speaking rates', *Journal of Speech and Hearing Research* **39**:1, 177–90.

Weismer, S. E., Evans, J. and Hesketh, L. J. 1999. 'An examination of verbal working memory capacity in children with specific language impairment', *Journal of Speech, Language, and Hearing Research* **42**:5, 1249–60.

Wetherell, D., Botting, N. and Conti-Ramsden, G. 2007. 'Narrative in adolescent specific language impairment (SLI): a comparison with peers across two different narrative genres', *International Journal of Language & Communication Disorders* **42**:5, 583–605.

Wetzel, W. F. and Molfese, D. L. 1992. 'The processing of presuppositional information contained in sentences: electrophysiological correlates', *Brain and Language* **42**:3, 286–307.

Whelan, B. M., Murdoch, B. E. and Bellamy, N. 2007. 'Delineating communication impairments associated with mild traumatic brain injury: a case report', *Journal of Head Trauma Rehabilitation* **22**:3, 192–7.

Whitworth, A., Perkins, L. and Lesser, R. 1997. *Conversation analysis profile for people with aphasia* (CAPPA), London: Whurr Publishers.

Williams, S. E., Li, E. C., Della Volpe, A. and Ritterman, S. I. 1994. 'The influence of topic and listener familiarity on aphasic discourse', *Journal of Communication Disorders* **27**:3, 207–22.

Wilson, B. A., Cockburn, J. and Halligan, P. 1987. *Behavioural inattention test*, Bury St. Edmunds, Suffolk, England: Thames Valley Test Company.

Wilson, B. M. and Proctor, A. 2000. 'Oral and written discourse in adolescents with closed head injury', *Brain and Cognition* **43**: (1–3), 425–9.

2002. 'Written discourse of adolescents with closed head injury', *Brain Injury* **16**:11, 1011–24.

Wilson, D. 2005. 'New directions for research on pragmatics and modularity', *Lingua* **115**:8, 1129–46.

Wilson, D. and Sperber, D. 1991. 'Inference and implicature', in S. Davis (ed.), *Pragmatics: a reader*, New York: Oxford University Press, 377–93.

Wimmer, H. and Perner, J. 1983. 'Beliefs about beliefs: representation and constraining function of wrong beliefs in young children's understanding of deception', *Cognition* **13**:1, 103–28.

Wing, L. and Gould, J. 1979. 'Severe impairments of social interaction and associated abnormalities in children: epidemiology and classification', *Journal of Autism and Developmental Disorders* **9**:1, 11–29.

Winner, E., Brownell, H., Happé, F., Blum, A. and Pincus, D. 1998. 'Distinguishing lies from jokes: theory of mind deficits and discourse interpretation in right hemisphere brain-damaged patients', *Brain and Language* **62**:1, 89–106.

Wiseman-Hakes, C., Stewart, M. L., Wasserman, R. and Schuller, R. 1998. 'Peer group training of pragmatic skills in adolescents with acquired brain injury', *Journal of Head Trauma Rehabilitation* **13**:6, 23–38.

World Health Organisation 1993. *International classification of diseases*, Geneva: WHO.

Wu, E. Q., Shi, L., Birnbaum, H., Hudson, T. and Kessler, R. 2006. 'Annual prevalence of diagnosed schizophrenia in the USA: a claims data analysis approach', *Psychological Medicine* **36**:11, 1535–40.

Yirmiya, N. and Shulman, C. 1996. 'Seriation, conservation, and theory of mind abilities in individuals with autism, individuals with mental retardation, and normally developing children', *Child Development* **67**:5, 2045–59.

Yirmiya, N., Erel, O., Shaked, M. and Solomonica-Levi, D. 1998. 'Meta-analyses comparing theory of mind abilities of individuals with autism, individuals with mental retardation, and normally developing individuals', *Psychological Bulletin* **124**:3, 283–307.

Yirmiya, N., Solomonica-Levi, D., Shulman, C. and Pilowsky, T. 1996. 'Theory of mind abilities in individuals with autism, Down syndrome, and mental retardation of unknown etiology: the role of age and intelligence', *Journal of Child Psychology and Psychiatry* **37**:8, 1003–14.

Young, E. C., Diehl, J. J., Morris, D., Hyman, S. L. and Bennetto, L. 2005. 'The use of two language tests to identify pragmatic language problems in children with autism spectrum disorders', *Language, Speech, and Hearing Services in Schools* **36**:1, 62–72.

Young, S. E., Smolen, A., Hewitt, J. K., Haberstick, B. C., Stallings, M. C., Corley, R. P. and Crowley, T. J. 2006. 'Interaction between MAO-A genotype and maltreatment in the risk for conduct disorder: failure to confirm in adolescent patients', *American Journal of Psychiatry* **163**:6, 1019–25.

Zaidel, E., Kasher, A., Soroker, N. and Batori, G. 2002. 'Effects of right and left hemisphere damage on performance of the "right hemisphere communication battery"', *Brain and Language* **80**:3, 510–35.

Zaidel, E., Kasher, A., Soroker, N., Batori, G., Giora, R. and Graves, D. 2000. 'Hemispheric contributions to pragmatics', *Brain and Cognition* **43**: (1–3), 438–43.

Zebenholzer, K. and Oder, W. 1998. 'Neurological and psychosocial sequelae 4 and 8 years after severe craniocerebral injury: a catamnestic study', *Wiener Klinische Wochenschrift* **110**:7, 253–61.

Zelazo, P. D., Burack, J. A., Benedetto, E. and Frye, D. 1996. 'Theory of mind and rule use in individuals with Down's syndrome: a test of the uniqueness and specificity claims', *Journal of Child Psychology and Psychiatry* **37**:4, 479–84.

Ziatas, K., Durkin, K. and Pratt, C. 2003. 'Differences in assertive speech acts produced by children with autism, Asperger syndrome, specific language impairment, and normal development', *Development and Psychopathology* **15**:1, 73–94.

Index

aetiology, 9, 44, 54, 62, 63, 69, 75, 79, 88

AIDS/HIV, 69, 182

alcohol, 63, 69, 85, 86, 117, 203, *See also* foetal alcohol (syndrome)

Alzheimer's disease, 6, 21, 22, 29, 37, 38, 85, 88, 89, 90, 93, 108, 109, 110, 111, 116, 117, 153, 186, 193, 194, *See also* dementia

amygdala damage, 115, 168

amyotrophic lateral sclerosis (ALS), 109, 117, *See also* motor neurone disease

anomia, 117, *See also* aphasia, word-finding deficit

aphasia
agrammatic, 3
anomic, 92, 105, 112, 113
Broca's, 94, 105, 112, 189
conduction, 112, 113
fluent, 18, 91, 92, 112, 194, 197
global, 112
jargon, 91
nonfluent, 18, 91, 92, 112, 250
transcortical motor, 105, 112
transcortical sensory, 112
Wernicke's, 112, 113

argumentation, 38, 39, 176, 246

Asperger's syndrome, 21, 39, 54, 56, 57, 58, 59, 60, 66, 81, 82, 95, 115, 121, 128, 130, 138, 169, 172, 184, 220, 224, *See also* autistic spectrum disorder (ASD)

assessment
formal, 177, 178, 209, 223
informal, 177

attention, 2, 4, 42, 51, 56, 61, 63, 65, 66, 74, 86, 96, 99, 108, 124, 125, 133, 136, 137, 176, 184, 195, 204, 214, 218, 235, 245, 249, 253, 254, 255

attention deficit hyperactivity disorder (ADHD), 42, 61, 62, 63, 64, 65, 66, 67, 83, 184, 213, *See also* emotional and behavioural disorder

Austin, J., 2, 9, 10, 11, 13, 36, 38, 219

autistic spectrum disorder (ASD)
Asperger's disorder, 49, 122, 135, *See also* Asperger's syndrome
atypical autism, 38, 81
autism, 11, 18, 21, 26, 33, 36, 48, 49, 54, 55, 56, 57, 58, 59, 60, 66, 67, 75, 79, 81, 82, 86, 87, 118, 119, 120, 121, 122, 123, 124, 125, 127, 128, 129, 130, 132, 133, 134, 135, 136, 137, 138, 139, 141, 168, 169, 176, 179, 181, 183, 184, 186, 190, 201, 202, 207, 208, 209, 214, 215, 220, 221, 222, 224, 226, 227, 241, 242, 247, 251, 254, 255
autistic disorder, 49, 54, 72, 81, 122, 183, 184
childhood disintegrative disorder (CDD), 54, 81
high-functioning autism (HFA), 25, 39, 55, 56, 58, 59, 78, 128, 137, 138, 172, 184, 220, 251
pervasive developmental disorder (PDD), 53, 54, 61, 62, 81, 135, 241
pervasive developmental disorder, not otherwise specified (PDD,NOS), 38, 49, 54, 56, 66, 67, 81, 183, 184
Rett's disorder, 54, 61, *See also* Rett's (syndrome)

belief
attribution, 30, 52, 53, 75, 99, 121, 161, 167, 207, 208
false, 30, 52, 53, 58, 75, 86, 111, 114, 115, 120, 121, 128, 129, 136, 163, 203, 207, 208, 215, 220, 221, 247, 251

brain
damage, 21, 47, 70, 90, 92, 94, 95, 98, 102, 104, 105, 110, 133, 134, 139, 151, 156
injury, 3, 5, 6, 8, 22, 28, 37, 38, 70, 88, 90, 104, 105, 106, 107, 178, 182, 191, 193, 195, 205, 206, 221, 230, 255
tumour, 88, 90, 91, 96, 97